Cerebral Protection in Cerebrovascular and Aortic Surgery

J. Ennker · J. S. Coselli
T. Treasure
Editors

Cerebral Protection in Cerebrovascular and Aortic Surgery

STEINKOPFF
DARMSTADT

Springer

Editors address:

J. Ennker M.D.
Heart Institute Lahr/Baden
Hobergweg 7
D-77933 Lahr
Germany

Joseph S. Coselli, M.D.
6560 Fannin, # 1144
Houston, TX 77030
USA

T. Treasure, M.D., MS, FRCS
St. George Hospital
Dept. of Cardiothoracic Surgery
Blackshow Road
London SW17 0QT
Great Britain

ISBN-13: 978-3-642-95989-9 e-ISBN-13: 978-3-642-95987-5
DOI: 10.1007/978-3-642-95987-5

Die Deutsche Bibliothek – CIP-Einheitsaufnahme

Cerebral protection in cerebrovascular and aortic surgery / J. Ennker ... ed. – Darmstadt : Steinkopff ; New York : Springer, 1997

NE: Ennker, Jürgen [Hrsg.]

Softcover reprint of the hardcover 1st edition 1997

Medical Editor: Beate Rühlemann – English Editor: James C. Willis – Production: Heinz J. Schäfer
Cover Design: Erich Kirchner, Heidelberg

Typesetting: Typoservice, Griesheim

Preface

The contributions in this book were originally presented in a symposium held in October 1995, at the Schloßhotel Bühlerhöhe in Baden-Baden, on the theme about "Cerebral Protection in Cerebrovascular and Aortic Surgery". The symposium was planned to combine the experience of prominent authorities in cerebral physiology, neurology and neurosurgery with the experience of international surgeons operating on the diseased aorta and its supraaortic vessels. The first part focuses on cerebral monitoring, cerebral physiology and neurological disorders after operations on the aorta and its supraaortic vessels. The second part concentrates on the surgical techniques and corresponding results of some of the most experienced surgeons from leading centers of the world.

The protection of the brain from hypoxic or ischemic injury is a major challenge during repair of aortic arch aneurysms and operations on the supraaortic vessels. Operations in this difficult field pose one of the most complicate technical challenges in surgery today.

The first successful replacement of an aortic arch aneurysma was carried out by DeBakey in 1957 (1) with an aortic homograft. For many years after this pioneering operation morbidity and mortality for the treatment of aortic pathology in the transverse arch location have remained unacceptably high. The early operations were carried out with one of the following two methods. One method was to establish circulation to the brachiocephalic vessels by placement of temporary bypass grafts originating off the proximal ascending aorta to be taken down at the completion of arch replacement. The second technique employed direct antegrade perfusion through the brachiocephalic vessels with the aid of cardiopulmonary bypass. In 1975, Griepp and coworkers (2) reported that the use of profound hypothermia and circulatory arrest for cerebral protection during aortic surgery provided a far simpler and safer technique for repair of aortic arch pathology. With popularization of profound hypothermia and deep circulatory arrest the results of aortic arch surgery improved. Nevertheless, in case of arrest times exceeding 60 minutes the incidence of neurological disorders and cerebral injury increased. This phenomenon was confirmed in clinical series by Griepp et al. 1991 (3) and supported by E. S. Crawford and coworkers in 1993 (5).

In an effort to prolong the safe period of hypothermic circulatory arrest Ueda and associates (6) reported the use of continuous retrograde cerebral perfusion via the superior vena cava in 1990. This technique was first described by Ochsner and Mills in 1980 (4) who installed retrograde perfusion for treatment of massive air embolism occurring during cardiopulmonary bypass. In 1982, Lemole and coworkers published a technique of intermittent retrograde cerebral perfusion during profound hypothermia and circulatory arrest it.

Today the technique of antegrade cerebral perfusion and the technique of retrograde cerebral perfusion are both in use. Among the most eminent surgeons of the antegrade perfusion technique are T. Kazui and J. Bachet who demonstrated their excellent results on neurologic outcome in their presentations. On the other hand J. Coselli presented his results with no neurological complication using, retrograde cerebral perfusion.

To answer the question of which concept is best to protect the brain during operations on the aortic arch many new studies have to be performed. The questions of safe duration for brain perfusion, range of perfusion pressure or use of a cerebroplegia with antiischemic drugs, still have to be answered.

We would like to thank the authors for their support and contributions. We are also indebted to Mrs. Ibkendanz and Mrs. Rühlemann and others from the Steinkopff Verlag for assembling and publishing this book. Our special gratitude goes to our coworker Stefan Bauer for his support in organizing the symposium and his share in the production of the book.

We hope that this book will serve as an useful synopsis of current knowledge of cerebral damage, cerebral protection and surgical management of pathology of the aortic arch and the supraaortic vessels.

Lahr, December 1996 J. Ennker

References

1. DeBakey ME, Cooley DA, Crawford ES, Morris GC (1957) Successful resection of fusiform aneurysm of the aortic arch with replacement by homograft. Surg Gynecol Obst 105: 656–664
2. Griepp RB, Stinson EB, Hollinsworth JF, Buehler D (1975) Prosthetic replacement of the aortic arch. J Thorac Cardiovasc Surg 70: 1051–1063
3. Griepp RB, Ergin MA, Lansman JL, Gall JD, Pogo G (1991) The physiology of hypothermic circulatory arrest. Semin Thorac Cardiovasc Surg 3: 188–193
4. Mills NL, Ochsner JL (1980) Massive air embolism during CPB: causes, prevention and management. J Thorac Cardiovasc Surg 80: 708–717
5. Svensson LG, Crawford ES, Rashkind SA et al. (1993) Deep hypothermia with circulatory arrest: determinants of stroke and early mortality in 656 patients. J Thorac Cardiovasc Surg 106: 19–31
6. Ueda Y, Miki S, Kusuhara K, Okita Y, Tahara T, Yamanaka K (1990) Surgical treatment of aneurysm of dissection involving the ascending aorta and aortic arch, utilizing circulatory arrest and retrograde cerebral perfusion. J Cardiovasc Surg (Torino) 31: 553–558

Contents

Cerebral protection in the pediatric age group

Neurophysiology, monitoring, cardiopulmonary bypass technique

Cerebral protection in aortic arch surgery

Protection, diagnosis and treatment of cerebral ischemia

Neuroprotection in cerebral ischemia

W. Paschen, K.-A. Hossmann

Max-Planck-Institute for Neurological Research, Department of Experimental Neurology, Köln, Germany

Introduction

The brain exhibits, in comparison with other organs, a high sensitivity to a critical reduction in blood flow. A few minutes after cessation of cerebral blood flow the tissue is depleted of primary and secondary energy compounds (glycogen, glucose and high energy phosphates such as adenosine triphosphate and phosphocreatine) due to the low energy reserves of the brain (34, 56). Such a situation occurs during cardiac arrest when blood flow to the brain stops completely. The occlusion of an intracerebral artery, in contrast, may cause a mild or severe reduction or even cessation of cerebral blood flow. The extent of this disturbance depends on the quality of collateral circulation and the local perfusion pressure. Whether these changes are critical for the survival of neurons depends on the duration and density of blood flow reduction. Different functions of neurons are affected at different threshold levels of cerebral blood flow: e.g., spontaneous electrical activity is already impaired when blood flow is reduced to about 60 % of control (26, 42), aerobic glucose metabolism is disturbed when blood flow is reduced to below 35 % of control (50), and at flow levels below about 20 % of control the tissue is depleted of ATP (50), the electrolyte homeostasis is disturbed (8–10), and cell death ensues unless blood flow is re-established. Interestingly, protein synthesis is suppressed already at blood flow levels of about 55 to 60 % of control, i.e., at considerably higher flow levels than those below which disturbances in energy metabolism take place (38).

In experimental studies, the strategy for protecting neurons from cell damage depends greatly on the model used for producing cerebral ischemia. The pathological process leading to ischemic cell death in models of focal and global cerebral ischemia is different from that occurring in permanent or reversible focal cerebral ischemia. Spreading depression for example, plays a major role in neuronal destruction in the penumbra of an ischemic focus (38) while after global cerebral ischemia spreading depression-like phenomena have not been observed, and the pathological process leading to ischemic cell damage is restricted to selectively vulnerable brain areas such as the hippocampal CA1-subfield where neuronal cell death occurs after a delay of about 3 days following cerebral ischemia (32). Exact knowledge of the pathological process leading to ischemic cell damage is the prerequisite for cause-related, direct therapeutical intervention. This paper, therefore, is designed to provide a comprehensive description of the pathophysiological and pathobiochemical disturbances induced by focal and global cerebral ischemia.

Focal cerebral ischemia

Pathophysiological and pathobiochemical disturbances

During severe focal cerebral ischemia of the cortex when blood flow is reduced below the critical level, spontaneous electrical activity is reduced briefly after vascular occlusion, as indicated by the diminution of EEG amplitude (26). The electrolyte homeostasis is maintained until the cells depolarize. The depolarization of the cells (terminal depolarization) is accompanied by massive electrolyte shifts from the intra- to the extracellular compartment (potassium ions) and vice versa (sodium and calcium ions) (3, 9, 10, 21). These changes are most dramatic for calcium ion activity, a difference of about 4 to 5 orders of magnitude developing between the extra- and intracellular compartments. Concomitant with the influx of calcium ions, the excitatory neurotransmitter glutamate is released from neurons into the synaptic cleft (55). Since the energy-requiring glutamate uptake systems cannot work during a state of energy depletion, extracellular glutamate levels are sharply increased, the extent of this increase depending on the density and duration of ischemia. It is therefore not surprising that in focal cerebral ischemia a sharp increase in extracellular glutamate levels is restricted to brain areas with flow rates below about 20 ml/100 g/min (54), i.e., a flow threshold below which the tissue is depleted of ATP (50).

The reduction of blood flow is not uniform after occlusion of a major cerebral artery within the ipsilateral hemisphere. The affected area can be differentiated into core tissue and penumbra: in the ischemic core cerebral blood flow is reduced below the threshold of ATP depletion and induction of disturbances in electrolyte homeostasis; in the penumbra, in contrast, ATP levels and electrolyte homeostasis are maintained for some time after vascular occlusion. Protein synthesis is, however, suppressed (38) and the tissue is, therefore, at risk as long as blood flow fails to improve. When the occlusion of the artery continues, the area of the tissue depleted of ATP increases: 12 h after vascular occlusion the threshold of cerebral blood flow causing ATP depletion increases (from about 19 ml/100 g/min immediately after vascular occlusion) to about 32 ml/100 g/min (38). This growth of the tissue area depleted of ATP probably results from spreading depression (SD) waves which are elicited by glutamate and potassium (released from the ischemic core) and then spread over the cortex (39). As discussed below, SD induces transient physiological and metabolic changes (16, 21, 37) which are tolerated by the intact brain (44), but not by the metabolically compromised tissue surrounding an ischemic core.

During SD a wave of electrical silence and cell depolarization moves over the cortex with a speed of about 3 mm/min. In addition, massive electrolyte shifts are induced as indicated by a sharp increase in extracellular potassium and decrease in calcium activity (21). Energy is required to reestablish electrolyte homeostasis. This increased energy demand causes a transient reduction in the levels of glucose and ATP and an acidic pH-shift (16, 37), indicative of partially anaerobic glucose metabolism. Further, cerebral blood flow, glucose utilization and pO_2 are transiently increased (4, 37). In control animals, SD waves can be elicited by different means: by chemical, physical or mechanical stress of the tissue.

In the penumbra of an ischemic core, SD-like waves are elicited spontaneously (4, 39), most probably by glutamate released into the extracellular space from energy-depleted neurons within the ischemic core. The hemodynamic and metabolic response to SD in the penumbra of an ischemic focus differs from that occurring in the control state: the duration of SD waves (as measured by direct current (DC) deflections) is significantly prolonged from 1.4 ± 0.5 min in the control brain to 5.2 ± 4.8 min in the periphery of ischemic brain lesions (4). In addition, cerebral blood flow (cortical laser-Doppler flow) is not increased in the penumbra during the passage of DC deflections and the pO_2 decreases rather than increases during this event (4). Thus, in the periphery of an ischemic core, the increased energy demand induced by spontaneously elicited SD waves is not matched by a concomitant increase in local cerebral blood flow and pO_2. It can, therefore, be assumed that within the penumbra metabolic disturbances intensify with each passage of SD waves, and that in focal cerebral ischemia the observed increase in the area of tissue undergoing ATP depletion with time (38) is caused by spontaneously elicited SD waves. In fact, in diffusion weighted images in models of focal cerebral ischemia the size of tissue exhibiting hyperdensity increases with each SD wave (Hoehn-Berlage et al., in preparation) and the size of the infarcts correlates closely with the number of DC-deflections after middle cerebral artery occlusion in rats (39).

Pharmacological intervention

Several strategies have been developed for the reduction of cell damage in focal cerebral ischemia by pharmacological intervention, their success depending on the feasibility of pretreatment. The major goal of pretreament is to prolong the neuronal survival time by protracting the time interval between onset of ischemia and terminal depolarization, and thus delaying the tissue depletion of high energy phosphates. Once the tissue is depleted of ATP and cells are depolarized, the pathological process leading to ischemic cell damage can be stopped by thrombolytic therapy, i.e., a recanalization of the occluded artery. Finally, cells in the penumbra of the ischemic core can be protected by reducing the energy demand of the tissue, e.g., by preventing spreading depression waves, or by counteracting with pathological disturbances induced by spreading depression.

The main routes of therapeutical intervention in focal cerebral ischemia have been summarized before (20, 28, 30, 35, 36, 47) and need not be repeated here. Among others, the following groups of compounds have been used as neuroprotective agents: glutamate antagonists, calcium antagonists, sodium-channel blockers, potassium-channel openers, free-radical scavengers, nitric oxide synthase inhibitors, protease inhibitors (for a review see (36)). In addition, hypothermia proved to have a robust neuroprotective effect (for a review see (35)).

Recently, interest has focused on spreading depression as a detrimental factor in focal cerebral ischemia (4, 39). As discussed above, spreading depression probably plays a major role in the pathological process leading to ischemic cell damage in the penumbra of an ischemic focus. Thus, agents decreasing the number of spreading depression waves, elicited spontaneously by glutamate released from the ischemic core, can cause a 75 % reduction in the size of neocortical infarct volume (39). Glutamate antagonists belonging to the N-methyl-D-aspartate (NMDA) and alpha-amino-3-hydroxy-5-methyl-isoxazole-4-propionate (AMPA)/ kainate receptor families were found to block spreading depression waves and to reduce the size of the infarct significantly (39). The possible mechanism by which suppression of peri-infarct depolarizations protects cells in the penumbra from damage has recently been elucidated (40): In untreated animals, breakdown of energy metabolism and protein synthesis occurred at flow values below about 15 and 50 ml/100 g/min (40). In MK-801-treated animals the perfusion threshold for inhibition of protein synthesis declined to 19 ml/100 g/min, whereas the flow threshold for inducing disturbances in energy-producing metabolism remained constant (40). Thus, metabolic disturbances (as indicated by the inhibition of protein synthesis) were absent in the penumbra of treated animals. Spontaneously elicited peri-infarct depolarizations have been observed in animals in models of focal cerebral ischemia (see above). Whether similar phenomena occur in human stroke has still to be established.

Transient global cerebral ischemia

Pathophysiological and pathobiochemical disturbances

Pathophysiological and pathobiochemical disturbances induced by global cerebral ischemia are almost identical to those observed in focal cerebral ischemia within the ischemic core. Here, blood flow is reduced below the threshold necessary to maintain energy state and electrolyte homeostasis so that within a few seconds after onset of ischemia, spontaneous electrical activity of the cerebral cortex ceases and phosphocreatine levels start to decline (34). About 2 min later the terminal depolarization of the cells takes place as indicated by a sharp decrease in extracellular calcium and sodium activity and increase in extracellular potassium activity (21, 22, 24). Within 3 to 5 min after onset of ischemia the tissue becomes depleted of primary and secondary energy reserves, exhibits a sharp increase in lactate levels and an acidic pH shift (49, 56) because the acidic equivalents produced during glucose metabolism cannot be cleared into the blood. In contrast to focal cerebral ischemia, the organism cannot survive global cerebral ischemia, unless the brain is recirculated.

In animal models of isolated global cerebral ischemia, in which the blood supply to the brain is arrested by occluding the respective arteries, recirculation is not a major problem even after ischemic periods of up to 1 h duration (23, 27, 29), because, after releasing the occluder, a sufficiently high perfusion pressure can be built up to flush the stagnant blood out of the vascular bed. During ischemia blood viscosity increases owing to the aggregation of blood corpuscles and a shift of water from blood into the brain along osmotic gradients (25). The viscosity changes produced by complete cerebral ischemia, as observed after isolated cerebral ischemia, are similar to those occurring after cardiac arrest. However, the perfusion pressure of the brain is higher after isolated ischemia, because, under these circumstances, the heart is not damaged.

One of the major complications arising after complete cerebral ischemia is the no-reflow phenomenon which is characterized by a lack of reperfusion (1). Areas with impaired vascular filling increase with the duration of ischemia (18). After isolated cerebral ischemia a homogenous reperfusion (without areas of no-reflow) was achieved after 30 min four-vessel occlusion in rats (52) and even after 1 h of complete global cerebral ischemia, providing the recirculation started with a hypertensive flush (23, 29). After cardiac arrest, however, areas of no-reflow developed during resuscitation after only 5 min of circulatory arrest (18) and the volume of the tissue showing no-reflow increased with longer durations of ischemia (18).

Energy metabolism and electrolyte homeostasis are restored within the first 30 min after global cerebral ischemia (56). The levels of energy metabolites stay high during the recovery phase as long as the cells are intact (2), but ATP and PCR levels decline after about 4 days of recirculation in selectively vulnerable brain structures such as the hippocampal CA1-subfield (see below) at the same time that cell damage is manifested morphologically (2, 32). Blood flow is considerably reduced for several hours after complete cerebral ischemia, a phenomenon termed post-ischemic hypoperfusion (29); some believe this hypoperfusion to be a cause of relative hypoxia and thus a possible risk factor in transient global cerebral ischemia (29). Furthermore, CO2-reactivity is abolished after transient global cerebral ischemia (29), suggesting that the blood flow is not coupled to glucose metabolism.

A characteristic feature of transient global cerebral ischemia is that the pathological process leading to ischemic cell damage is restricted to selectively vulnerable brain regions. After forebrain ischemia of only 5 min, cells of the hippocampal CA1-subfield are almost completely destroyed, a process which is morphologically manifested with a delay of about 3 days after vascular occlusion (32). This phenomenon is not restricted to animal experiments, because even in humans the hippocampal CA1-subfield is particularly sensitive to transient global cerebral ischemia, when caused by cardiac arrest followed by resuscitation (51). In experimental studies, when the period of global cerebral ischemia is extended to 30 min, neuronal cell damage is also evident in the lateral striatum (53). The cerebral cortex, however, is remarkably resistant to transient cerebral ischemia and cell damage is minor in this region even after complete cerebral circulatory arrest of up to 1-h duration (27).

The mechanisms of ischemic cell damage induced by transient global cerebral ischemia have not been fully elucidated. It has been proposed that the sharp increase in intracellular calcium levels plays a pivotal role in the pathological process, where voltage-gated and agonist-operated calcium channels and a release of calcium from intracellular stores contribute to the rise in intracellular calcium activity during ischemia (57). The main route for the influx of calcium into the cell by agonist-operated channels is the glutamate-operated channel of the NMDA type which gates both monovalent and divalent cations; the non-NMDA glutamate receptor channel, in contrast, have only a low calcium conductance under physiological conditions in most of the neurons (42). Further, it has been assumed that the calcium overload of neurons during ischemia activates several calcium-dependent processes, such as lipolysis and proteolysis, and secondary reactions such as the formation of free radicals which finally destroy the integrity of cellular membranes (57).

The observation that glutamate is neurotoxic in vivo under certain experimental conditions (46), that glutamate is released from neurons into the synaptic cleft during ischemia (5) and that, in primary neuronal tissue culture, cell death can be induced with glutamate (providing the experiments are performed in the absence of serum (13)), have been taken as evidence that ischemic cell death is an excitotoxic process triggered by glutamate released during ischemia . However, this is still a matter of debate (for a recent review see 30), and the observation that non-NMDA antagonists are neuroprotective even when applied several hours after cerebral ischemia (see below) argue against the hypothesis that ischemically released glutamate plays a major role in the pathological process leading to neuronal damage after transient global cerebral ischemia.

One of the common responses to severe metabolic stress as produced by transient global cerebral ischemia is a depression of overall protein synthesis (6, 15). Immediately after cerebral ischemia polyribosomes disaggregate and protein synthesis is severely inhibited throughout the forebrain (15), most probably because the initiation process is blocked (15). Polyribosomes reaggregate and protein synthesis recovers in non-vulnerable brain structures such as the cortex, but polyribosomal disaggregation and suppresion of protein synthesis persist in the vulnerable hippocampal CA1-subfield (7). Whether the post-ischemic inhibition of protein synthesis is per se a pathological process contributing to the development of ischemic cell damage or whether it is only an epiphenomenon without any direct effect on cell integrity after ischemia has still to be established.

Pharmacological intervention

The form of therapeutic intervention most dramatically affecting cell survival after transient global cerebral ischemia is hypothermia (for a review see (35). Even mild reduction of body temperature by only 2 °C had a neuroprotective effect when applied during ischemia (12). Hypothermia can also mitigate neuronal damage when applied several hours after transient global cerebral ischemia: a significant reduction of cell death has been achieved with hypothermia induced 12 h after forebrain ischemia (14). Hyperthermia exacerbates the pathological process (41), so that, in animals in which brain temperature increases spontaneously after ischemia, cell damage can be blocked by keeping the tissue normothermic during early recirculation after ischemia (33).

The protective effect of mild hypothermia is so strong that, in experimental studies designed to limit ischemic cell damage pharmacologically, brain temperature has to be carefully controlled to distinguish any specific protective effect of the drug under trial from an unspecific temperature effect. In fact, it was found that the beneficial effect of the NMDA-receptor antagonist MK-801 on cell damage in the hippocampal CA1-subfield of gerbils (19) was produced by hypothermia and not by blocking of the NMDA-receptor (11): when brain temperature was carefully controlled during the experiment, MK-801 failed to be neuroprotective in this model.

The neuroprotective efficicacy of various groups of pharmacological compounds in different models of transient global cerebral ischemia has been reviewed before (28, 30, 35). As stated earlier (28), calcium antagonists have little or no effect on the damage produced by global cerebral ischemia, and the observed improvements can be explained by the vasoactive properties of the drugs. The protective potency of different NMDA and non-NMDA glutamate receptor antagonists on neuronal injury of the hippocampal CA1-subfield has been reviewed recently (30). Interestingly, in all but one of the studies employing the non-NMDA glutamate receptor antagonist NBQX, this drug was found to inhibit the development of ischemic cell damage in the CA1-subfield, and a significant effect could be achieved in most of the experimental series even when application of the compound was delayed until 24 h after transient ischemia (54). These results, therefore, indicate that if glutamate contributes to the pathological process leading to cell death, it does so postischemically

Perspective

The most marked neuroprotective effect is achieved by inducing hypothermia in different models of transient or permanent focal and transient global cerebral ischemia, as discussed above. One neuron-produced compound has attracted particular attention recently, as a putative factor in the development of ischemic cell damage: nitric oxide (NO), the product of nitric oxid synthase (NOS) reaction. The use of NOS inhibitors has generated widely disparate findings (for a review see (17)), because NO has diverse physiological functions. However, experiments with different models of ischemia in neuronal NOS knock-out animals showed that cell damage was significantly reduced in animals lacking neuronal NOS, thus confirming a role of neuronal NO in brain pathology during and after ischemia (31, 48).

References

1. Ames A, Wright L, Kowada M, Thurston JM, Majeno G (1968) Cerebral ischemia. The no-reflow phenomenon. Am J Pathol 52: 437–453
2. Arai H, Passonneau JV, Lust WD (1986) Energy metabolism in delayed neuronal death of CA1 neurons of the hippocampus following transient ischemia in the gerbil. Metabol Brain Dis 1: 263–278

3. Astrup J, Symon L, Branston NM, Lassen NA (1977) Cortical evoked potential and extracelluar K^+ and H^+ at critical levels of brain ischemia. Stroke 8: 51–57
4. Back T, Kohno K, Hossmann K-A (1994) Cortical negative DC deflections following middle cerebral artery occlusion and KCl-induced spreading depression: Effect on blood flow, tissue oxygenation, and electroencephalogram. J Cereb Blood Flow Metabol 14: 12-19
5. Benveniste H, Drejer J, Schousboe A, Diemer NH (1984) Elevation of the extracellular concentrations of glutamate and aspartate in rat hippocampus during transient cerebral ischemia monitored by intracerebral microdialysis. J Neurochem 43: 1369–1374
6. Bodsch W, Takahashi K, Barbier A, Grosse Ophoff B, Hossmann K-A (1985) Cerebral protein synthesis and ischemia. Prog Brain Res 63: 197–210
7. Bonnekoh P, Kuroiwa T, Oschlies U, Hossmann KA (1992) Barbiturate promotes post-ischemic reaggregation of polyribosomes in gerbil hippocampus. Neurosci Lett 146: 75–78
8. Branston NM, Syman L, Crockard HA, Pasztor E (1974) Relationship between the cortical evoked potential and local cortical blood flow following acute middle cerebral artery occlusion in the baboon. Exp Neurol 45: 195–208
9. Branston NM, Strong AJ, Symon L (1976) Different flow thresholds for failure of evoked response and increase in extracellular potassium activity during progressive ischaemia in cerebral cortex. J Physiol (Lond) 263: 139P–140P
10. Branston NM, Strong AJ, Symon L (1977) Extracellular potassium activity, evoked potential and tissue blood flow: Relationship during progressive ischaemia in baboon cerebral cortex. J Neurol Sci 32: 305–321
11. Buchan A, Pulsinelli WA (1990) Hypothermia but not the N-methyl-D-aspartate antagonist, MK-801, attenuates neuronal damage in gerbils subjected to transient global ischemia. J Neurosci 10: 311–316
12. Busto R, Dietrich WD, Globus MY-T, Valdès I, Scheinberg P, Ginsberg MD (1987) Small differences in intraischemic brain temperature critically determine the extent of ischemic neuronal injury. J Cereb Blood Flow Metabol 7: 729–738
13. Choi DM, Maulucci-Gedde M, Krieglstein AR (1987) Glutamate neurotoxicity in cortical cell culture. J Neurosci 7: 357–368
14. Coimbra C, Wieloch T (1994) Moderate hypothermia mitigates neuronal damage in the rat brain when initiated several hours following transient cerebral ischemia. Acta Neuropathol 87: 325–331
15. Cooper HK, Zalewska T, Kawakami S, Hossmann K-A (1977) The effect of ischemia and recirculation on protein synthesis in the brain. J Neurochem 929–934
16. Csiba L, Paschen W, Mies G (1985) Regional changes in tissue pH and glucose content during cortical spreading depression in rat brain. Brain Res 336: 167–170
17. Dawson DA (1994) Nitric oxide and focal cerebral ischemia: Multiplicity of actions and diverse outcome. Cerebrovasc Brain Metabol Rev 6: 299–324
18. Fischer M, Hossmann K-A (1995) No-reflo after cardiac arrest. Intens Care Med 21: 132–141
19. Gill R, Foster AC, Woodruff GN (1988) MK-801 is neuroprotective in gerbils when administered during the post-ischemic period. Neurosci 25: 847–855
20. Hacke W, Niedermaier N, Wildemann B (1994) Thrombolytic therapy in acute ischemic stroke – an update. In: Kriegelstein J, Oberpichler-Schwenk H (eds) Pharmacology of cerebral ischemia. Medpharm Scientific Publishers, Stuttgart, pp 617–624
21. Hansen AJ, Zeuthen T (1981) Extracellular ion concentrations during spreading depression and ischemia in the rat brain cortex. Acta Physiol Scand 113: 437–445
22. Harris RJ, Symon L, Branston NM, Bayhan M (1981) Changes in extracellular calcium activity in cerebral ischemia. J Cereb Blood Flow Metabol 1: 203–209
23. Hossmann K-A, Lechtape-Grüter H, Hossmann V (1973) The role of cerebral blood flow for the recovery of the brain after prolonged ischemia. Z Neurol 204: 281–299
24. Hossmann K-A, Sakaki S, Zimmermann V (1977) Cation activities in reversible ischaemia of the cat brain. Stroke 8: 77–81
25. Hossmann K-A, Takagi S (1979) Osmolality of the brain in cerebral ischemia. Exp Neurol 51: 124–131
26. Hossmann K-A, Schuier FJ (1980) Experimental brain infarcts in cats. I. Pathological observations. Stroke 11: 583–592
27. Hossmann K-A, Schmidt-Kastner R, Grosse Ophoff B (1987) Recovery of integrative nervous functions after one hour global cerebro-circulatory arrest in normothermic cat. J Neurol Sci 77: 305–320
28. Hossmann K-A (1989) Calcium antagonists for the treatment of brain ischemia: A critical apprisal. In: Kriegelstein J (ed) Pharmacology of cerebral ischemia. Wissenschaftliche Verlagsgesellschaft, Stuttgart, pp 53–63
29. Hossmann K-A (1990) Hemodynamics of post-ischemic reperfusion of the brain. In: Weinstein PR, Faden AI (eds). Protection of the brain from ischemia. Williams & Wilkins, Baltimore, pp 21–26
30. Hossmann K-A (1994) Mechanisms of ischemic injury: is glutamate involved? In: Kriegelstein J, Oberpichler-Schwenk H (eds) Pharmacology of cerebral ischemia. Medpharm Scientific Publishers, Stuttgart, pp 239–251

31. Huang Z, Huang PL, Panahian N, Dalkara T, Fishman MC, Moskowitz MA (1994) Effects of cerebral ischemia in mice deficient in neuronal nitric oxide synthase. Science 265: 1883–1885
32. Kirino T (1982) Delayed neuronal death in the gerbil hippocampus following ischemia. Brain Res 239: 57–69
33. Kuroiwa T, Bonnekoh P, Hossmann K-A (1990) Prevention of postischemic hyperthermia prevents ischemic injury of CA1 neurons in gerbils. J Cereb Blood Flow Metabol 10: 550–556
34. Lowry OH, Passonneau JV, Hasselberger FY, Schulz DW (1964) Effects of ischemia on known substrates and cofactors of the glycolytic pathway in brain. J Biol Chem 239: 18–30
35. Maher J, Hachinski V (1993) Hypothermia as a potential treatment for cerebral ischemia. Cerebrovasc Brain Metabol Rev 5: 277–300
36. Meldrum BS (1995) Cytoprotective therapies in stroke. Curr Opinion Neurol 8: 15–23
37. Mies G, Paschen W (1984) Regional changes of blood flow, glucose, and ATP content determined on brain sections during a single passage of spreading depression in rat brain cortex. Exp Neurol 84: 249–258
38. Mies G, Ishimaru S, Xie Y, Seo K, Hossmann K-A (1991) Ischemic thresholds of cerebral protein synthesis and energy state following middle cerebral artery occlusion in rat. J Cereb Blood Flow Metabol 11: 753–761
39. Mies G, Iijima T, Hossmann K-A (1993) Correlation between peri-infarct DC shifts and ischaemic neuronal damage in rat. NeuroReport 4: 709–711
40. Mies G, Kohno K, Hossmann K-A (1993) MK-801, a glutamate antagonist, lowers flow threshold for inhibition of protein synthesis after middle cerebral artery occlusion of rat. Neurosci Lett 155: 65–68
41. Minamisawa H, Smith M-L, Siesjö BK (1990) The effect of mild hyperthermia and hypothermia on brain damage following 5, 10, and 15 min of forebrain ischemia. Ann Neurol 28: 26–33
42. Monaghan DT, Bridges RJ, Cotman CW (1989). The excitatory amino acid receptors: their classes, pharmacology, and distinct properties in the function of the central nervous system. Ann Rev Pharmacol Toxicol 29: 365–402
43. Moraweth RB, Crowell RH, DeGirolami U, Marcoux FW, Jones TH, Halsey JH (1979) Regional cerebral blood flow thresholds during cerebral ischemia. Fed Proc Fed Am Soc Exp Biol 38: 2493–2494
44. Needergaard M, Hansen AJ (1988) Spreading depression is not associated with neuronal injury in the normal brain. Brain Res 449: 395–398
45. Nicholson C (1980) Measurement of extracellular ions in the brain. Trends Neurosci 3: 216–218
46. Olney JW (1969) Brain lesions, obesity, and other disturbances in mice treated with monosodium glutamate. Science 164: 719–721
47. Overgaard K (1994) Thrombolytic therapy in experimental stroke. Cerebrovasc Brain Metabol Rev 6: 257–286
48. Panahian N, Yoshida T, Huang PL, Hedley-Whyte T, Fishman M, Moskowitz MA (1995) Attenuated hippocampal damage after global cerebral ischemia in knock-out mice deficient in neuronal nitric oxide synthase. J Cereb Blood Flow Metabol 15 (Suppl 1): S5
49. Paschen W, Djuricic B, Mies G, Schmidt-Kastner R, Linn F (1997) Lactate and pH in the brain. Association and dissociation in different pathological states. J Neurochem 48: 154–159
50. Paschen W, Mies G, Hossmann K-A (1992) Threshold relationship between cerebral blood flow, glucose utilization, and energy metabolites during development of stroke in gerbils. Exp Neurol 117: 325–333
51. Petito CK, Feldmann E, Pulsinelli WA, Plum F (1987) Delayed hippocampal damage in human following cardiorespiratory arrest. Neurol 37: 1281–1286
52. Pulsinelli WA, Levy DE, Duffy TE (1982) Regional cerebral blood flow and glucose metabolism following transient forebrain ischemia. Ann Neurol 11: 499–509
53. Pulsinelli WA, Brierley JB, Plum F (1982) Temporal profile of neuronal damage in a model of transient forebrain ischemia. Ann Neurol 11: 491–498
54. Sheardown MJ, Suzdak PD, Nordholm L (1993) AMPA, but not NMDA, receptor antagonism is neuroprotective in gerbil global ischemia, even when delayed 24 h. Eur J Pharmacol 236: 347–353
55. Shimada N, Graf R, Rosner G, Wakayama A, George CP, Heiss W-D (1989) Ischemic flow threshold for extracellular glutamate release in cat cortex. J Cereb Blood Flow Metabol 9: 603–606
56. Siesjö BK (1978) Brain energy metabolism. Wiley, New York
57. Siesjö BK (1981) Cell damage in the brain: A speculative synthesis. J Cereb Blood Flow Metabol 1: 155–185

Authors' address:
Priv.-Doz. Dr. rer. nat. W. Paschen
Max-Planck-Institut
für Neurologische Forschung
Gleueler Str. 50
50931 Köln
Germany

PET, MRI, and MRS for imaging of functional brain disorders

K. Herholz, H. Lanfermann

Max-Planck-Institut für neurologische Forschung, Neurologische Klinik und Klinik und Poliklinik für diagnostische Radiologie der Universität zu Köln

Introduction

Since the development of computed tomography (CT) by Hounsfield and Ambrose rapid further diversification of tomographic methods occurred. CT is extremely useful for clinical diagnosis of structural brain lesions and is widely available today. In recent years, new methods were developed that, in addition to imaging of brain structure, also permit tomographic imaging of brain function and its alterations (Fig. 1).

The most versatile technique for functional brain imaging is positron emission tomography (PET). By the use of very short-lived isotopes, a large variety of physiological pro-

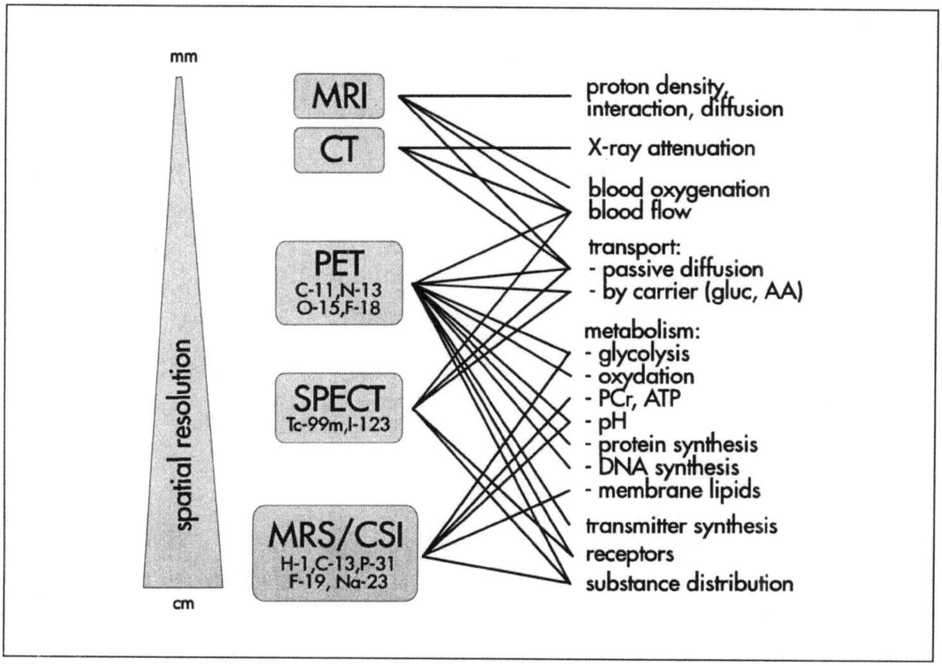

Fig. 1. Scheme of computed tomography methods, indicating spatial resolution and physical or physiological parameters that determine image intensity (see text for explanation of abbreviations).

cesses can be measured locally. Single photon emission computed tomography (SPECT) is another isotope technique for imaging of cerebral blood flow, but metabolic imaging is not possible.

Magnetic resonance imaging employs neither external (x-rays) nor internal (radio-isotopes) radiation, but uses magnetic resonance phenomena of the natural nuclei (in most instances H-1) that make up normal and pathological tissue. It is most frequently used for imaging of normal and pathological morphology, but some new developments also permit imaging of brain function (functional MRI, fMRI). Magnetic resonance spectroscopy analyzes small shifts in resonance frequencies that are due to the interaction of nuclei with their neighbors. The concentrations of some of the most abundant biochemical substrates present in normal and pathological tissue can be analyzed by this technique with a spatial resolution on the order of 1 ccm.

In the first part of this brief review, the most important technical aspects of PET, MRI and MRS will be discussed to lay the ground for understanding of their potential to image brain dysfunction. In the second part, the most important aspects of the pathophysiology of hypoxic and ischemic brain damage that can be studied with PET, MRI, and MRS will be described.

PET

With PET, positron emitting isotopes (^{11}C, ^{13}N, ^{15}O, ^{18}F) with half-life times of 2 to 110 min are used to label biochemical tracers (Table 1). Medical cyclotrons are used most frequently to produce these isotopes. Coupling of an isotope to a physiological tracer and preparation as an injectable radiopharmaceutical requires a specialized laboratory (44).

Table 1. Selected Isotopes and Tracers for PET

Isotope	Measurement	Tracer
^{11}C (20,4)*	pH	carbon dioxide, DMO
	blood flow	butanol, fluoromethane
	glucose consumption	glucose, deoxyglucose
	amino acid uptake	valine, leucine, tyrosine
	D2 receptors	raclopride, spiperone
	serotonine receptors	ketanserine, altanserine
	opiate receptors	carfentanyl, diprenorphine
	benzodiazepine rec.	flumazenil
^{15}O (2,05)*	oxygen consumption	O_2 gas
	blood flow	water, carbondioxide, butanol
	blood volume	carbon monoxide
^{18}F (109,7)*	blood flow	fluoromethane
	glucose consumption	2-fluoro-2-deoxyglucose
	amino acid uptake	fluorotyrosine
	dopamine synthesis	fluorodopa
	D2/S2 receptors	spiperone
	opiate receptors	cylofoxy

*) Half-life time in minutes

After intravenous injection or inhalation of the tracer, its distribution in the brain is imaged with a positron emission tomograph. The positrons emitted by the isotope annihilate with electrons after a free path length of up to 2 mm, thereby emitting two gamma rays of 511 kev energy at an angle of 180 degree to each other. These gamma rays are detected by coincidence detector rings in the tomograph. In many tomographs, coincidence detection is limited to planes within adjacent detector rings, but very recently also three-dimensional coincidence detection became available (46), improving effective sensitivity approx. three- to four-fold. Current tomographs provide a spatial resolution of about 4 to 5 mm in all three dimensions. Corrections for random coincidences, scatter and attenuation can be performed with high accuracy, thus permitting quantitative measurements of local isotope activities in tissue.

Measurement of CBF

For assessment of ischemic or hypoxic brain damage, the physiological parameters cerebral blood flow (CBF), cerebral metabolic rate of oxygen ($CMRO_2$) and cerebral metabolic rate of glucose (CMRGlu) are of most interest. Their measurement is based on mathematical physiological models.

For measurement of CBF freely diffusible tracers are used, most frequently ^{15}O water. The most straightforward approach is the intravenous bolus injection of ^{15}O-water (36). At arrival of the bolus in the brain, its initial distribution mainly depends on local blood flow because diffusion distances are small enough not to limit tracer distribution. Tissue tracer activity equilibrates with venous activity. The differential equations describing this process lead to an operational equation that relates local CBF with the time-course of arterial tracer activity (measured by continuous blood sampling from the radial artery) and local tissue activity (measured by the tomograph). By this technique local and global CBF can be measured.

For assessment of focal functional brain impairment or stimulation, measurement of global CBF (in absolute units, i.e. in ml blood per 100 g tissue per min) may not be necessary. Arterial blood sampling is not required for measurement of local CBF changes (relative to other brain regions with normal CBF). In this case, a completely non-invasive technique is sufficient (10).

At very high blood flow levels some underestimation of CBF occurs with ^{15}O-water (approximately 15 % at true CBF of 100 ml/100 g/min), because it is not completely freely diffusible. This problem can be overcome by tracers ^{15}O-butanol or ^{18}F-fluoromethane, but these tracers are more difficult to synthesize and, in the case of fluoromethane, application of the gaseous tracer to subjects is inconvenient. Therefore, the ^{15}O water bolus technique is preferred currently, because it provides reasonable accuracy and good practicability.

Noninvasive CBF measurements are often used in functional activation studies. The increase of local CBF that is elicited in brain areas that are functionally active is detected by comparison with a resting or reference measurement. Most studies of normal brain function employed stereotactic or nonlinear standardization of brain size and shape for pixel-wise averaging over several individuals (11, 14, 32) to improve the sensitivity for signal detection and statistical analysis. With 3D coincidence detection, sensitivity is high enough to perform activation studies of higher brain functions in single individuals with multiple replication of activation and resting states.

Measurement of metabolism

Measurement of $CMRO_2$ requires the inhalation of ^{15}O-oxygen gas. The distribution of the tracer in brain depends on delivery by CBF and on local oxygen consumption. The metabolic end product is ^{15}O-CO_2 and ^{15}O-water, which is washed out by CBF. To acount for delivery of the tracer, wash-out of metabolic products and correction for recirculating ^{15}O-water, CBF must be known and is therefore generally measured immediately before or after measurement of $CMRO_2$. For quantitative calculations, the single-bolus inhalation method and the operational equation developed by Mintun et al. (33) is usually preferred. Experiments that were done on older tomographs with low count-rate capabilites employed a steady-state model that was described by Frackowiak et al. (12). Yet, this approach yields less accurate results than Mintun's method.

For measurement of CMRGlu, intravenous injection of ^{18}F-2-fluoro-2-deoxy-D-glucose (FDG) (37) is the standard technique. It is based on experimental work by Sokoloff et al. (42), who demonstrated that deoxy-glucose is transported and phosphorylized by hexokinase in the brain similar to glucose. It accumulates there because, in contrast to glucose, very little further metabolism occurs, and the hexokinase reaction in the brain is essentially unidirectional. Again, from the appropriate differential equations with empirical correction factors to account for the different enzyme affinities of deoxy-glucose and glucose (lumped constant), an operational equation is derived which relates CMRGlu to the time-course of arterial tracer activity and tissue activity, measured by the tomograph. Since the peripheral extraction fraction of deoxy-glucose is low, sampling of arterialized venous blood is sufficient to determine the arterial concentration, thus permitting completely non-invasive measurement. The time required for sufficient tracer accumulation is usually 30 to 60 min. With some measurement protocols the whole time-course of tracer accumulation over approx. 60 min is recorded by the tomograph, but for most purposes recording times of 10 to 20 min in the tomograph (starting 30 to 40 min after injection) are sufficient.

MRI

The nuclei of hydrogen (^1H) are single protons which have a spin and an associated magnetic momentum. In a strong external magnetic field (typical magnetic field strength for clinical applications is 0.15 to 2 Tesla) these spins tend to align with the external field and, after a certain time, reach a steady-state of magnetization. By application of an electromagnetic wave impulse with appropriate frequency some of the nuclei are excited. This excitation disappears again with time constants T_1 (due to spin-lattice interactions) and T_2 (spin-spin interactions) by emission of an electromagnetic signal which is recorded by the tomograph. Superposition of gradient magnetic fields to the stationary field permits localization and tomographic reconstruction of the signal based on small shifts in resonance frequency and phase (29).

Frequently used excitation sequences generate images that are dominated by proton density, T_1, or T_2. T_2-weighted images show stationary fluids and most pathological alterations, e.g. infarcts, inflammatory foci, demyelination, and tumors, with high signal intensity and are therefore included in most clinical standard imaging protocols. Low signal intensity is obtained in moving fluids, and in the basal ganglia and the cerebellar dentate nuclei, probably due to their iron content. Proton-density and T_1-weighted images can contribute to lesion differentiation. Paramagnetic substances, e.g. methemoglobin (degradation product from intracerebral hematomas) and Gd-containing contrast agents, shorten T_1 considerably and produce high signal in T_1-weighted images. Another important feature of most T_1-weighted images is a good contrast between normal gray and white matter, providing rich anatomical detail. Inversion recovery images also show detailed anatomy, but are not sensitive to many pathological changes.

Typical recording times for images with conventional equipment are in the order of 5 to 20 min. With recent techniques for volume excitation (e.g., FLASH, FFE, (13)) one brain study can be performed within a few minutes. With special hard- and software for echo planar imaging (EPI), recording times for single slices are reduced to the order of milliseconds (43), thus, the complete brain can be studied within less than 1 min.

Further recent developments include diffusion-weighted imaging that shows brain areas in which diffusion of water is more restricted than in other areas with high signal. This is of particular interest for imaging of brain infarcts a few hours after onset of ischemia (31).

Functional MRI (fMRI) shows CBF-dependent signal changes. The blood oxygenation-level dependent (BOLD) method uses a small shortening of effective tissue T_2 that is due to the presence of paramagnetic deoxyhemoglobin in capillary and venous blood (34). As explained later, deoxyhemoglobin levels often decline in functionally activated brain areas. By pixel-wise comparison of images obtained during activated and resting state, functionally activated brain areas can be localized. Often multiple scans are obtained during activated and resting states with high temporal resolution.

MRS

In biochemistry, MRS is often used for chemical analysis of small in vitro probes. It is based on small shifts of resonance frequency (in the order of 1/1000000, i.e. 1 ppm) that is caused by the chemical bonds to other nuclei. The technique can be integrated into magnetic resonance tomographs to examine biochemical tissue composition in vivo, although the volume resolution (typically in the order of 1 ccm) is much lower than with MRI. In addition to protons, several other nuclei can be analyzed with MRS (Table 2), of which only ^{31}P was included in clinical studies as yet.

Proton MR spectra of the normal brain show at least three distinct peaks: choline, creatine (including phosphocreatine), and N-acetyl asparate (NAA). NAA is of particular interest in studies of brain damage, because it is a by-product of neuronal metabolism and may therefore probably be used as an indicator of the density of viable neurons (5, 15). A large signal from water can be suppressed by various technical means (9). Some pathological processes, i.p. recent infarcts and most brain tumors contain increased lactate levels that are detected as a double peak at 1.3 ppm. Extracerebral lipids from the galea would appear at approx. the same frequency and must be excluded by appropriate localization techniques. Minor peaks of glutamin and glutamate, taurine, myo-inositol and glucose have been identified in human brain in vivo (16).

Phosphorus MR spectra include peaks representing phosphomonoesters, anorganic phosphate (P_i), phosphodiesters, phosphocreatin, and three peaks from energy-rich phosphonucleotides. They therefore represent tissue energy state that may be impaired after an

Table 2. Nuclides for magnetic resonance imaging and spectroscopy

Nucleus	Resonance frequency at 1 Tesla (MHz)	Relative natural abundance (%)	Relative sensitivity sensitivity
^{1}H	42.58	99.98	1
^{13}C	10.71	1.11	0.0096
^{19}F	40.05	100	0.83
^{23}Na	11.26	100	0.093
^{31}P	17.23	100	0.066

ischemic insult. Also phosphomono- and -diesters may be changed in pathological tissue, such as malignant brain tumors (18). The location of the P_i peak depends on intracellular pH, and thus permits detection of intracellular acidosis (e.g., in recent ischemia) or alkalosis (e.g., in reperfused infarcts and most brain tumors).

Representation of the spatial variation of the intensity of selected peaks as low-resolution images is known as chemical-shift imaging (CSI). Such images can be superimposed onto high-resolution MRI images, thus combining structural and functional biochemical information (Fig. 2).

Acute ischemia

Cerebral blood flow (CBF) is severely reduced in acute cerebral ischemia. Animal experiments and human PET data indicate that function is impaired at CBF values of approx. 20 ml/100 g/min, and irreversible damage is caused within minutes (at normal body temperature) by cortical CBF values below 12 ml/100 g/min (review by Heiss (19)). Absolute regional CBF can currently be measured with good spatial resolution with PET, employing freely diffusible tracers and arterial blood sampling.

Assessment of tissue viability is a very important issue in acute ischemia. Arterial collaterals, e.g. the Circle of Willis and leptomeningeal anastomoses, can provide CBF above 12 ml/100 g/min in vascular borderzones even after complete occlusion of a major artery. Survival of tissue then depends on quick restoration of perfusion, e.g., by thrombolysis (8). Yet, reperfusion of irreversibly damaged tissue bears the danger of a massive space-occupying hemorrhage. Therefore, practicable and fast imaging techniques to identify critically perfused but viable tissue are needed urgently.

A simple compensatory mechanism to survive impaired CBF is an increase of the oxygen extraction fraction (OEF), which is normally around 40 to 50 %. The condition of "misery perfusion", i.e. severe reduction of CBF, relative preservation of oxygen metabolism ($CMRO_2$) indicating tissue viability, and increased OEF has been demonstrated repeatedly with PET in acute brain infarcts (2, 17, 22, 50) up to 24 h in the borderzone of completed ischemic infarcts, and in rare cases even later. Yet, the complicated PET techniques are not practical for widespread use in acute stroke.

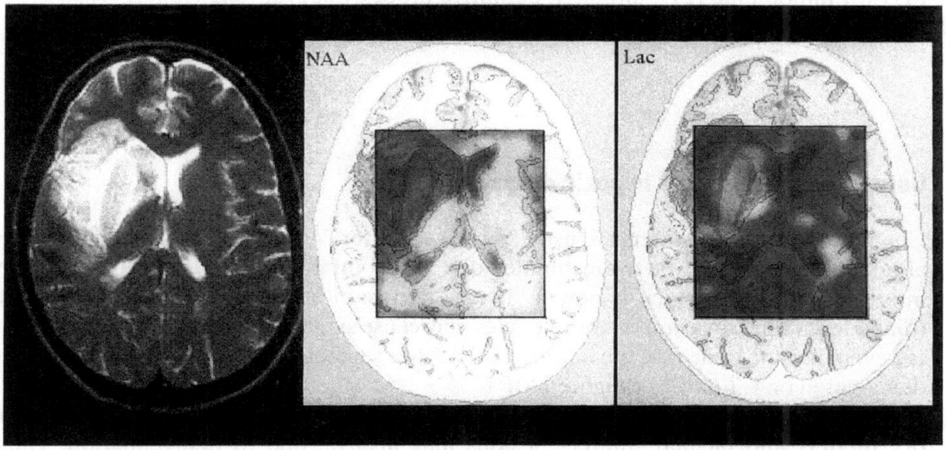

Fig. 2. T_2-weighted MRI (left) and CSI (rectangular color display area superimposed onto MRI contours) of NAA (middle) and lactate (right) in a recent MCA infarct. In the infarct, MRI signal intensity is increased, NAA is lacking (green color), and lactate is increased (orange and yellow colors).

After a severe ischemic insult, cytotoxic (intracellular) edema develops, probably due to the breakdown of ion gradients. If it is very severe, it can be seen a few hours after onset of ischemia as diffuse hypointensity on CT and "loss of the insular ribbon" (47). Better sensitivity is provided by a new MRI technique: diffusion-weighted imaging (48). Its signal depends on the reduction of the apparent diffusion coefficient of water protons that is probably due to intracellular edema and shrinkage of extracellular space. Yet, it is not yet entirely clear whether this phenomenon may be partially reversible and whether mild edema is compatible with tissue viability.

The lack of oxygen often leads to an increase in non-oxidative glycolysis, which is possible because the normal glucose extraction fraction is much lower (approx. 10 %), and production of lactate. Increased glycolysis in recent ischemic infarcts has been measured with PET (51), and the accumulation of lactate has been demonstrated with proton MRS (4, 6, 28, 40). In acute stroke this is accompanied by intracellular acidosis, which can be measured by ^{31}P MRS, and may contribute to neuronal damage (41). After a few days, ischemic infarcts may still contain lactate, probably due to invasion by macrophages, but are often alkalotic (26).

Severe depletion of energy stores indicates irreversible tissue damage (25). Energy-rich phosphates phosphocreatine and ATP can be measured with ^{31}P MRS, but low spatial resolution and long data acquisition times limit its clinical practicability in acute stroke.

NAA is an intermediate product of neuronal metabolism (5) and may prove to be a valuable indicator of neuronal viablity, which can be measured with proton MRS. Its spatial distribution and depletion in completed infarcts was recently demonstrated with CSI (Fig. 2) (28).

In the following days after an acute ischemic stroke, tissue damage may still progress in the infarct borderzones. This has been demonstrated with PET (22) and with proton MRS (40). The responsible pathophysiological mechanisms are not entirely clear and may include calcium influx, neurotoxic excitation and alterations of gene expression and protein synthesis (25). Some drugs may reduce delayed neuronal death, as demonstrated with

PET for nimodipine (21), although definitive proof by appropriate clinical studies is still lacking.

Completed ischemic or hypoxic damage

Completed ischemic infarcts are usually well seen after 24 h on CT and T_2-weighted MRI, although their size may be overestimated due to peri-infarct edema. In the following days, infarct reperfusion (which is now a "luxury perfusion"), extravasation of erythrocytes (diapedesis), and invasion of granulocytes may cause signal changes on MRI and blurring (or even disappearence) of the infarct on CT. After several weeks, infarcts are usually well demarcated on CT and T_2-weighted MRI.

MRI is particularly sensitve to detect white-matter lesions. In addition to partial territory infarcts and lacunar infarcts, lesions may also be due to demyelination, gliosis, enlarged perivascular (Virchow-Robin) spaces, and inflammatory processes. Minor lesions are often found in healthy elderly individuals, and their frequency is correlated with vascular risk factors (30). Only large or very widespread lesions lead to significant cortical dysfunction and mild cognitive impairment. Yet, small strategic lesions affecting the pyramidal tract can cause spastic paresis. MRI may also demonstrate Wallerian degeneration of fiber tracts after a focal brain lesion (35).

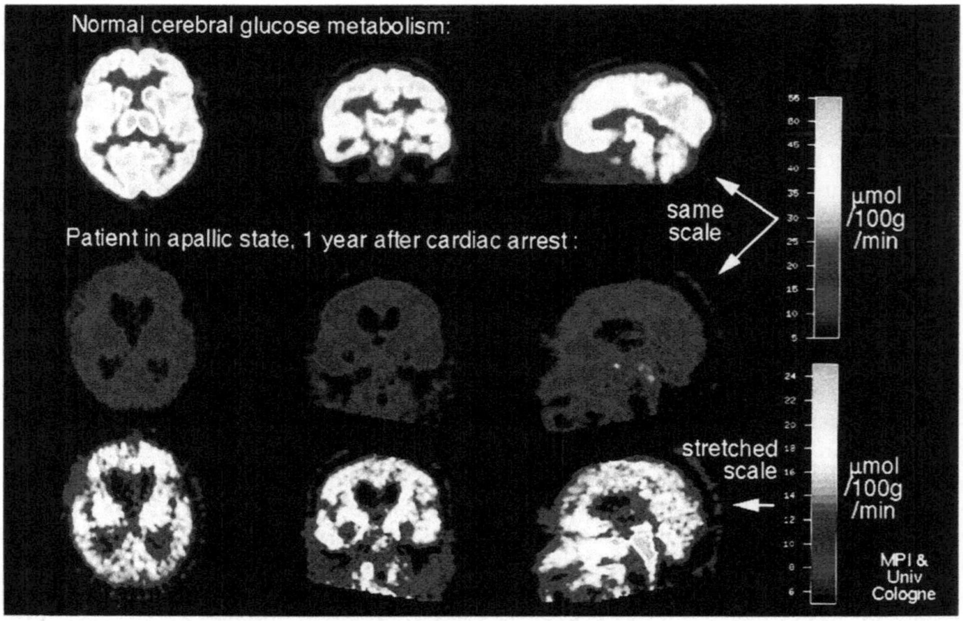

Fig. 3. Cerebral glucose metabolism measured with PET (transaxial, coronal, and sagittal slices) extremely low values in a patient in apallic state (middle row) compared to normal (top row). With adjustment of the color scale (bottom row), it is evident that brainstem and cerebellar vermis (red color) are less affected than the other brain structures.

Small cortical infarcts can be difficult to detect on CT and MRI, because there is little signal difference to CSF. In the subacute phase, application of contrast agents can demonstrate a typical gyral pattern of contrast enhancement. In the chronic phase, focal atrophy may be the only residual finding. PET images of CMRGlu have a high sensitivity to detect cortical lesions (20), which typically occur as multiple scattered foci in cortical multi-infarct dementia (3).

Most lesions cause functional impairment of remote brain areas which can be demonstrated on PET images of CBF and CMRGlu, and also with SPECT. The most conspicuous finding is crossed cerebellar diaschisis (1), most often due to frontal or parietal lesions which affect the cortico-ponto-cerebellar projections. Lesions of the basal ganglia often cause cortical dysfunction. It could be demonstrated, for instance, that the severity of aphasia is highly correlated with metabolic impairment of posterior superior temporal cortex (Wernicke's area), even if the ischemic infarct is located in the basal ganglia (27). Studies during language stimulation have demonstrated that contralateral temporal cortex or ipsilateral thalamus and frontal cortex may show compensatory activation in patients with aphasia due to lesions of superior temporal cortex (23, 49).

After diffuse hypoxic damage, cerebral energy metabolism may be impaired globally, as demonstrated with PET (7, 39, 45). Extent and intensity of metabolic impairment may vary considerably, and reductions of CMRGlu to 30 to 50 % of normal values are typical for patients in coma or persistent vegetative state. Sometimes, brainstem and cerebellum are relatively spared (Fig. 3). Cardiac arrest or severe circulatory failure may also lead to infarcts of the basal ganglia (38) or to neuronal loss in cortical vascular boderzones and hippocampus (Fig. 4).

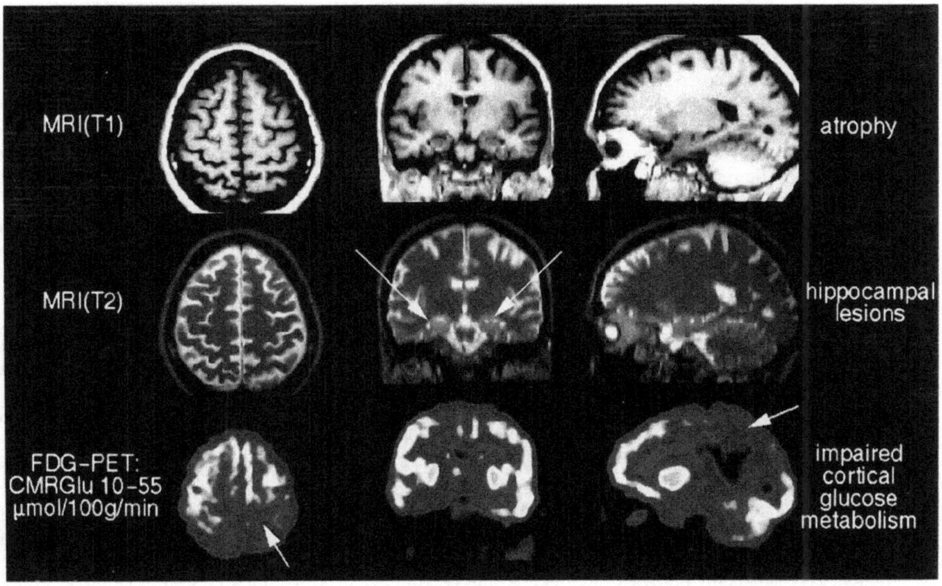

Fig. 4. MRI (slice thickness 2.5 mm) and FDG PET of long-distance runner with amnesic syndrome after repeated collapses and exsiccosis (corresponding transaxial, coronal and sagittal slices). MRI shows global atrophy and lacunar lesions in hippocampal structures (arrows in middle row). PET demonstrates reduced parietal glucose metabolism (arrows in bottom row).

Conclusion

Modern functional imaging techniques have improved our ability to detect acute and chronic neuronal damage. In addition, they can demonstrate impairment of specific aspects of brain perfusion and metabolism after an ischemic or hypoxic insult. This increases our understanding of the pathophysiology of neuronal damage and may help to improve prevention and treatment.

References

1. Baron JC, Bousser MG, Comar D, Duquesnoy N, Sastre J, Castaigne P (1980) Crossed cerebellar diaschisis in human supratentorial brain infarction. Transactions of the American Neurological Association 105: 459–61
2. Baron JC, Bousser MG, Rey A, Guillard A, Comar D, Castaigne P (1981) Reversal of focal "misery-perfusion syndrome" by extra-intracranial arterial bypass in hemodynamic cerebral ischemia. A case study with 15O positron emission tomography. Stroke 12 (4): 454–9
3. Benson DF, Kuhl DE, Hawkins RA, Phelps ME, Cummings JL, Tsai SY (1983) The fluorodeoxyglucose 18F scan in Alzheimer's disease and multi-infarct dementia. Archives of Neurology 40 (12): 711–4
4. Berkelbach van der Sprenkel JW, Luyten PR, van Rijen PC, Tulleken CA, den Hollander JA (1988) Cerebral lactate detected by regional proton magnetic resonance spectroscopy in a patient with cerebral infarction. Stroke 19 (12): 1556–60
5. Birken DL, Oldendorf WH (1989) N-acetyl-L-aspartic acid: a literature review of a compound prominent in 1H-NMR spectroscopic studies of brain. (Review). Neuroscience & Biobehavioral Reviews 13 (1): 23–31
6. Bruhn H, Frahm J, Gyngell ML, Merboldt KD, Hanicke W, Sauter R (1989) Cerebral metabolism in man after acute stroke: new observations using localized proton NMR spectroscopy. Magnetic Resonance in Medicine 9 (1): 126–31
7. De Volder AG, Michel C, Guerit JM, Bol A, Georges B, de Barsy T, Laterre C (1994) Brain glucose metabolism in postanoxic syndrome due to cardiac arrest. Acta Neurologica Belgica 94 (3): 183–9
8. del Zoppo GJ, Pessin MS, Mori E, Hacke W (1991) Thrombolytic intervention in acute thrombotic and embolic stroke. (Review). Seminars in Neurology 11 (4): 368–84
9. den Hollander JA (1987) Practical in vivo human MR spectroscopy. Budinger TF, Margulis AR, editors. Medical magnetic resonance imaging and spectroscopy. Primer supplement. Society of Magnetic Resonance in Medicine, Berkeley. p. 53–62
10. Fox PT, Mintun MA, Raichle ME, Herscovitch P (1984) A noninvasive approach to quantitative functional brain mapping with H2 (15)O and positron emission tomography. Journal of Cerebral Blood Flow & Metabolism 4 (3): 329–33
11. Fox PT, Perlmutter JS, Raichle ME (1985) A stereotactic method of anatomical localization for positron emission tomography. Journal of Computer Assisted Tomography 9 (1): 141–53
12. Frackowiak RS, Lenzi GL, Jones T, Heather JD (1980) Quantitative measurement of regional cerebral blood flow and oxygen metabolism in man using 15O and positron emission tomography: theory, procedure, and normal values. Journal of Computer Assisted Tomography 4 (6): 727–36
13. Frahm J, Haase A, Matthaei D (1986) Rapid three-dimensional MR imaging using the FLASH technique. Journal of Computer Assisted Tomography 10 (2): 363–8
14. Friston KJ, Frith CD, Liddle PF, Frackowiak RS (1991) Comparing functional (PET) images: the assessment of significant change. Journal of Cerebral Blood Flow & Metabolism 11 (4): 690–9
15. Gill SS, Small RK, Thomas DG, Patel P, Porteous R, Van Bruggen N, Gadian DG, Kauppinen RA, Williams SR (1989) Brain metabolites as 1H NMR markers of neuronal and glial disorders. NMR in Biomedicine 2 (5–6): 196–200
16. Gyngell ML, Michaelis T, Horstermann D, Bruhn H, Hanicke W, Merboldt KD, Frahm J (1991) Cerebral glucose is detectable by localized proton NMR spectroscopy in normal rat brain in vivo. Magnetic Resonance in Medicine 19 (2): 489–95
17. Hakim AM, Evans AC, Berger L, Kuwabara H, Worsley K, Marchal G, Biel C, Pokrupa R, Diksic M, Meyer E et al. (1989) The effect of nimodipine on the evolution of human cerebral infarction studied by PET. (Review). Journal of Cerebral Blood Flow & Metabolism 9 (4): 523–34

18. Heindel W, Bunke J, Glathe S, Steinbrich W, Mollevanger L (1988) Combined 1H-MR imaging and localized 31P-spectroscopy of intracranial tumors in 43 patients. Journal of Computer Assisted Tomography 12 (6): 907–16
19. Heiss WD (1992) Experimental evidence of ischemic thresholds and functional recovery. (Review). Stroke 23 (11): 1668–72
20. Heiss WD, Herholz K, Bocher-Schwarz HG, Pawlik G, Wienhard K, Steinbrich W, Friedmann G (1986) PET, CT, and MR imaging in cerebrovascular disease. Journal of Computer Assisted Tomography 10 (6): 903–11
21. Heiss WD, Holthoff V, Pawlik G, Neveling M (1990) Effect of nimodipine on regional cerebral glucose metabolism in patients with acute ischemic stroke as measured by positron emission tomography. Journal of Cerebral Blood Flow & Metabolism 10 (1): 127–32
22. Heiss WD, Huber M, Fink GR, Herholz K, Pietrzyk U, Wagner R, Wienhard K (1992) Progressive derangement of periinfarct viable tissue in ischemic stroke. Journal of Cerebral Blood Flow & Metabolism 12 (2): 193–203
23. Herholz K, Karbe H, Ghaemi M et al. (1995) Compensatory activations of frontal and thalamic regions in subacute aphasia during word repetition. Journal of Cerebral Blood Flow & Metabolism 15: (Suppl. 1) S186
24. Hossmann KA (1993) Disturbances of cerebral protein synthesis and ischemic cell death. (Review). Progress in Brain Research 96: 161–77
25. Hossmann KA (1994) Viability thresholds and the penumbra of focal ischemia (see comments). (Review). Annals of Neurology 36 (4): 557–65
26. Hugg JW, Duijn JH, Matson GB, Maudsley AA, Tsuruda JS, Gelinas DF, Weiner MW (1992) Elevated lactate and alkalosis in chronic human brain infarction observed by 1H and 31P MR spectroscopic imaging. Journal of Cerebral Blood Flow & Metabolism 12 (5): 734–44
27. Karbe H, Herholz K, Szelies B, Pawlik G, Wienhard K, Heiss WD (1989) Regional metabolic correlates of Token test results in cortical and subcortical left hemispheric infarction. Neurology 39 (8): 1083–8
28. Lanfermann H, Kugel H, Heindel W, Herholz K, Heiss WD, Lackner K (1995) Metabolic changes in acute and subacute cerebral infarctions: findings at proton MR spectroscopic imaging. Radiology 196 (1): 203–10
29. Lauterbur PC (1973) Image formation by induced local interactions: examples employing nuclear magnetic resonance. Nature 242: 438–9
30. Meyer JS, Kawamura J, Terayama Y (1992) White matter lesions in the elderly. (Review). Journal of the Neurological Sciences 110 (1–2): 1–7
31. Minematsu K, Li L, Fisher M, Sotak CH, Davis MA, Fiandaca MS (1992) Diffusion-weighted magnetic resonance imaging: rapid and quantitative detection of focal brain ischemia. Neurology 42 (1): 235–40
32. Minoshima S, Koeppe RA, Frey KA, Kuhl DE (1994) Anatomic standardization: linear scaling and non-linear warping of functional brain images. Journal of Nuclear Medicine 35 (9): 1528–37
33. Mintun MA, Raichle ME, Martin WR, Herscovitch P (1984) Brain oxygen utilization measured with O-15 radiotracers and positron emission tomography. Journal of Nuclear Medicine 25 (2): 177–87
34. Ogawa S, Lee TM, Nayak AS, Glynn P (1990) Oxygenation-sensitive contrast in magnetic resonance image of rodent brain at high magnetic fields. Magnetic Resonance in Medicine 14 (1): 68–78
35. Orita T, Tsurutani T, Izumihara A, Kajiwara K (1994) Early, evolving Wallerian degeneration of the pyramidal tract in cerebrovascular diseases: MR study. Journal of Computer Assisted Tomography 18 (6): 943–6
36. Raichle ME, Martin WR, Herscovitch P, Mintun MA, Markham J (1983) Brain blood flow measured with intravenous H2(15)O. II. Implementation and validation. Journal of Nuclear Medicine 24 (9): 790–8
37. Reivich M, Kuhl D, Wolf A, Greenberg J, Phelps M, Ido T, Casella V, Fowler J, Hoffman E, Alavi A et al. (1979) The (18F) fluorodeoxyglucose method for the measurement of local cerebral glucose utilization in man. Circulation Research 44 (1): 127–37
38. Roine RO, Raininko R, Erkinjuntti T, Ylikoski A, Kaste M (1993) Magnetic resonance imaging findings associated with cardiac arrest. Stroke 24 (7): 1005–14
39. Rudolf J, Beil C, Heiss WD (1993) Regional cerebrla glucose metabolism in postanoxic syndrome: evidence for prognostic sensitivity? Journal of Cerebral Blood Flow & Metabolism 13: (Suppl. 1) S391
40. Saunders DE, Howe FA, van den Boogaart A, McLean MA, Griffiths JR, Brown MM (1995) Continuing ischemic damage after acute middle cerebral artery infarction in humans demonstrated by short-echo proton spectroscopy. Stroke 26 (6): 1007–13
41. Siesjo BK, Katsura K, Kristian T (1995) The biochemical basis of cerebral ischemic damage. (Review). Journal of Neurosurgical Anesthesiology 7 (1): 47–52
42. Sokoloff L, Reivich M, Kennedy C, Des Rosiers MH, Patlak CS, Pettigrew KD, Sakurada O, Shinohara M (1977) The (14C) deoxyglucose method for the measurement of local cerebral glucose utilization: theory, procedure, and normal values in the conscious and anesthetized albino rat. Journal of Neurochemistry 28 (5): 897–916

43. Stehling MK, Turner R, Mansfield P (1991) Echo-planar imaging: magnetic resonance imaging in a fraction of a second. (Review). Science 254 (5028): 43–50
44. Stocklin G (1992) Tracers for metabolic imaging of brain and heart. Radiochemistry and radiopharmacology. (Review). European Journal of Nuclear Medicine 19 (7): 527–51
45. Tommasino C, Grana C, Lucignani G, Torri G, Fazio F (1995) Regional cerebral metabolism of glucose in comatose and vegetative state patients. Journal of Neurosurgical Anesthesiology 7 (2): 109–16
46. Townsend DW, Geissbuhler A, Defrise M, Hoffman EJ, Spinks TJ, Bailey DL, Gilardi MC, Jones T (1991) Fully 3-dimensional reconstruction for a PET camera with retractable septa. IEEE Transactions on Medical Imaging 10 (4): 505–12
47. von Kummer R, Meyding-Lamade U, Forsting M, Rosin L, Rieke K, Hacke W, Sartor K (1994) Sensitivity and prognostic value of early CT in occlusion of the middle cerebral artery trunk. Ajnr: American Journal of Neuroradiology 15 (1): 9–15
48. Warach S, Gaa J, Siewert B, Wielopolski P, Edelman RR (1995) Acute human stroke studied by whole brain echo planar diffusion-weighted magnetic resonance imaging. Annals of Neurology 37 (2): 231–41
49. Weiller C, Isensee C, Rijntjes M, Huber W, Muller S, Bier D, Dutschka K, Woods RP, Noth J, Diener HC (1995) Recovery from Wernicke's aphasia: a positron emission tomographic study. Annals of Neurology 37 (6): 723–32
50. Wise RJ, Bernardi S, Frackowiak RS, Legg NJ, Jones T (1983) Serial observations on the pathophysiology of acute stroke. The transition from ischaemia to infarction as reflected in regional oxygen extraction. Brain 106 (Pt 1): 197–222
51. Wise RJ, Rhodes CG, Gibbs JM, Hatazawa J, Palmer T, Frackowiak RS, Jones T (1983) Disturbance of oxidative metabolism of glucose in recent human cerebral infarcts. Annals of Neurology 14 (6): 627–37

Authors' address:
Prof. Dr. med. K. Herholz
Neurologische Universitätsklinik zu Köln
und Max-Planck-Institut für neurologische Forschung
Josef-Stelzmann-Str. 9
D-50931 Köln
Germany

Expression of ICAM-1 and VCAM-1 on endothelial cells after global cerebral ischemia and reperfusion in the rat

W. Harringer, X.-M. You, G. Steinhoff, U. Linstedt[1], A. Haverich

Department of Cardiovascular Surgery and [1]Department of Anesthesia, Christian-Albrechts University Kiel, Kiel, Germany

Introduction

Hypothermic circulatory arrest has been widely adopted in cardiovascular surgery to facilitate correction of congenital and acquired lesions. However, the central nervous system (CNS), is exquisitely sensitive to anoxic insults associated with cerebral ischemia during circulatory arrest. Additional to the abnormalities of the blood flow, metabolism and function of the brain during ischemia and reperfusion, leukocyte-mediated tissue damage will continue despite restoration of blood flow (1 – 3). This may promote the cerebral ischemia/reperfusion injury and contribute to the long-term neurological and neuropsychological consequences of circulatory arrest (4). ICAM-1 and VCAM-1, the members of supergene family, are inducible ligands expressed on endothelial cells. After exposure to cytokines, they bind to the receptors LFA-1 and VLA-4 on leukocytes. It has become clear that ICAM-1 and VCAM-1 play important roles in leukocyte adherence to endothelium and leukocyte transmigration to inflammation sites (5).

The expression of ICAM-1 and VCAM-1 after global cerebral ischemia and reperfusion is not known yet. In the present study, a rat model with global cerebral ischemia (6) was used to study the intensity and the time pattern of endothelial ICAM-1 and VCAM-1 expression.

Materials and methods

Male Wistar rats weighing between 280 – 350 grams were used in the present study. Animals were investigated in seven experimental groups (each group $n = 5$): control, sham-operation, ischemia without recovery and ischemia with 6 h, 1 day, 3 days and 7 days reperfusion. A previously published four-vessel occlusion model (6) was modified with rats undergoing 15 min of cerebral ischemia under anesthesia. EEG and somato-sensory evoked potentials (SSEP) were used to monitor brain activity. Only animals with complete loss of SSEP and a flat EEG during ischemia were studied further. Animals were sacrificed after a reperfusion interval of 6 h, 1 day, 3 days and 7 days. The brains were then removed and immediately cryopreserved in liquid nitrogen. Frozen section (7 μm thick) were performed at following brain levels (7): from bregma 1.7 mm to −0.3 mm, bregma −1.8 mm, bregma −2.8 mm and bregma −3.8 mm. Monoclonal antibodies of ICAM-1 (1A29, Osaka, Japan) and VCAM-1 (1E5, Biogen, Boston USA) were used for immunohistochemistry and the slides were stained with standard indirect immonoperoxidase.

Expression of ICAM-1 and VCAM-1 on endothelial cells was quantitatively evaluated by counting the percentage of positive arterioles, capillaries and venules, as has been previously described (8):

$$\frac{\text{Number of vessels stained positive for ICAM-1 or VCAM-1}}{\text{Total number of arterioles (capillaries or venules)}} \times 100\ \%$$

We recorded and averaged stained vessels in six randomly selected fields with × 100 magnification for each brain section.

Results

Expression of ICAM-1 and VCAM-1 on arterial, venous and capillary endothelial cells is depicted in Table 1. Both adhesion molecules showed very low expression levels on arterial and venous endothelial cells in the control group. Capillary endothelial cells of the control group were absolutely negative for ICAM-1 or VCAM-1. ICAM-1 expression slightly increased on arterial and venous endothelia and significantly increased on capillary endothelia after 15 min global ischemia without reperfusion. The percentage of positive vessels for ICAM-1 increased continuously after reperfusion and reached its peak 24 h after reperfusion. ICAM-1 expression began to decline slowly after day 1 but still remained on a significantly higher level on day 7, when compared to the control group. VCAM-1 was expressed in a similar pattern as ICAM-1. In contrast to ICAM-1, VCAM-1 expression on vascular endothelium had a significant increase after 15 min ischemia without reperfusion. The percentage of positive vessels also increased rapidly but reached its peak already 6 h after reperfusion (Fig. 1).

Table 1. Expression of ICAM-1 and VCAM-1 on endothelial cells of arteries, veins and capillaries

	ICAM-1 (%)			VCAM-1 (%)		
	Arteries	Veins	Capillaries	Arteries	Veins	Capillaries
Control	8.8±3.3	4.4±2.3	0	6.2±3.1	2.2±0.8	0
Sham operation	7.6±1.2	3.8±1.8	0	4.8±2.0	2.7±1.2	0
No recovery	8.2±3.3	9.4±4.1	7.5±2.8[1]	14.4±3.8[1]	11.2±3.2[1]	8.8±4.1[2]
Reperfusion						
6 h	62.8±8.7[2]	60.3±10.4[2]	71.4±11.2[2]	53.3±11.6[2]	66.4±8.7[2]	61.2±10.7[2]
Day 1	88.7±14.2[2]	90.5±13.2[2]	98.4±7.7[2]	57.7±14.6[2]	63.1±15.8[2]	62.2±11.4[2]
Day 3	74.4±15.4[2]	80.8±12.7[2]	62.4±12.0[2]	43.8±12.5[2]	56.8±8.6[2]	41.4±10.7[2]
Day 7	54.5±17.7[2]	50.5±13.2[2]	46.2±11.7[2]	34.4±10.4[2]	38.9±12.3[2]	28.4±8.7[2]

1 $p < 0.05$ vs. control group
2 $p < 0.01$ vs. control group

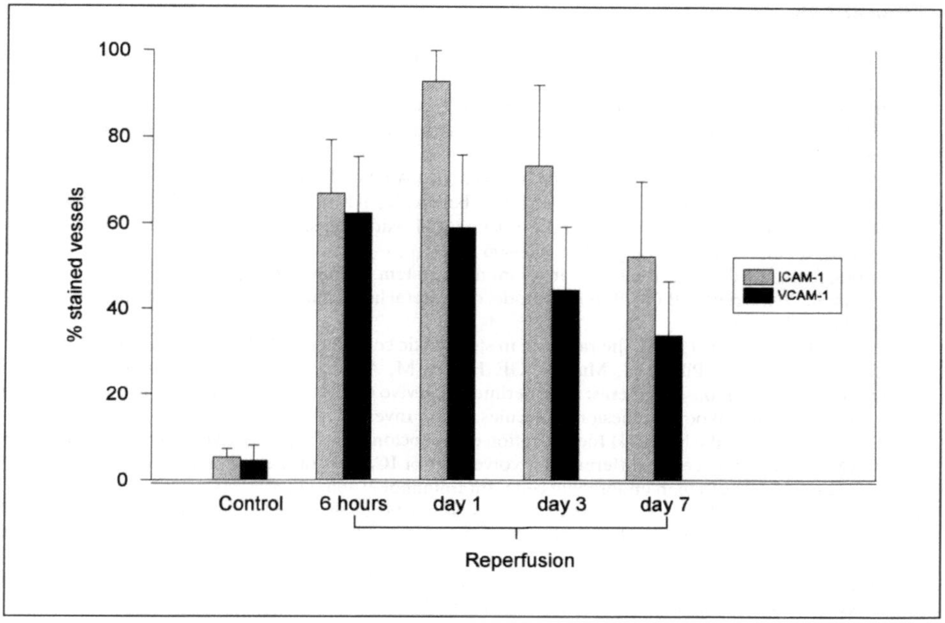

Fig. 1. Time pattern of ICAM-1 and VCAM-1 expression

Discussion

There is no (on capillary endothelium) or very low expression (only in large vessels endothelium) of ICAM-1 and VCAM-1 in normal rat brains, in accordance with previous reports in other animal models (8, 9). VCAM-1 expression on endothelial cells appeared to reach its peak earlier after reperfusion, indicating a more sensitive response to ischemic damage. Additionally, on capillary endothelial cells, both ICAM-1 and VCAM-1 were induced earlier than on arterial and venous endothelium. Significant expression of ICAM-1 and VCAM-1 on endothelial cells could be detected starting after 6 h of reperfusion until day 7. Even after 1 week following ischemia a significantly higher expression could be detected when compared to normal rat brains. In vitro, increased expression of ICAM-1 during hypoxia and reoxygenation in human brain endothelial cells has been reported (11). ICAM-1 and VCAM-1 are important receptors for leukocyte adhesion to endothelium as substantial part of an inflammatory response. Leukocyte migration into and accumulation in ischemic areas of myocardium as well as in areas of cerebral infarctions has been demonstrated (12, 13). Our study suggests that high levels of ICAM-1 and VCAM-1 expression induced by ischemia and reperfusion may lead to a significantly increased binding of leukocytes through their ligand receptors LFA-1 and VLA-4 on these adhesion molecules. Consequently, leukocytes adhere to the endothelium and will migrate into the injured tissue and may promote late cerebral damage. This offers a possible therapeutical option to modify cerebral reperfusion injury by blocking adhesion molecules with antibodies.

References

1. Hernandez L, Grisham M, Twohig B (1987) Role of neutrophils in ischemia reperfusion induced microvascular injury. Am J Physiol 253: H699–H703
2. Barone FC, Schmidt DB, Hillegass LM, Price WJ, White RF, Feuerstein GZ, Clark RK, Lee EV, Griswold DE, Sarau HM (1992) Reperfusion increases neutrophils and leukotriene B4 receptor binding in rat focal ischemia. Stroke 23: 1337–1348
3. Harlan J (1985) Leukocytes-endothelial interaction. J Am Soc Hemato 65: 513–525
4. Greeley WJ, Bracey VA, Ungerleider RM, Greibel JA, Kern MH, Boyb JL, Reves JG, Piantadosi (1991) Recovery of cerebral metabolism and mitochondrial oxidation state is delayed after hypothermic circulatory arrest. Circulation suppl III: 400–406
5. Springer TA (1990) Adhesion receptors of immune system. Nature 346: 425–434
6. Pulsinelli WA, Brierley B (1979) A new model of bilateral hemispheric ischemia in the unanesthetized rat. Stroke 10: 267–272
7. Paxinos G, Watson C (1986) The rat brain in stereotaxic coordinates. 2ed. Acedemic Press. Sidney
8. Yan HC, Juhasz I, Pilwski J, Murphy GF, Herlyn M, Albelda SM (1993) Human/severe combined immunodeficient mouse chimeras: an experimental in vivo model system to study the regulation of human endothelial cell-leukocyte adhesion molecules. J Clin Invest 91: 986–996
9. Tamatani T, Miyasaka M (1993) Identification of monoclonal antibody reactive with the rat homologue of ICAM-1, and evidence for differential involvement of ICAM-1 in the adherence of resting versus activated lymphocytes to high endothelial cells. Int Immunol 2: 166–172
10. Zhang RL, Chopp M, Li Y, Zaloga C, Jiang N, Jones ML, Miyasaka M, Ward PA (1994) Anti-ICAM-1 antibody reduces ischemic cell damage after transient middle cerebral artery occlusion in the rat. Neurology 44: 1747–1751
11. Hess DC, Zhao W, Carroll J, McEachin M, Buchanan (1994) Increased expression of ICAM-1 during reoxygenation in brain endothelial cells. Stroke 25: 1463–1468
12. Dreyer WJ, Michael LH, West MS, Smith CW, Rothlein R, Rossen RD, Anderson DC, Entman ML (1991) Neutrophil accumulation in ischemic canine myocardium. Circulation 84: 400–411
13. Yamasaki Y, Matsuo Y, Matsuura N, Onodera H, Itoyama Y, Kogure K (1995) Transient increase of cytokine-induced neutrophil chemoattractant, a member of the interleukin-8 family, in ischemic brain areas after focal ischemia in rats. Stroke 26: 318–323

Authors' address:
Wolfgang Harringer, M.D.
Department of Cardiovascular Surgery
Christian-Albrechts University Kiel
Arnold-Heller-Straße 7
24105 Kiel, Germany

Cerebral protection during neurosurgical operations

J. Hamer

Department of Neurosurgery, University of Heidelberg, Germany

Introduction

The neurosurgeon is not infrequently confronted with cerebral complications after cadiovascular surgery. This is mainly due to intracranial hematoma which developed after cardiac emboli, cerebral infarction and secondary hemorrhage or to the sometimes disastrous effects of anticoagulants. Cerebral protection is therefore a challenge to both the cardiovascular surgeon and the neurosurgeon. Neuroprotection encompasses three aspects:

1) Neuromonitoring for early detection of factors which cause "secondary brain trauma" (see Table 1)
2) Pharmacological therapy to raise the threshold of ischemic damage (see Table 2)
3) Preliminary procedures to prevent a primary lesion during neurosurgical dissection.

With regard to ischemic brain damage it seems appropriate to briefly emphasize the different thresholds of cell dysfunction with decreasing cerebral blood flow (CBF). This will clearly show how narrow the borders are between survival and death of cerebral tissue. Nevertheless, this narrow gap offers the unique possibility of saving life and even neurophysiological function.

Table 1. Neuromonitoring

Neuromonitoring
ICP-Measurement
Trans / intracranial Ultrasound
Evoked Potentials
Near infrared Spectroscopy (NIRS)
Cerebral venous oxygen saturation

Table 2. Pharmacological Therapy

Pharmacological Therapy
Reduction of cerebral metabolism
Buffering of tissue acidosis
Prevention of damage to cellular membranes (phospholipids)
Antagonization of the influence of excitotoxic amino-acids

Threshold of ischemia

The normal blood flow of the human brain is about 50 ml/100 g/min. A decrease to half of the normal value leads to unconsciousness, and a further fall to 20 – 18 ml abolishes neurophysiological function and brings about an isoelectric EEG. But this does not yet mean cell death. The integrity of cell structure is preserved, although physiological membrane activity has ceased. With a further drop of cerebral circulation, a few ml of blood flow will now decide whether the brain tissue will be irreversibly destroyed or not. Below a flow of 12 ml, loss of cellular ion homeostasis will occur with influx of calcium and sodium into the cell, the ATP energy stores of the cells are exhausted, proteinsynthesis is inhibited and lipid peroxidation further enhances the damage to the cell membrane (19, 20).

This narrow range of low flow values where the tissue is put at risk of infarction (which, however, has not yet occurred), has been termed the penumbra-zone of ischemic lesions. It becomes evident that therapeutic activities may be successful and rewarding even in these highly dangerous limits. Thus, a small augmentation of blood flow by raising cerebral perfusion pressure can increase the threshold for permanent ischemic lesion. In neurosurgical practice the predominant factor for disturbed cerebral blood flow is raised intracranial pressure (ICP). ICP is also the most frequent cause for what has been called secondary brain trauma.

Secondary brain trauma

In many cases of primary lesion either due to trauma, bleeding or to stroke, further life-threatening deterioration with secondary damage may follow. These secondary lesions are mainly caused by the following factors:

1) Decrease of cerebral perfusion pressure (CPP)
2) Respiratory disturbances (hypoxemia and hypercarbia)
3) Hyperthermia

The cerebral perfusion pressure is calculated as the difference of the mean arterial pressure and intracranial pressure. This perfusion pressure is of outstanding importance for neurosurgical decision-making during intensive care management and in the operating theatre. It has been shown that the intrinsic autoregulatory mechanism which maintains cerebral blood flow over a relatively wide range of falling or raising systemic arterial blood pressure is also active, to a certain degree, in the presence of increasing intracranial pressure (12). Thus, a decrease of CPP is not immediately linked with disturbed cerebral circulation. The lower limit, however, is 70 mm Hg. Below this value, CBF drops critically. It is therefore obvious that all measures which decrease intracranial pressure or which raise the level of blood pressure are of paramount importance for restoring sufficient flow above the critical level. Combating raising intracranial pressure in the presence of ischemic swelling, tumor progression or head trauma is practically the most important task in preventing further damage to the brain tissue.

The dangerous influence of respiratory disturbances to the brain is two-fold: Even moderate systemic hypoxemia may markedly aggravate the extent of already damaged brain parenchyma and, due to the very strong vasodilatatory effect of raised aPC02 on cerebral resistant vessels, hypercarbia following lung contusion or hypoventilation after fractures of the ribs, increases cerebral blood volume and, according to the exponential function of the intracranial volume-pressure relationship (14), a steep rise in ICP will follow. This exponential relationship also explains why the induction of normoventilation or moderate artificial hyperventilation may rapidly lower the intracranial pressure. The deleterious effect of hyperthermia on the injured brain is explained by its undue acceleration of metabolism. In the course of primary hypoperfusion and low CPP-values, a fatal vicious circle may come into play with increase of brain lactacidosis which further raises ICP by cerebral vasoparalysis.

Neuromonitoring

Monitoring intracranial pressure is an essential measure with regard to cerebral protection. Continuous registration of the intracranial pressure curve by miniaturized, extradurally implanted pressure transducers offer the possibility to detect an early rise in ICP and to control therapeutical procedures. Episodic pressure changes with sudden steep increases of ICP lasting for 10 min or even half an hour (so-called plateauwaves A according to Lundberg (15) are well known to the neurosurgeon. In unconscious patients where the common clinical warning symptoms cannot be safely detected, ICP-monitoring is the only efficacious way to check the intracranial pressure. Trans- und intracranial ultrasound (Fig. 1) play a major role in patients with severe subarachnoid hemorrhage (SAH) due to a rupture of an arterial aneurysm in the Circle of Willis. The accumulation of blood in the subarachnoid space of the basal cisterns is the most important risk factor for cerebral vasospasm with following ("delayed") ischemic deficit. The danger of ischemia is very high at the end of the first week after bleeding and in the following days. Early detection of beginning vasoconstriction is therefore essential for successful therapy. Besides calcium-channel blockers (nimodipine) which are generally administered immediately after the diagnosis of SAH, the so-called triple H-therapy (i.e. hypervolemia, induced arterial hypertension and hemodilution) is started in cases with continuously raising blood velocities in the basal cerebral arteries. A prerequisite of this aggressive therapy is of course the microsurgical clipping of the aneurysm. During intra-operative exposing of the cerebral arteries and dissection, the neurosurgeon controls the maneuver of clip-application by direct ultrasound investigation. This helps him to eliminate inadequate partial or even complete occlusion of major vessels or important branches of the arteries.

The continuous registration of somatosensory-, visual- or auditory-evoked potentials is more or less a standard procedure in certain intracranial operations, in particular in skull base surgery and during working in eloquent areas of the brain. It has also been used for intraoperative "brain-mapping". Although not a completely reliable method, it may minimize the risk of permanent lesions to the brain during difficult dissection on cranial nerves and the brain stemm. For topical orientation, however, monitoring of evoked potential is increasingly being replaced by modern neuronavigation systems which represent a remarkable advance in neurosurgery.

Near-infrared spectroscopy (NIRS) and jugular oximetry provide valuable information about global cerebral oxygenation (8, 10, 18, 22). NIRS registrates the changing levels of oxygenated hemoglobin, deoxyhemoglobin and cell-oxidized cytochrome aa3. This method has been used as intraoperative monitoring in carotid endarterectomy and in sur-

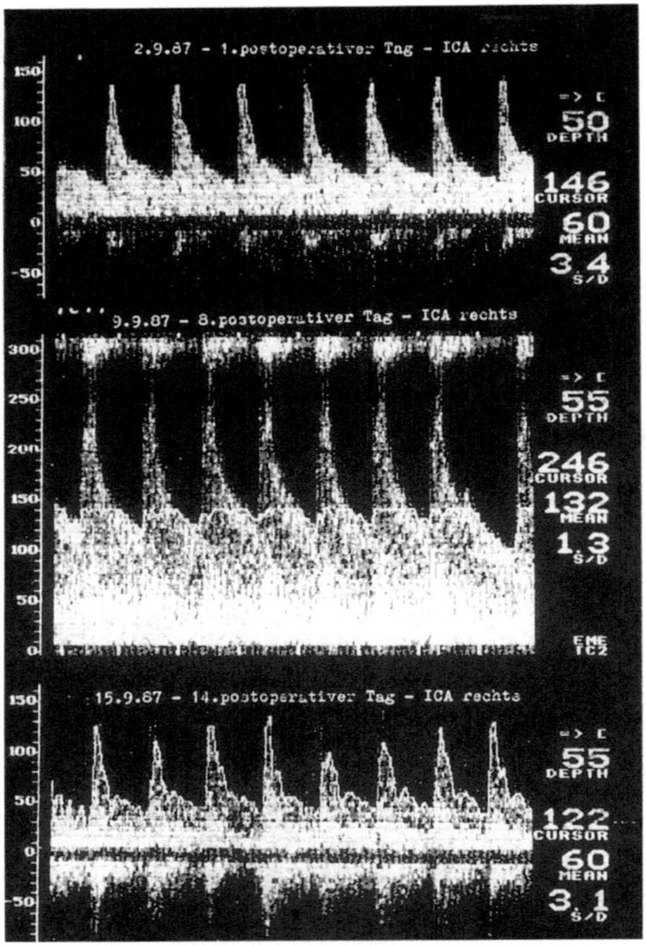

Fig. 1. Transcranial ultrasound in a case with severe SAH and progressive cerebral vasospasm (note the markedly increased blood velocity in the carotid artery on day 8 after aneurysmal rupture).

gical procedures performed under deep hypothermia and circulatory arrest (7, 13). In brain surgery this method has not yet become of major interest. However, as a transcranial, non-invasive bedside technique in the intensive care unit, it is increasingly employed and its reliability in clinical practice is being tested. The same holds true for cerebral venous oximetry by placing a fiber optic catheter into the jugular bulb. During neurosurgical procedures this method is very rarely used, but in comatose patients with severe head injury and in stroke cases this in vivo estimation of jugular venous oxygen saturation in combination with pulse oximetry offers useful information about the autoregulatory status of the brain and the coupling or uncoupling of flow and metabolism (6).

Pharmacological therapy

A marked reduction of cerebral metabolism is achieved by barbiturates and hypothermia. Special interest has recently be focused on controlled cranial cooling. But methodological and technical problems are not yet sufficiently solved and larger clinical experience is still lacking. The administration of barbiturates (Thiopental), however, is a widely used emergency measure in severe intracranial hypertension. In cases with rapidly rising intracranial pressure which is not influenced by other therapeutical efforts, a test loading dose of 250 – 500 mg is given slowly intravenously. If ICP decreases within the next minutes after injection, a continuous infusion (5 mg/kg body weight/per hour) is instituted. The effect of falling ICP is explained by diminished intracranial blood volume following the reduction of brain metabolism.

A similar effect can be obtained by buffering tissue lactacidosis. The accumulation of lactate in the course of enhanced glycolysis dilates the resistant vessels of the brain and induces vasoparalysis with increased blood volume. THAM (Tris-hydroxy-methyl-amino-methane) is administered, and one starts with a test dosis of 1 mval/kg body weight. The drug is given over a period of 10 min. If ICP responds to this measure, a permanent infusion with 2 – 4 mval/per hour is instituted. The borderline for base excess should be +3 and pH should not increase above 7.5. The use of both drugs in this clinical setting absolutely necessitates the preliminary implantation of an intracranial pressure transducer for checking the efficiency of the therapy. Furthermore, artificial ventilation is mandatory. Because of the very dangerous side-effects of high dosis of barbiturates this therapy is to be limited and should not be performed longer than 2 or 3 days.

To prevent further damage to cellular membranes, a new drug, Tirilazad-Mesylate, has recently been tested in stroke patients and in cases with SAH (11). In the last group a beneficial effect has been noticed in the European-Australian multicenter study which included 1023 patients. The international multicenter study in stroke cases, however, has shown no promising results of this so-called inhibitor of lipid peroxidation, and has therefore been interrupted. It seems noteworthy to point out that phenobarbital is also a free-radical scavenger, and that other well-known substances such as vitamin C and E or bromocriptine are potent antioxidants. But a remarkable breakthrough in therapeutic efforts with these radical scavengers has not yet been obtained.

Much interest has been devoted in recent years to excitatory aminoacids, in particular to glutamate which is an important neurotransmitter and which rapidly accumulates in cerebral ischemia and leads to lipid peroxidation. Substances are currently tested to block glutamate receptors, predominantly the subtypes AMPA and NMDA (3, 4, 16). The beneficial effect of calcium channel-blockers (nimodipine) in stroke patients has not yet been unequivocally demonstrated. However, in cases with SAH, as mentioned above, the early application of nimodipine has proven to lower the incidence of delayed ischemic deficits. The initial dosis is 1 mg in the first and second hour, and further administration continues then with 2 mg under very careful controlling of the systemic arterial blood pressure.

Peri- and intra-operative neuroprotection

In neurosurgical practice, the major interest of intra-operative neuroprotection is focused on cases with cerebral angiomas, arterial aneurysms and highly vascular tumors. Advancement in interventional neuroradiology has proven to be a considerable help for the neurosurgeon. In more or less large cerebral arterio-venous malformations the first deliberate step of therapy is endovascular embolization to reduce the size of high flow area. This is a very efficient cerebral protection with regard to following microsurgical extirpation of the angioma. With increasing experience, neuroradiological intervention succeeds in more and more completely occluding A-V-malformations. Embolization is also very helpful in meningiomas and hemangiopericytomas which generally constitute the most vascularized brain tumors. Dissection is facilitated, blood loss is minimal, and the duration of operation has become markedly shorter.

Many aneurysms are now safely excluded from arterial circulation by the microneurosurgical technique. However, some giant aneurysms still offer problems during dissection. This pertains in particular to large aneurysms of the carotid and the basilar artery.

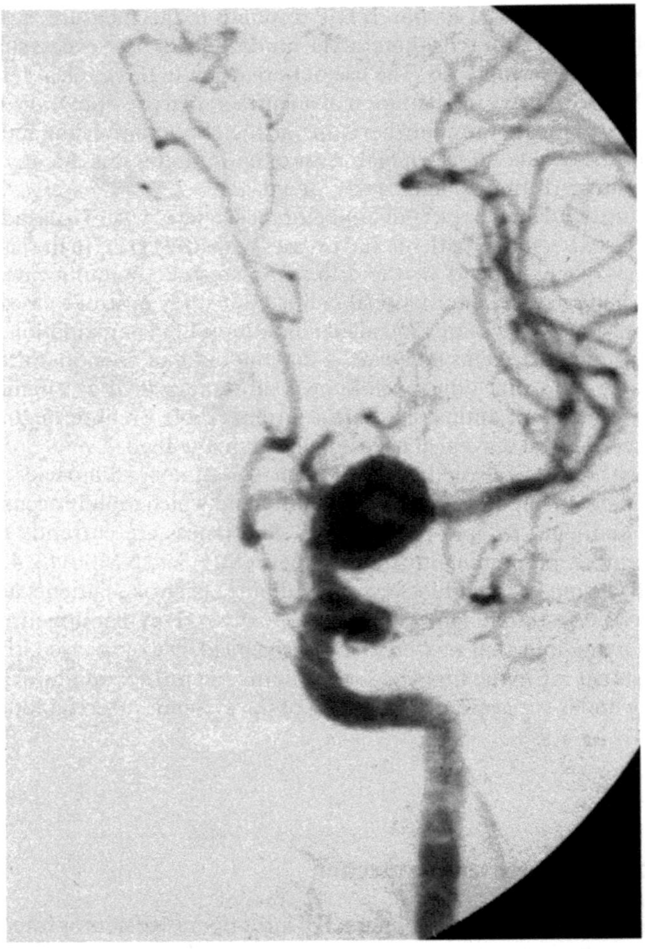

Fig. 2. Cerebral subraction angiography with a large ("giant") paraclinoidal carotid aneurysm.

In selected cases these aneurysms have been attacked with the help of the cardiovascular surgeon under circulatory arrest and hypothermia (2, 5, 21, 23). The progress in endovascular catheter techniques has reduced the need for this aggressive procedure. Larger paraclinoidal carotid aneurysms (see Fig. 2) with a particularly broad base can now be clipped with the support of the balloon-catheter “Trapping-Evacuation”-Technique (1). A double-lumen balloon-catheter is inserted in the petrous segment of the carotid artery (see Fig. 3). The artery is temporarily occluded by inflation of the balloon and a microsurgical clip is instantly placed on the distal part of the intracranial carotid artery just beyond the giant aneurysm. With continuously retrograde sucking of blood from the distal vessel, the aneurysm is evacuated and collapses. Under these temporary circumstances, a permanent clip can be put on the sluggish sack of the aneurysm. After complete exclusion of the aneurysm from the carotid flow, the distal clip is removed and the balloon deflated. This maneuver is done under a single bolus injection of thiopental (150 – 200 mg).

Finally, a very old neurosurgical procedure which has been largly abandoned in modern neurosurgery is to be mentioned in the context with cerebral protection. This is decompressive osteoclastic craniotomy, a method which has been reserved in recent decades only for selected cases of irreversibly high intracranial pressure after head trauma. A surprising revival came with the world-wide development of aggressive neurological intensive care therapy in stroke patients. Modern neuro-imaging has convincingly shown that in many cases of complete embolic occlusion of the middle cerebral artery or in patients with cervical carotid artery dissection massive intracranial brain shift develops in the first 6 to 12 h after vascular accidents. The mortality from cerebral herniation is high in these cases. The same holds true for patients with swelling of the brain from encephalitis, in particular

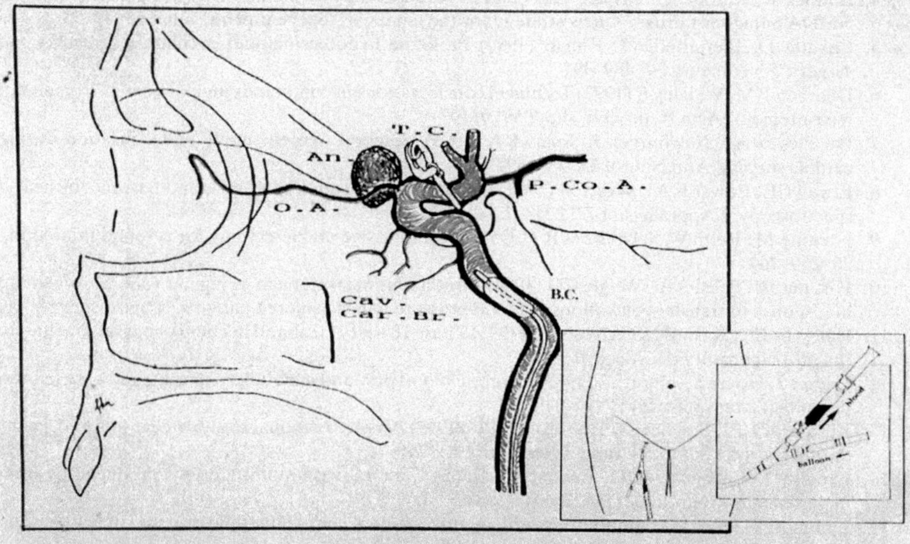

caused by herpes simplex infection. In these cases early cranial decompression is of paramount importance and lifesaving. Recent encouraging results have even shown that neurological function can be improved and progression of the lesion may be stopped (9, 17). In this sense, decompressive craniotomy is also neuroprotective. The rationale of this procedure is to gain space for the brain. This is achieved by craniotomy and a dural plasty. The resected bone is preserved and replaced some weeks later. Theoretical calculations from spherical and cylindrical bodies clearly suggest that a considerable space will only be gained if the diameter of the osteoclastic defect is larger than 10 cm. For this reason, the neurosurgeon should be aware of planning a large hemispheric trepanation. Solely local decompression over the area of infarction will prove to be less successful, and a good outcome can hardly be expected. An oldfashioned operative procedure may thus unfairly be disfavored in the future. The crucial point is the time of intervention. Early detection of brain shift is essential, and in our opinion, operation should be done before clinical symptoms of cerebral herniation (i.e. pupillary disturbances, coma) have developed. With deliberate early surgery, the results are rewarding.

References

1. Albert FK, Forsting M, Aschoff A (1993) Clipping of proximal paraclinoid aneurysms with support of the balloon catheter "Trapping-Evacuation"-Technique. Acta Neurochir 125: 138–141
2. Brawanski A, Ullrich OW, Hartung U (1992) Circulatory arrest and hypothermia in the treatment of cerebral aneurysms. Advances in Neurosurgery Vol. 20, Piscol K, Klinger M, Brock M (eds.) Springer Verlag Berlin–Heidelberg, pp 91–95
3. Buchan AM, Xue D, Huang ZG (1991) Delayed AMPA receptor blockade reduces cerebral infarction induced by focal ischemia. Clin Neurosci Neuropathol 2: 473–476
4. Bullock R, Kuroda Y, Teasdale GM (1992) Prevention of post-traumatic excitotoxic brain damage with NMDA antagonist drugs: A new strategy for the nineties. Acta Neurochir, suppl 55: 49–55
5. Chyatte D, Elefteriades J, Kim B (1989) Profound hypothermia and circulatory arrest for aneurysm surgery. J Neurosurg 70: 489–491
6. Dearden NM, Widgley S (1993) Technical considerations in continuous jugular venous oxygen saturation measurement. Acta Neurochir, suppl 59: 91–97
7. Du Plessis AJ, Newburger J, Jonas RA (1995) Cerebral oxygen supply and utilization during infant cardiac surgery. Ann Neurol 37: 488–497
8. Elwell CE, Edwards AP, Wyatt JS (1994) Quantification of adult cerebral hemodynamics by near-infrared spectroscopy. J Appl Physiol 77: 2753–2760
9. Forsting M, Reith W, Schäbitz WR (1995) Decompressive cranio-ectomy for cerebral infarction. Stroke 26: 259–264
10. Fortune JB, Feustel PJ, Weigle CG (1994) Continuous measurement of jugular venous oxygen saturation in response to transient elevations of blood pressure in head-injured patients. J Neurosurg 80: 461–468
11. Haley Jr. EC, Kassell NF, Alves WM (1995) Phase II-trial of tirilazad in aneurysmal subarachnoid hemorrhage. J Neurosurg 82: 786–790
12. Hamer J, Hoyer S, Alberti E (1973) Cerebral blood flow and metabolism in acute increase in intracranial pressure. Acta Neurochir 28: 95–110
13. Kirkpatrick PJ, Smielewski P, Whitfield PC (1995) An observational study of near-infrared spectroscopy during carotid endarterectomy. J Neurosurg 82: 756–763
14. Langfitt TW, Weinstein JD, Kassell NF (1965) Cerebral vaso-motorparalysis produced by intracranial hypertension. Neurology 15: 622–641
15. Lundberg N (1960) Continuous recordings and control of ventricular fluid pressure in neurosurgical practice. Acta Psychiatr Neurol Scand 36, suppl 149: 1–193
16. Nellgard B, Wieloch T (1992) Postischemic blockade of AMPA but not NMDA receptors mitigates neuronal damage in rat brain following transient severe cerebral ischemia. J Cereb Blood Flow Metabol 12: 2–11

17. Schwab S, Rieke K, Aschoff A (1995) Kraniektomie bei raumfordernden Mediainfarkten. Nervenarzt 66: 430–437
18. Sheinberg M, Kanter MJ, Robertson CS (1992) Continuous monitoring of jugular venous oxygen saturation in head-injured patients. J Neurosurg 76: 212–217
19. Siesjö BK (1992) Pathophysiology and treatment of focal cerebral ischemia. Part I: pathophysiology. J Neurosurg 77: 169–184
20. Siesjö BK (1992) Pathophysiology and treatment of focal cerebral ischemia. Part II: mechanisms of damage and treatment. J Neurosurg 77: 337–354
21. Silverberg GD, Reitz BA, Ream AK (1981) Hypothermia and cardiac arrest in the treatment of giant aneurysms of the cerebral circulation and hemangioblastoma of the medulla. J Neurosurg 55: 337–346
22. Slavin KV, Dujouny M, Ausman J (1994) Clinical experience with transcranial cerebral oximetry. Surg Neurol 42: 531–539
23. Spetzler RF, Hadley MN, Rigamonti D (1988) Aneurysms of the basilar artery treated with circulatory arrest, hypothermia, and barbiturate cerebral protection. J Neurosurg 68: 868–879

Authors address:
Prof. Dr. med. J. Hamer
Neurochirurgische Universitätsklinik Heidelberg
Im Neuenheimer Feld 400
69120 Heidelberg
Germany

Intensive care of acute ischemic stroke*

W. Hacke, S. Schwab, M. De Georgia

Department of Neurology, University of Heidelberg, Germany

Introduction

This work addresses the everyday situation in stroke assessment and treatment. It does not consider the problem of global ischemia but presents an overview of the current status in the treatment of acute ischemic stroke, with special respect to what happens in cardiology and in cardiosurgical patients with an acute stroke.

Stroke is not uncommon among patients undergoing cardiac surgery, cardiovascular surgery or in cardiology. The reason for that is quite simple: Stroke ischemic heart disease have almost the same risk factor profile. In addition cardiac disease are major risk factors for stroke and vice versa, stroke and TIA's are major risk factors for myocardial infarction. Diagnostic procedures in cardiology and cardiac surgery carry a high risk of brain embolism. Anticoagulation and thrombolitic therapy in myocardiac infarction may cause intracranial bleeding. Embolic stroke is the most frequent stroke that we encounter in Etiology of Stroke in cardiac patients. Hemodynamic stroke is a rare event and it's occurance has been overestimated for many years. Hemorrhagic stroke is something that especially our cardiology colleagues are afraid of when they look at the miss of thromboly *tic* therapy in cardiology. The main safty concern is the incidence of hemorrhagic stroke events in cardiology trials, the incidence of hemorrhagic stroke. It is interesting that the more neurologists become involved in the safety monitoring of stroke events in cardiology trials, the incidence of stroke in those trials goes up. This is probably due to the fact, that have not been reported or not recognised in the past. If one considers, that almost 5 % of patients with myocardial infarction will suffer a stroke within the subsequent 2 or 3 weeks, the incidences reported in major trials which are as low as 0.5 % cannot reflect the real world simulation.

How to diagnose stroke? If the patient is awake, it should not be a major problem to realize that the patient has a stroke. An acute stroke is something that every physician should be able to recognize. Unfortunately this is not always the case. A severe hemispheric syndrome with a hemiparalysis and maybe aphasia is something that one should not miss. During an operation it is more difficult to realize that the patient had a stroke. The main hint for that is that the patient seems not to wake up properly, fails to wean from the ventilator, and is unconscious. One can diagnose a hemiparesis in an unconscious or/and uncooperative patient by the way the patient reacts to painful stimuli. This again is not well known to many cardiologists. In one of the recent trials, every stroke has to be recorded and stroke scales had to be filled out. Frequently it is noted in the stroke sheets that the patient "cannot be evaluated because the patient is unconscious" – it can be and should be evaluated. Sometimes, in about 20 % of the embolic events, not the hemispheric circula-

* First published in Cerebrovasc Dis 1994, 4: 385–392

tion but the brain stem or cerebellar circulation is involved. Basilar artery occlusion due to the embolism is one of the most difficult diagnosis to make, because it has a very mixed pattern oculomotor symptoms, diplopia, ataxia, sensory, disturbance and crossed symptoms with facial palsy on one side and hemiparesis on the other side. Embolic stroke happens spontaneously, mostly in patients with arterial fibrillation, with heart valve disease with atrial or ventricular thrombi, and is increasingly diagnosted in patients with a foramen ovale. Embolism during cardiac catherization is not infrequent, or if it happens, the best thing to do is to leave the introduction sheets in and send the patient over to neurology or neuro-radiology to perform whatever treatment is available.

Recent developments in the pathophysiology, diagnosis, and treatment of acute ischemic stroke have made neurological critical care medicine one of the fastest growing fields in clinical neurology. In this article, we will review the basic approach to evaluation and management of critically ill patients with acute stroke. Clinical evaluation of patients with acute cerebrovascular diseases in the emergency department should focus on four major questions: (a) Is there a life-threatening condition? (b) Is there a severe underlying disease? (c) Are there signs of increased intracranial pressure (ICP)? and (d) What is the patient's prognosis (that is, chance of survival or severity of the expected neurologic deficit)? The first and most important step in the emergency department is always to stabilize the patient's condition with regard to airway, breathing, and circulation. Breathing abnormalities, hypertension, cardiac dysfunction, and electrolyte disturbances are all early complications of acute stroke which may require immediate assessment and therapy. There should be no significant delay between admission to the emergency department, initial diagnostic work-up and transfer to the neurocritical care unit.

Airway management, pulmonary function, and cardiac care

Intubation and ventilatory support

Respiratory problems are uncommon in the first few hours after acute stroke though they are a major cause of illness and death in critically ill patients (1). Adequate ventilation and oxygenation are important for preserving metabolic turnover in the marginal zone of ischemia, the so-called penumbra (2, 3).

Patients with extensive hemispheric or vertebrobasilar territory infarctions, seizures, or massive intracranial or subarachnoid hemorrhages usually have impaired consciousness and are at particular risk for aspiration. They may require immediate airway management similar to patients with severe hypoxemia and hypercarbia. Initial orotracheal intubation is preferred to nasotracheal intubation because of the high incidence of sinusitis (table 1).

Intubation of neurocritically ill patients is associated with several specific problems. For example, laryngoscopy and intubation often lead to a substantial hemodynamic response, and some anesthetic agents may increase ICP. We suggest short-acting agents, such as thiopental (3–5 mg/kg), etomidate (0.3–0.5 mg/kg) or propofol (1.5–3 mg/kg), be used with a depolarizing neuromuscular blocking agent, such as succinylcholine (1.2 mg/kg), to blunt the ICP response.

Patients with acute stroke often require prolonged ventilatory support. Although positive end-expiratory pressure may be useful to treat diverse pulmonary problems including

Table 1. Indication for endotracheal intubation (3)

Blood gas analysis	pO2 < 50–60 mm Hg pCO2 > 50–60 mm Hg Vital capacity < 500–800 ml
Signs of respiratory distress	Tachypnea (rate > 30 breaths/min) Dsypnea Use of accessory muscles
Coma High risk for aspiration Maintenance of stable airways	

pneumonia, pulmonary edema and adult respiratory distress syndrome, the resulting increase in intrathoracic pressure may lead to a rise in ICP (4).

Neurogenic pulmonary edema may develop rapidly in patients with subarachnoid hemorrhage, seizures and dysautonomia. It is characterized by protein-rich alveolar fluid, but the pathophysiologic mechanisms are not clear. A combination of factors such as left atrial hypertension, systemic hypertension and increased sympathetic activity may be involved (5).

Tracheotomy

With the development of high-volume, low-pressure cuffs, the risk of tracheal stenosis after prolonged orotracheal or nasotracheal intubation has markedly decreased. Nevertheless, prolonged intubation (longer than 2–3 weeks) may cause laryngeal damage and subsequent difficulty speaking. In general, tracheotomy should be performed whenever the benefits of better patient mobility and earlier weaning outweigh the risks and complications of the procedure (table 2).

Cardiac care

Lesions of the central nervous system may cause two major cardiac complications: arrhythmias and repolarization disturbances with increased cardiac enzyme levels. Patients with subarachnoid hemorrhage, seizures and head trauma are at particular risk for these complications (6). As in neurogenic pulmonary edema, increased sympathetic drive with elevated catecholamine levels may play an important role. For prevention and treatment, benzodiazepines, barbiturates, beta-blockers, calcium channel blockers, and free-radical scavengers have all been tried but none has been tested prospectively.

Table 2. Indications for tracheotomy

Coma for > 14 days
Bronchial toilet
Laryngeal obstruction
Prolonged weaning
Interference with early rehabilitation due to intubation

Hypertension, metabolic disturbances and prophylaxis

Deep-vein thrombosis

Most patients with acute ischemic stroke present initially with hypertension. Whether or not to treat the hypertension in the acute setting continues to be debated (2, 3, 7–9). We take a conservative approach to the treatment of hypertension in acute stroke. Blood pressure generally decreases in the first 24–48 h without treatment. In addition, autoregulation is impaired in acute stroke such that cerebral blood flow is passively dependent on arterial pressure. Thus, a significant reduction in mean arterial pressure (MAP) can compromise ischemically threatened tissue (10). Systolic blood pressure should not be lowered below 160 mm Hg and, in patients with an intracerebral mass, cerebral perfusion pressure (CPP = MAP – ICP) should not fall below 60 mm Hg. Specific guidelines are given in table 3.

Sodium nitroprusside and hydralazine are cerebral vasodilators that increase cerebral blood flow, impair autoregulation and increase ICP. ACE inhibitors are currently not recommended because of their often extensive activation of the renin system (11). Anti-adrenergic agents such as clonidine or short acting alpha-beta-blockers such as labetalol (continuous i.v. infusion 2 mg/min) are recommended.

A central venous catheter provides direct information on the intravascular volume (central venous pressure) and is a safe route for the administration of large volumes of fluids, parenteral nutrition and medication. The safest approach is via the cubital vein. When multilumen catheters are needed, the subclavian or internal jugular vein approach is recommended. Internal jugular vein catheters may impede central venous drainage and should be avoided in patients with incresed ICP. Occasionally, a pulmonary artery catheter (Swan-Ganz, see Monitoring below) is necessary to obtain information on cardiac output,

Table 3. Treatment of hypertension in acute stroke

Condition	Action
Heidelberg regimen (3)	
1 Systolic BP < 220 mm Hg and diastolic BP < 110 mm Hg	do not treat
2 Systolic BP > 220 mm Hg and/or diastolic BP 110–120 mm Hg on repeated measurements	(a) nifidepine 10 mg s.l.[1] (b) clonidine 0.075 mg s.c. (c) urapidil 12.5 mg i.v.
3 Diastolic BP > 120 mm Hg or systolic BP slightly increased on repeated measurements 15 min apart	nitroglycerin 5 mg i.v. or 10 mg orally
Cincinnati regimen (8)	
1 Systolic BP < 120 mm Hg or diastolic BP < 120 mm Hg	do not treat
2 Systolic BP > 230 mm Hg and/or diastolic BP 120–140 mm Hg on repeated measurements	(a) labetolol 10 mg i.v. (may be repeated if necessary. Maximum dose 160 mg)[2] (b) nifedipine 10 mg s.l.
3 Diastolic BP > 140 mm Hg or systolic BP slightly increased on repeated measurements 15 min apart	sodium nitroprusside 2 mg/kg/min (dose may be doubled after 3–5 min)

[1] Caution: Nifedipine may cause too rapid a decline in BP.
[2] Not available in Germany.

and right and left ventricular diastolic function. The best approach is via the right internal jugular vein or left subclavian vein.

Electrolyte and glucose metabolism

Hyponatremia frequently develops in critically ill patients. Most have hypotonic hyponatremia, that is an excess of total body water relative to sodium. They may be hypovolemic (e.g., gastrointestinal and renal losses), hypervolemic (e.g., congestive heart failure, liver failure, nephrotic syndrome), or isovolemic (e.g., SIADH). Hypovolemic patients should be treated with isotonic saline while hypervolemic and isovolemic patients should be treated with free water restriction. Treatment with hypertonic saline should be reserved for symptomatic patients (e.g., mental status changes or seizures) and those with sodium concentrations < 120 mEq/l (with the goal of raising the concentration to 125 mEq/l). Rapid correction of hyponatremia should be avoided because it can precipitate central pontine demyelinization (12). Hypertonic hyponatremia occasionally develops in patients receiving mannitol or glycerol therapy as in those with marked hyperglycemia. Hypernatremia may result from osmotic diuresis, gastrointestinal losses, and insensible losses from skin and lungs. Hypokalemia may result from diuretic therapy, gastrointestinal losses, certain antibiotics, and alkalosis. In a critical care unit, at least daily monitoring of potassium levels is necessary and 20–60 mEq/l should be added daily to parenteral nutrition.

Hyperglycemia occurs frequently in patients with acute stroke. Because hyperglycemia increases cerebral infarct size (13), levels over 250–300 mg/dl should be treated by subcutaneous injection or continuous intravenous infusion of insulin. In patients with acute stroke, parenteral nutrition should not contain more than 40 g glucose/day.

Prophylaxis of deep-vein thrombosis

Patients with acute stroke are at high risk of developing deep vein thrombosis (DVT) and pulmonary embolism. We recommended prophylaxis with low-dose heparin (5,000 IU s.c.

Table 4. Treatment strategies for raised ICP (3)

Without ICP monitoring	
Osmotherapy	Glycerol 10 %: 4 x 125 or 250 ml Mannitol 20 %: 4–6 x 100 ml
Controlled hyperventilation	Controlled mandatory ventilation No PEEP (if possible) pCO_2: 28–35 mm Hg
With ICP monitoring	
Barbiturates	Thiopental bolus of 0.25–0.5 g up to 1 g/10 kg/day (exact hemodynamic monitoring with Swan-Ganz catheter preferable)
THAM-buffer solution	Base excess < + 10 mEq (administration via central venous line)

every 12 h) and graduated elastic compression stockings for all patients with acute stroke. Patients in whom CT scan reveals large intracranial hemorrhage and selected neurosurgical patients (e.g., patients with cranial or spinal trauma) should receive intermittent pneumatic compression instead of heparin. Those with documented DVT should be treated with full anticoagulation. If anticoagulation is contraindicated, an inferior vena cava "Greenfield filter" can be implanted to reduce the risk of pulmonary embolism.

Brain edema and increased intracranial pressure

Brain edema is the most frequent complication of any acute brain injury. Cerebral blood flow is reduced by compression of adjacent brain tissue and secondary neuronal damage occurs. An ICP monitoring device may be helpful to detect increasing ICP, judge effectiveness of therapy and recognize iatrogenic errors that may increase ICP, for example excessive free water administration. All patients should be well sedated, since coughing and elevated intra-abdominal pressure increase ICP. Procedures such as endotracheal suctioning, turning the patient, and central venous catheterization have also been shown to considerably raise ICP. The patient should be positioned upright at approximately 20–30 °C (15). Because fever increases cerebral blood flow and raises ICP, antipyretics and cooling blankets should be used liberally. Moreover, animal experiments show that hypothermia reduces infarct volume and may decrease ICP in patients with head trauma (16, 17).

Hyperventilation induces serum and CSF alkalosis and vasoconstriction, thereby reducing cerebral blood flow and cerebral blood volume. In most patients, an initial reduction of arterial pCO_2 to 28–33 mm Hg lowers ICP by 25–30 % (18). This can be achieved by increasing the ventilation rate while maintaining a constant tidal volume. Reduction of cerebral blood flow may be dangerous if mean arterial pressure and cerebral perfusion pressure are low. In addition, because of compensation of CSF alkalosis, hyperventilation becomes less effective after hours. Rebound vasodilation and increase in ICP can occur if normoventilation is resumed too rapidly.

Low-molecular hypertonic solutions as glycerol, mannitol and sorbitol are used frequently to reduce brain water content by producing an osmolar gradient between brain and plasma and drawing water from brain tissue into plasma. Serum osmolality should be increased initially to between 295 and 305 mosm/l. Glycerol can either be given intravenously (125 or 250 ml of a 10 % solution over 1 h four times daily) or orally (50 ml of a 80 % solution four times daily). Onset of action is not rapid. Glycerol is metabolized by glycolysis within brain tissue and is cleared by the kidney. Volume overload, hemolysis and electrolyte disturbances are frequent problems associated with glycerol treatment (19, 20). Renal function and central venous pressure must be carefully monitored in patients with underlying cardiac disease and the glucose load must be reduced during full-dose glycerol treatment. Mannitol 20 % (0.25–0.5 g/kg every 4–6 h) is an osmotic diuretic with a faster onset of action. It is the therapy of choice in first-time pupil dilatation in patients with space occupying MCA infarctions and may reverse early signs of herniation. However, because equilibration between brain osmolality and plasma osmolality occurs, mannitol loses its therapeutic effect after a few days. A reverse osmotic drive resulting in a marked rebound phenomenon may occur if treatment with mannitol is suddenly discontinued or reduced too rapidly (21). Mannitol is cleared by the kidney. Electrolyte disturbances, renal dysfunction, and hypovolemia are known complications. Loop diuretics may decrease intracranial pressure by removing water from edematous brain. Diuretics alone have not been tested for the control of ICP though in addition to osmotic agents they may be helpful.

Tris-hydroxy-methyl-aminomethane (THAM) is a solution that decreases ICP by inducing vasoconstriction, increasing the capacity of CSF to buffer pH changes and neutralizing acidosis-mediated vasodilatation. A test dose of 60 mmol of THAM in 100 ml in 5 % dextrose can be infused over 45 min. If effective, ICP should fall by 10–15 mm Hg. THAM can then be infused at a rate of 3 mmol/h. A central venous catheter should be used since it causes severe tissue necrosis. THAM is nephrotoxic and should only be used when all other conservative therapies have failed (22).

In patients with head trauma, short-acting barbiturates such as thiopental lead to a prompt and significant reduction of cerebral blood flow and ICP (23). The effect is short acting so its use must be restricted to acute crises. Barbiturate therapy has also been frequently used in patients with malignant ischemic brain edema. Complications, including hypotension, depression of cardiac contractility, and predisposition to infections, limit its routine use. Patients may require circulatory support.

General anesthesia reduces cerebral blood volume and central venous pressure. However, inhalative agents such as halothane, trichlorethylene, or methoxyflurane may increase ICP and should be avoided. Nitrous oxide has only a minimal effect on ICP. Propofol (dosage 5–50 μg/kg/h as a continuous drip) is now recommended for sedation because it has only minimal cardiodepressive effects and reduces ICP (24).

Monitoring of critically ill patients in the intensive care unit

Blood pressure, cardiac function (ECG) and breathing should be monitored in all critically ill patients. Blood pressure can be monitored either by an arterial cannula (preferably at the radial artery) or a blood pressure cuff (dynamometry). Oxygenation can be assessed noninvasively with pulse oximetry or with arterial blood gas analysis from the arterial line. Ventilation can be assessed by measuring forced vital capacity and negative inspiratory force. All patients should have a central venous catheter. Pulmonary artery catheterization (Swan-Ganz) is sometimes necessary for monitoring cardiac output and fluid therapy.

Intracranial pressure monitoring

ICP monitoring helps to provide data for rational treatment. ICP devices can be epidural, subdural, intraparenchymal, or intraventricular. They are either fluid-coupled (ventricular catheter, subarachnoid bolt) or non fluid-coupled (fiberoptic, pneumatic devices). No system works completely satisfactorily. Main disadvantages are unreliable measurements and risk of infections. We prefer pneumatic devices for epidural ICP monitoring because they are easy to handle and give exact measurements (26) (table 5).

Electrophysiologic monitoring

Median nerve somatosensory evoked potentials (MSEP) with both spinal and cortical leads, brain stem auditory-evoked potentials (BAEP), and less frequently, visual-evoked

Table 5. ICP monitoring devices

ICP monitor	Advantage	Disadvantage
Ventricular catheter	drainage and exact measurements	surgery, high infection rate
Subarachnoid bolt	low infection rate, not invasive	often no exact monitoring possible, obstruction of device
Pneumatic device	accurate measurement	expensive, dislocation possible
Fiberoptic device	accurate measurements, subdural, intraparenchymal, and intraventricular location	no further calibration possible, breakage risk

and middle latency acoustic potentials may be used to monitor therapy in the critical care unit even in sedated patients. BAEP and MSEP are helpful when deciding how aggressively patients with basilar thrombosis, space-occupying cerebellar lesions, or severe hemispheric stroke should be treated. Alterations of BAEP and MSEP in patients with cerebellar infarction indicate the need for neurosurgical intervention even if patients are awake and alert (27). EEG monitoring is rarely performed in the setting of acute stroke. It is useful for monitoring barbiturate induced coma. Spectral features and measures of period and amplitude may give furter information.

Vascular and neuroradiological monitoring

Transcranial Doppler ultrasound is a useful tool for assessment of vasospasm in subarachnoid hemorrhage or recanalization in patients with ischemic stroke. Cerebral oxygen consumption can be monitored using a jugular bulb catheter or near infrared laser spectroscopy. However both methods still need validation in larger series (28). Most patients will acute cerebrovascular disease undergo repeated MRI and CT scans. Patients with spaceoccupying lesions often require daily scans in the first few days after admission.

Intensive care management of acute ischemic stroke

Because there is no proven treatment strategy for acute ischemic stroke, intensive care focuses mainly on respiratory and cardiac complications and nursing care. Patients with some stroke subtypes, such as acute proximal middle cerebral artery occlusion, acute basilar thrombosis, or space-occupying cerebellar infarction, almost always require immediate neurocritical care (table 6).

Table 6. Indications for ICU treatment of acute cerebral ischemia

Progressing symptoms, crescendo TIA
Fluctuating, hemodynamically induced infarction
Embolic intracranial ICA/MCA occlusion
Endocarditis with septic cerebral emboli
Arterial dissection plus embolism
Thrombolytic or proposed hypervolemic therapy

Acute middle cerebral artery stroke

Most patients present with severe hemiparesis or hemiplegia. In the first hours after onset of symptoms, level of consciousness is normal or only slight depressed. Forced conjugate eye deviation often implies a large infarct. Prognosis is correlated with the severity of the initial neurologic deficit. Hemiplegia, forced eye deviation, and decreased level of consciousness indicate a poor outcome. The diagnosis of acute intracranial ICA or MCA occlusion is made either by ultrasound or angiography. CT scan often reveals early signs of infarction within the first 2–3 h (29). The "dense middle cerebral artery" sign is present in 50 % of acute ICA/MCA occlusions. Other signs such us effacement of the cortical sulci, compression of the insular cistern, loss of internal capsule definition, or focal loss of white/gray matter contrast may be observed.

Intravenous or local thrombolysis may be performed within 6 h after onset of symptoms following protocols of controlled trials. A final statement about the safety and effectiveness of thrombolytic therapy cannot be made until the results of the major ongoing randomized trials are available (30, 31). The use of full-dose heparin anticoagulation for acute ischemic stroke continues to be controversial (31–34). The rationale for early anticoagulation is the inhibition of local thrombus propagation and growth and prevention of embolism (either artery to artery or cardiac embolism). A beneficial effect of early anticoagulation has never been shown prospectively, however, and it is not clear whether the risk of parenchymal hemorrhage outweighs the presumed benefits. In Europe, full-dose heparin anticoagulation is frequently used immediately after stroke if a possible cardioembolic source is present (33). In North America, anticoagulation is often postponed for 48–72 h in patients with large infarcts (35). Anticoagulation is probably not indicated for lacunar stroke. Within the first 24 h, cerebral edema becomes a serious complication of large MCA infarcts. Alertness, pupillary reaction, and neurologic status should be carefully monitored. Serial CT scans may demonstrate increasing edema formation which may require ICP monitoring and treatment (31).

Decompressive surgery

In some patients, cerebral edema after ischemic stroke may become life threatening. Early surgical intervention may be life saving if the CT scan reveals signs of malignant MCA infarction. This will be the topic of a forthcoming editorial.

Acute basilar artery thrombosis

All patients with acute basilar artery occlusion should be treated in an intensive care unit. In those with impaired consciousness, immediate endotracheal intubation and sedation is necessary. Predictors of a good outcome include young age, presumed embolic occlusion, preserved collateral circulation, only slightly impaired consciousness, and preserved sensory-evoked potentials. We treat these patients with local intra-arterial thrombolysis using urokinase (dose 1 million IU/h). Although not yet tested against placebo-controlled, randomized trials, survival rates from open trials indicate that thrombolytic therapy may be life saving (36). Our patients are fully anticoagulated with heparin after thrombolysis. Repeat CT scans after angiography are done to exclude intracerebral hemorrhage and to reveal major cerebellar infarction.

Cerebellar infarction

In general, patients with cerebellar infarction due to occlusion of basilar artery branches have a good clinical outcome even without aggressive treatment. However, in some patients, perischemic edema causes occlusive hydrocephalus or brain stem compression with rapid deterioration of brain stem functions. Therefore, close clinical monitoring and often serial CT scans are needed to estimate the severity of obstructive hydrocephalus. Neurocritical care is necessary if the CT scan reveals signs of increased pressure in the posterior fossa. In comatose patients, decompressive surgery of the posterior fossa (with or without removal of infarcted cerebellar tissue) is significantly better than ventriculostomy alone (37–39).

Hypertensive-hypervolemic therapy in progressing stroke

Hypertensive-hypervolemic therapy has been widely advocated for therapy of vasospasm after subarachnoid hemorrhage (40). This concept has been adopted for the treatment of progressing stroke due to hemodynamic failure of blood supply and for brain trauma. We use this strategy in patients with severe hemodynamic stenosis and reversible neurologic symptoms and in patients with marginal cerebral perfusion pressure due to increased ICP, low MAP, or both. Plasma expanders are infused aiming at a central venous pressure of 8 mm Hg and an arterial systolic blood pressure of up to 180 mm Hg. In addition, vasopressor agents may be necessary to achieve a higher MAP (table 7). Although the benefit of this therapy has not been proven by randomized studies, the rate of permanent ischemic deficits following subarachnoid hemorrhage seems to be lower. Complications include pulmonary and cerebral edema, myocardial infarction, and the risk of secondary intracerebral hemorrhage.

Table 7. Hypertensive-hypervolemic therapy

Other measures

A team of nurses, speech and physical therapists, and doctors is needed for optimal performance in the ICU. Physical and speech therapy must be started early in the critical care unit. Relatives of patients must be included in both the decision-making process and care for the patient.

References

1. Bounds JV, Wiebers DO, Whisnant JP, Okazaki H (1981) Mechanisms and timing of deaths from cerebral infarction. Stroke 19: 1119–1124
2. Brott T, Fieschi C, Hacke W (1994) General therapy of acute ischemic stroke; in Hacke W (ed): Neurocritical care. Berlin, Springer, pp 552–577
3. Hacke W, del Zoppo GJ, Furlan A, von Kummer R (1994) Ischemic stroke; in Hanley DF (ed): Principles and Practices in Neurocritical Care. Baltimore, Williams & Wilkins
4. Aidinis SJ, Lafferty J, Shapiro HM (1976) Intracranial response to PEEP. Anesthesiology 45: 275–286
5. Malik AB (1985) Mechanisms of neurogenic pulmonary edema. Circ Res 57: 1–18
6. Samuels MA (1993) Cardiopulmonary aspects of acute neurologic disease; in Ropper AH (ed): Neurological and Neurosurgical Intensive Care, ed 3. New York, Raven Press, pp 103–120
7. Yatsu FM, Zivin J (1985) Hypertension in acute ischemic strokes. Not to treat. Arch Neurol 42: 999–1000
8. Brott T, MacCarthey EP (1989) Antihypertensive therapy in stroke; in Fischer M (ed): Medical Therapy of Acute Stroke. New York, Dekker, pp 117–143
9. Spence JD, Del Maestro RF (1985) Hypertension in acute ischemic stroke: Treat. Arch Neurol 42: 1000–1002
10. Powers WJ (1993) Acute hypertension after stroke: The scientific basis for treatment decisions. Neurology 43: 461–467
11. Strandgaard S, Paulsen OB (1992) Regulation of cerebral blood flow in health and disease. J Cardiovasc Pharmacol 19 (suppl 6): 89–93
12. Sterns RH, Riggs JE, Schochet S (1986) Osmotic demyelination syndrome following correction of hyponatriemia. N Engl J Med 314: 1535–1542
13. Wagner KR, Kleinholz M, de Courten-Myers GM, Myers RE (1992) Hyperglycemic versus normoglycemic stroke: Topography of brain metabolites, intracellular pH, and infarct size. J Cereb Blood Flow Metab 12: 213–222
14. Scurr JH, Coleridge-Smith PD, Hasty JH (1987) Regimen for improved effectiveness of intermittent pneumatic compression in deep venous thrombosis prophylaxis. Surgery 102: 817–820
15. Feldmann Z, Kanter MJ, Robertson CS et al. (1992) Effect of head elevation on intracranial pressure, cerebral perfusion pressure, and cerebral blood flow in head-injured patients. J Neurosurg 76: 207–211
16. Ginsberg M, Sternau L et al. (1992) Therapeutic modulation of brain temperature: Relevance to ischemic brain injury. Cerebrovasc Brain Metab Rev 4: 189–225
17. Marion D, Obrist W, Carlier P et al. (1993) The use of moderate therapeutic hypothermia for patients with severe head injuries: A preliminary report. J Neurosurg 79: 354–362
18. Marshall LF, Smith RW, Shapiro HM (1979) The outcome of aggressive treatment in severe head injuries. I. The significance of intracranial pressure monitoring. J Neurosurg 50: 20–30
19. Yu YL, Kumana CR, Lauder IJ et al. (1992) Treatment of acute cerebral hemorrhage with intravenous glycerol. A double-blind, placebo controlled, randomized trial. Stroke 23: 967–971
20. Frank MS, Nahata MC, Hilty MD (1981) Glycerol: A review of its pharmacology, pharmacokinetics, adverse reactions, and clinical use. Pharmacotherapy 1: 147–160
21. Kaufmann AM, Cardoso ER (1992) Aggravation of vasogenic edema by multiple-dose mannitol. J Neurosurg 77: 584–589
22. Wolf A, Levi L, Marmorou A et al. (1993) Effect of THAM upon outcome in severe head injury: A randomized prospective clinical trial. J Neurosurg 78: 54–59
23. Eisenberg HM, Frankowski RF, Contant CF et al. (1988) High dose barbiturate control of elevated intracranial pressure in patients with severe head injury. J Neurosurg 69: 15–23
24. Harris CE, Grounds RM, Murray AM, Lumley J, Royston D, Morgan M (1990) Propofol for longterm sedation in the intensive care unit. Anaesthesia 45: 366–372
25. Zander JF, Bourke DL (1994) Pain relief and sedation; in Hacke W, Hanley DF, Einhäupl K et al. (eds): Neurocritical Care. Berlin, Springer, pp 116–124

26. Schnitzer MS, Aschoff AA (1994) Intracranial pressure monitoring; in Hacke W (ed): Neurocritical Care. Berlin, Springer, pp 90–97
27. Krieger D, Adams H, Rieke K, Schwarz S, Forsting M, Hacke W (1992) Prospective evaluation of the prognostic significance of evoked potentials in acute basilar occlusion. Crit Care Med 21: 1169–1174
28. Stocchetti N, Pararella A, Bridelli F et al. (1994) Cerebral venous oxygen saturation studied with bilateral samples in the internal jugular veins. Neurosurgery 34: 38–44
29. Kummer R von, Meyding-Lamade U, Forsting M et al. (1994) Sensitivity and prognostic value of early CT in occlusion of the middle cerebral artery trunk. AJNR 15: 9–15
30. Del Zoppo GJ, Pessin MS, Mori E, Hacke W (1991) Thrombolytic intervention in acute thrombolytic and embolic stroke. Semin Neurol 11: 368–384
31. Furlan AJ, Busse O, Ringelstein RB (1994) Special aspects in the treatment of severe hemispheric infarction; in Hacke W (ed): Neurocritical Care. Berlin, Springer
32. Miller VT, Hart RG (1988) Heparin anticoagulation in acute brain ischemia. Stroke 19: 403–406
33. Phillips SJ (1989) An alternative view of heparin anticoagulation in acute focal brain ischemia. Stroke 20: 295–298
34. Easton CJ, Pessin MS (1990) Anticoagulation. Is there still a role in atherothrombotic stroke? Stroke 21: 820–823
35. Cerebral Embolism Task Force (1989) Cardiogenic brain embolism (second report). Arch Neurol 46: 727–735
36. Hacke W, Zeumer H, Ferbert A et al. (1988) Intraarterial thrombolytic therapy improves outcome in patients with acute vertebrobasilar occlusive disease. Stroke 19: 1216–1222
37. Rieke K, Krieger D, Adams HP, Aschoff A, Meyding-Lamada U, Hacke W (1993) Therapeutic strategies in space-occupying cerebellar infarction based on clinical, neuroradiological and neurophysiological data. Cerebrovasc Dis 3: 45–55
38. Heros RC (1992) Surgical treatment of cerebellar infarction. Stroke 23: 937–938
39. Chen HJ, Lee TC, Wei CP (1992) Treatment of cerebellar infarction by decompressive suboccipital craniectomy. Stroke 23: 957–961
40. Awad IA, Carter P, Spetzler RF, Medina M, Williams FW (1987) Clinical vasospasm after subarachnoid hemorrhage: Response to hypervolemic hemodilation and arterial hypertension. Stroke 18: 365–372

Authors address:
Werner Hacke, MD
Department of Neurology
University of Heidelberg
Im Neuenheimer Feld 400
69120 Heidelberg
Germany

Cerebral protection in Cerebrovascular Surgery

Anesthesia in cerebrovascular surgery

A. Thiel, G. Hempelmann

Department of Anaesthesiology and Intensive Care Medicine, Justus-Liebig-University, Gießen, Germany

Introduction

Cerebrovascular surgery focuses on the prevention of ischemic stroke by removing embolic sources and/or restoring decreased blood flow to the brain. For this purpose, most often carotid endarterectomy or extra-intracranial bypassing are performed. There are, however, two main controversies regarding these operative procedures: First, it has been seriously questioned in the past whether the surgical strategy can improve neurologic outcome compared to conservative therapy. Second, temporary shunting during carotid endarterectomy remains a matter of intensive debate, and the question "to shunt or not to shunt" is far from being answered. It has become clear now from the European and North-American multi-center studies (5, 14) that carotid endarterectomy reduces stroke risk in symptomatic patients with high-grade carotid stenoses while extra-intracranial bypass procedures have yielded discouraging results (4). As carotid endarterectomy is the most frequent procedure within cerebrovascular surgery, this chapter emphasizes the anesthetic considerations related to this type of surgery.

Preoperative assessment

Ischemic cerebral vascular disease may have various etiologies, atherosclerosis, however, is a common one. Therefore, patients presenting with symptoms of ischemic syndromes like transient ischemic attacks (TIA), amaurosis fugax, reversible neurologic deficits (RIND), or completed stroke should be carefully assessed regarding the whole cardiovascular system. Risk factors for stroke include smoking, obesity, family history of stroke, diabetes, arterial hypertension, and increased plasma fibrinogen levels (12). In addition, the cardiac situation of the patient should be evaluated. Chronic atrial fibrillation, mitral valve prolapse or annulus calcification can be responsible for cardioembolic events which account for approximately 15 % of ischemic strokes. More important, the anesthetist should look for signs or symptoms of coronary artery disease which will be found in about one-third of patients scheduled for carotid surgery (8).

When assessing the patient with ischemic cerebral vascular disease preoperatively, the anesthetist should be aware of the fact that myocardial infarction is the most frequent cause for perioperative and late death following carotid endarterectomy. Hypertension doubles the risk of stroke (12). However, aggressive treatment of elevated blood pressure immediately prior to surgery is not recommended because cerebral perfusion pressure may reach critical limits in some patients. A history of smoking is common, so problems associated with chronic obstructive pulmonary disease are likely to occur intraoperatively. Apart from the usual preoperative diagnostic measures (clinical evaluation, electrocardiogram, chest x-ray, spirometry, laboratory analyses, ultrasonography of the brain-supplying arteries), a short neurologic re-examination just before surgery should be added.

Choice of anesthetic technique

On the day of surgery, the patient should receive her or his morning cardiovascular medication except for digitalis and diuretics. For anxiolysis, benzodiazepines may be given orally but patients should be sedated only lightly to allow neurologic judgement just prior to induction of anesthesia.

Based on the preoperative considerations, the anesthetic regimen aims at minimizing potential cerebral ischemia, monitoring the brain to detect ischemia, and avoiding unstable cardiovascular conditions. Ventilation conditions, fluid replacement, and head and neck position should be selected that will not compromise cerebral blood flow and perfusion pressure. Essentially, the patient will benefit from any technique that might protect the brain and the heart, and both regional and general anesthesia may be performed according to the patient's individual risk profile.

When applied by experienced hands, cervical epidural anaesthesia or the combination of deep and superficial cervical nerve block can be used safely in cooperative patients to provide anesthesia during carotid endarterectomy (15). The main advantages of regional anesthetic techniques are that the neurologic state of the patient can be assessed throughout the operative procedure, and general anesthetics can be avoided. However, there are strong arguments against regional anaesthesia for carotid surgery. Most anesthetists are not familiar with these techniques, and cervical block has a high failure rate (20 %). Surgery under regional anesthesia may be uncomfortable for a number of patients which will result in a high rate of tachycardia and/or hypertension. Intervention with vasoactive drugs and/or sedatives will be necessary in a considerable number of procedures to provide stable cardiovascular conditions. Over-sedation may mimic or, even worse, hide a deterioration of neurologic state after carotid clamping. Ventilation cannot be controlled. Agitation, loss of cooperation or consciousness may afford induction of general anesthesia, and endotracheal intubation can be extremely difficult under these circumstances. For these reasons, most carotid endarterectomies are performed under general anesthesia.

The anesthetist should use general anesthetics which are as advantageous as possible for both the brain and the heart. Basically, all intravenous anesthetics may be used for induction except for ketamine because of its cardiovascular stimulating properties. Barbiturates are the agents of choice for induction as they will decrease cerebral oxygen demands. The role of propofol in this setting remains to be fully evaluated. Post-induction hypotension as well as hypertension following laryngoscopy or intubation are critical conditions which should be treated immediately by given short-acting vasopressors, or antihypertensive substances, respectively.The hypertensive response to intubation stress may be avoided by lidocain, the short-acting beta-blocker esmolol, or a potent opioid like alfentanil. Muscle relaxation can be achieved with any non-depolarizing blocker, e.g., vecuronium or pipecuronium which seem preferable because of lacking cardiovascular side-effects. Suxamethonium should be used with care in hemiplegic patients because serum potassium levels may rise dramatically which can result in significant cardiac dysrhythmias.

For maintenance of anesthesia, halogenated agents like halothane, enflurane, or isoflurane are frequently applied as they allow rapid awakening and early assessment of neurologic state, postoperatively. All three agents increase cerebral blood flow (CBF) and decrease cerebral metabolism. Recent studies suggest that isoflurane is advantageous when compared with enflurane or halothane because isoflurane reduces the frequency of cerebral ischemia during carotid surgery (13). Changes in the electroencephalogram (EEG) indicating ischemia will occur if regional cerebral blood flow (rCBF) is reduced to 18 – 20 ml/100 g/min. This is also true for patients undergoing carotid endarterectomy anesthetized with halothane/nitrous oxide. If isoflurane/nitrous oxide was applied instead, a significantly lower limit of rCBF was tolerated (10 ml/100 g/min) until ischemic EEG changes were seen (11). At equianesthetic concentrations, cerebral metabolism is more suppressed by isoflurane than by halothane. Isoflurane, in contrast to halothane, does not increase CBF at a concentration of 1.0 MAC, so an increase of intracranial pressure is unlikely. Therefore, some degree of cerebral protection is provided by isoflurane which makes it an excellent anesthetic for cerebrovascular surgery. Neurologic outcome, however, is not affected by the choice of agent (11).

Volatile anesthetics may be critical in patients who suffer also from severe coronary artery disease. Here, a balanced technique using opioids like fentanyl or alfentanil, and benzodiazepines seems more adequate for cardiac reasons but recovery from anesthesia will be prolonged and postoperative neurologic assessment delayed. Nitrous oxide should be used with care as it may cause considerable myocardial depression in patients with severe cardiac diseases. However, the incidence of myocardial infarction as the most frequent cause of perioperative mortality did not differ significantly between patients given halothane, enflurane, or isoflurane (2), and there is no evidence that a balanced technique should improve outcome in endarterectomy patients.

Ventilation remains a matter of debate. Hypercapnia is obsolete as intracerebral "steal" may occur which diverts blood flow from ischemic to unaffected areas of perfusion. In addition, high tensions of carbon dioxide induce undesirable cardiac arrhythmias. Hypocapnia, in contrast, may be advantageous by producing an inverse "steal" phenomenon. Excessive hyperventilation (arterial $pCO2 < 25$ mmHg) should be avoided as the concomitant CBF reduction may reach critical levels. As a result, most anesthetists choose normoventilation or moderate hyperventilation for endarterectomies.

Prior to induction of anesthesia, fluid volume of the patient should be balanced by an infusion of 500 ml crystalloid solution. In fluid-depleted patients, additional colloids may be helpful to avoid significant blood pressure decreases after induction. Patients may also profit from colloids (e.g., hydroxy ethyl starch) because of their rheologic properties, and infusion of these substances should be completed before carotid clamping.

Monitoring

The electrocardiogram (ECG) must be monited continuously. As ischemic heart disease is not uncommon in carotid patients, simultaneous registration of leads II and V5 is recommended. Arterial blood pressure must be measured directly via an intravascular catheter placed under local anesthesia. A large-bore venous cannula serves for rapid fluid replacement if neccessary. A central venous line or a pulmonary artery catheter is not indicated unless the patient presents with severe cardiac problems. Peripheral pulse-oxymetry should be used in every case. If general anesthesia is applied, ventilation is assessed by capnometry and intermittent arterial blood gas analyses. Monitoring should also include body temperature. While placing the patient's head for surgery, care should be taken because extreme rotation may compromise blood supply via the vertebral arteries.

Control of arterial blood pressure and avoidance of hypo- and hypertensive episodes, though not easy to achieve, are essential throughout the operative procedure. Hypotension lowers cerebral perfusion pressure and may result in critical cerebral hypoperfusion and neurologic deficits. It is of note that cerebral autoregulation pressure limits are shifted to higher levels in chronic hypertensive patients. Systolic pressure should always exceed 100 mmHg, and a decrease > 40 mmHg compared with the smallest preoperative pressure should be strictly avoided. With the carotid artery clamped, induced hypertension is often recommended in that mean arterial pressure should be elevated 20 – 30 mmHg. This approach has been seriously questioned in recent reviews (6, 19) because hypertension increases myocardial work load and oxygen consumption. Those who favor induced hypertension should reduce anesthetic depth rather than inject vasopressors because the latter technique increases the incidence of myocardial ischemia (20).

Detection of cerebral ischemia

Current surgical technique requires temporary occlusion of carotid artery blood flow to the brain. Several monitoring techniques have been used in the anesthetized patient to assess adequacy of cerebral perfusion and to support the decision for, or against, temporary shunting. Methods include assessment of cerebral function (e.g., EEG, somatosensory evoked potentials) or cerebral perfusion (e.g., internal carotid artery stump pressure, rCBF, transcranial Doppler sonography (TCD)).

Spontaneous activity of the cerebral cortex is registered by the EEG. Ischemia will be detected with a high sensitivity, but specifity is considerably lower. Ischemic changes may not be detected in patients with residual deficits (16, 17). Many factors, including general anesthetics, interfere with monitoring so that interpretation is best under steady-state conditions. Computer-aided EEG methods allow data reduction without altering sensitivity.

Somatosensory evoked potentials after median nerve stimulation (SEP) are comparable to the EEG with regard to sensitivity. Carefully conducted clinical studies (3, 18) suggest that SEP reflect ischemia also with a high specifity which would make the method superior to EEG monitoring. Notably, false-negative SEP results (i.e., new postoperative neurologic deficits despite unchanged SEP intraoperatively) have not been reported yet for carotid surgery. As with the EEG, general anesthetics may affect SEP waveforms. Nitrous oxide decreases cortical SEP amplitude by 50 % without affecting latencies. Halothane, enflurane, and isoflurane depress amplitude and increase latencies in a dose-dependent manner with isoflurane having the most pronounced effect.

Stump pressure measurement remains a common procedure after carotid clamping. Values below 50 – 60 mmHg are considered critical, i.e., reflecting inadequate collateral flow. There are, however, only poor correlations between stump pressure and rCBF in anesthetized patients (10), and stump pressure cannot reliably predict neurologic deteriorations (9).

The gold standard to assess cerebral perfusion is the measurement of global or regional cerebral blood flow (CBF) by the washout characteristics of inert gases or radioactive substances. The correlation between CBF and EEG changes is good. Main drawbacks of this method are that measurements are time-consuming, expensive, and can only be performed in specialized institutions.

Transcranial Doppler sonography (TCD) measures blood flow velocity in basal cerebral arteries. In contrast to CBF measurements, the method is noninvasive and provides continuous data. Since 1985, the number of TCD reports concerning carotid surgery has rapidly increased. The correlation between relative changes of rCBF and middle cerebral artery (MCA) flow velocity has well been established (1). Carotid clamping decreases flow velocity to a variable extent. If flow velocity in the MCA is reduced to less than 40 % of the preclamping value, SEP changes indicating ischemia are likely to occur (21). There is growing interest in TCD as a sensitive method to detect circulating cerebral emboli (7).

In contrast to cardiovascular and respiratory monitoring, methods determining cerebral function and/or perfusion have not yet become accepted standards of intraoperative care. The main reason is that clear evidence is lacking whether or not "cerebral monitoring" decreases the rate of perioperative neurologic complications. Future multi-center studies including thousands of patients would be necessary to answer this question. However, there is a strong trend visible as an increasing number of institutions apply neurophysiologic monitoring during carotid endarterectomy. The insertion of a temporary shunt by itself carries the risk of neurologic sequelae, and reliable monitoring allows shunt restriction to cases with critically reduced cerebral perfusion after clamping. Most patients tolerate carotid clamping without ischemic changes. Here, the anaesthetic regimen may primarily focus on the cardiovascular risk factors which are most important for long-term prognosis.

Postoperative problems

Considerable variations of arterial blood pressure are common in the immediate postoperative course and can result in severe cardiovascular and/or neurologic complications. It is therefore recommended to have patients in an intensive or intermediate care unit for monitoring and stabilization of hemodynamics. The etiology of cardiovascular problems may be multi-fold including postoperative pain, agitation, dysfunction of the carotid sinus baroreceptor reflexes, or new neurologic deficits. Selection of appropriate therapy should be based on these considerations.

If hypertension continues despite adequate pain relief, and in the absence of other factors that could explain an increase in blood pressure, short-acting antihypertensive drugs given by infusion are the treatment of choice. Substances commonly used include beta-blockers such as labetolol or esmolol, calcium channel blockers, urapidil, or sodium nitroprusside. The initial intravenous therapy should be changed to longer acting substances if required after a 24 – 28 h period after surgery.

Hypotension may occur unexpectedly and must be treated as carefully as hypertensive episodes. Absolute or relative hypovolemia, prolonged effects of anesthetics or sedatives, over-treatment with antihypertensives, and carotid sinus reponses may represent etiologic factors. Therapy includes correction of intravascular volume and vasoconstrictors given in incremental doses until hemodynamics have stabilized.

New neurologic deficits will occur in up to 7 % of patients. Symptoms may be present immediately after recovery from anesthesia but will develop later in the postoperative period in more than half of the cases. Cerebral ischemia due to carotid clamping, embolization of particles, early carotid thrombosis, poor control of blood pressure and hyperperfusion syndrome are the main pathogenetic factors. Early onset of symptoms right after surgery often requires immediate operative re-exploration. Peripheral nerve injury (N. vagus, N. facialis, N. hypoglossus) and wound hematoma may occur in 5 – 15 % of cases. In rare cases, operative evacuation of a large hematoma may be indicated. Here, the anesthetist must be aware that intubation is difficult and should be performed by fiberoptic bronchoscopy in the awake state.

References

1. Bishop CCR, Powell S, Rutt D, Browse NL (1986) Transcranial Doppler measurement of middle cerebral artery blood flow velocity: A validation study. Stroke 17: 913–915
2. Cucchiara RF, Sundt TM, Michenfelder JD (1988) Myocardial infarction in carotid endarterectomy patients anaesthetized with halothane, enflurane, or isoflurane. Anaesthesiology 69: 783–784
3. Dinkel M, Kamp HD, Schweiger H (1991) Somatosensorisch evozierte Potentiale in der Karotischirurgie. Anaesthesist 40: 72–78
4. EC/IC Bypass Study Group (1985) Failure of extracranial-intracranial arterial bypass to reduce the risk of ischemic stroke. N Engl J Med 313: 1191–1200
5. European Carotid Surgery Trialists Collaborative Group (1991) MRC European Carotid Surgery Trial: interim results of symptomatic patients with severe (70 – 99 %) or with mild (0 – 29 %) carotid stenosis. Lancet 337: 1235–1243
6. Garrioch MA, Fitch W (1993) Anaesthesia for carotid artery surgery. Br J Anaesth 71: 569–579
7. Gaunt ME, Martin PJ, Smith JL, Rimmer T, Cherryman G, Ratliff DA, Bell PRF, Naylor AR (1994) Clinical relevance of intraoperative embolization detected by transcranial Doppler ultrasonography during carotid endarterectomy. Br J Surg 81: 1435–1439
8. Hertzer NR, Beven EG, Young JR, O'Hara PJ, Ruschhaupt WF, Graor RA, deWolfe VG, Maljovec LC (1984) Coronary artery disease in peripheral vascular patients. Ann Surg 199: 223–233
9. Kwaan JHM, Peterson GJ, Conolly JE (1980) Stump pressure: An unreliable guide for shunting during carotid endarterectomy. Arch Surg 115: 1083–1085
10. McKay RD, Sundt TM, Michenfelder JD, Gronert GA, Messick JM, Sharbrough FW, Piepgras DG (1976) Internal carotid artery stump pressure and cerebral blood flow during carotid endarterectomy. Anaesthesiology 45: 390–399
11. Messick JM, Casement B, Sharbrough FW, Milde LN, Michenfelder JD, Sundt TM (1987) Correlation of regional cerebral blood flow (rCBF) with EEG changes during isoflurane anaesthesia for carotid endarterectomy: critical rCBF. Anaesthesiology 66: 344–349
12. Messick JM, Sundt TM (1990) Ischemic cerebral vascular disease. In: Cucchiara RF, Michenfelder JD, Clinical Neuroanaesthesia. Churchill Livingstone, New York, p 255–283
13. Michenfelder JD, Sundt TM, Fode N, Sharbrough FW (1987) Isoflurane when compared to enflurane and halothane decreases the frequency of cerebral ischemia during carotid endarterectomy. Anaesthesiology 67: 336–340
14. North American Symptomatic Carotid Endarterectomy Trial Collaborators (1991) Beneficial effect of carotid endarterectomy in symptomatic patients with high-grade stenosis. N Engl J Med 325: 445–453
15. Palmer MA (1989) Comparison of regional and general anaesthesia for carotid endarterectomy. Am J Surg 157: 329–330
16. Rampil IJ, Holzer JA, Quest DO, Rosenbaum SH, Correll JW (1983) Prognostic value of computerized EEG analysis during carotid endarterectomy. Anaesth Analg 62: 186–192
17. Rosenthal D, Stanton PE, Lamis PA (1981) Carotid endarterectomy. The unreliability of intraoperative monitoring in patients having had stroke or reversible ischemic neurologic deficit. Arch Surg 116: 1569–1575
18. Russ W, Fraedrich G, Hehrlein FW, Hempelmann G (1988) Intraoperative somatosensory evoked potentials as a prognostic factor of neurologic state after carotid endarterectomy. Thorac cardiovasc Surgeon 33: 392–396
19. Seubert C, Lehmann A, Gust R, Böhrer H (1994) Anästhesie in der Carotischirurgie. Anästhesiol Intensivmed Notfallmed Schmerzther 29: 195–202

20. Smith JS, Roizen MF, Cahalan MK, Benefiel DJ, Beaupre PN, Sohn YJ, Byrd BF, Schiller NB, Stoney RJ, Ehrenfeld WK, Ellis JE, Aronson S (1988) Does anaesthetic technique make a difference? Augmentation of systolic blood pressure during carotid endarterectomy: Effects of phenylephrine versus light anaesthesia and of isoflurane versus halothane on the incidence of myocardial ischemia. Anaesthesiology 69: 846–853
21. Thiel A, Russ W, Zeiler D, Dapper F, Hempelmann G (1990) Transcranial Doppler sonography and somatosensory evoked potential monitoring in carotid surgery. Eur J Vasc Surg 4: 597–602

Author's address:
PD Dr. A. Thiel
Abt. für Anaesthesiologie und
Operative Intensivmedizin
Rudolf-Buchheim-Straße 7
D-35385 Gießen
Germany

Neuromonitoring during carotid artery surgery: Somatosensory evoked potentials versus transcranial Doppler sonography

M. Dinkel, H. Langer, H. Loerler, J. Pflumm, J. Schüttler, H. Schweiger[1]

Clinic of Anesthesiology, University of Erlangen-Nürnberg, Germany
[1]Department of Vascular Surgery, Herz- und Gefäßklinik Bad Neustadt / Saale, Germany

In the recent past, various multi-center studies comparing the outcome of surgical and conservative management of high grade carotid artery stenosis were performed. In brief, the generally acknowledged result of these investigations has been that patients with high grade symptomatic or asymptomatic carotid artery stenosis will particularly benefit from carotid endarterectomy if the rate of perioperative strokes is as low as possible. It is therefore of prime importance during carotid artery surgery to prevent persistent neurological deficits which are especially tragic and devastating and thus raise questions about the value of carotid artery surgery in general (7, 8, 18).

Pathogenesis of neurological deficits

The pathogenesis of perioperative strokes can be reduced to three major mechanisms. Firstly, there is cerebral embolization of debris during manipulation of the carotid artery or shunt insertion. In most instances, this can be avoided by restrictive shunt use and a meticulous surgical technique. Secondly, cerebral hyperperfusion after release of the cross-clamp is a factor which can almost always be successfully dealt with by rigorous control of blood pressure. Last but not least, there is cerebral ischemia due to insufficient collateral blood flow after carotid clamping which is a main cause of strokes in the perioperative period (3, 12).

Unfortunately, in the preoperative period neither the neurological history nor angiographic examinations enable us to identify patients at risk of ischemia due to insufficient collateral perfusion (6). Nor is this achievable by means of transcranial Doppler sonography (TCD) even though theoretically this should be possible if there is evidence of impaired cerebrovascular reactivity, i.e. limited or no rise of blood flow velocity in the middle cerebral artery during carbon dioxide testing (2, 15, 21). In their series of 93 procedures, Thiel and co-workers had to establish that 12 out of 13 patients with critical hypoperfusion and pathological somatosensory evoked potentials (SEP) during surgery showed preoperative normal carbon dioxide reactivity, which would imply intact collateral perfusion. On the other hand, some 11 out of 80 patients with obvious patent collateral vessels and normal SEP response revealed pathological cerebrovascular reactivity (21).

Neuromonitoring: Essential considerations

These observations underline the fact that, at the moment, impending intraoperative ischemia due to poor intracerebral collateral circulation cannot be identified preoperatively. The list of intraoperatively applicable measures to produce a net increase in collateral perfusion during the clamping period is short and features the use of a temporary intraluminal shunt and induced hypertension. However, the risks associated with the use of either of these measures are not negligible. Shunt placement may not only cause dislodgement and cerebral embolization of debris but may also convey a false sense of security if blood flow through the shunt is inadequate. Induced hypertension incurs the increased risk of myocardial infarction in patients whose coronary reserve is already on the brink of compensation. Finally, in anesthetized patients the effectivity of these measures can only be verified after emergence from anesthesia – at a moment when therapeutic intervention will frequently no longer be successful (3, 6, 12).

For these reasons, a net reduction of neurological complications is to be expected if one succeeds in detecting critical ischemia early in the procedure and in selectively applying protective measures with instantaneous verification of their effectivity. To this end, we require a very sensitive monitor that identifies all patients with critical clamp-related hypoperfusion which renders them dependent on temporary shunting (Table 5). A suitable monitor must also have a high specificity in order to detect all patients with sufficient collateral circulation. This will result in a marked reduction of the complications of shunt insertion and induced hypertension. Furthermore, in order to be suitable for clinical routine application, a potential monitoring technique has to fulfill essential practical requirements (Table 5).

Monitoring the awake patient and its limitations

One technique that meets nearly all requirements of an ideal monitor is clinical assessment of the awake patient during surgery under local anesthesia. However, the ability to continuously monitor neurological functions during surgery without any expense and extra effort, which is the main advantage of local anesthesia, is compromised by the fact that patients often become agitated and need to be sedated, making a reliable differentiation between ischemia and drug-related neurological dysfunction not always possible. Moreover, other factors such as lack of control of vital parameters could worsen neurological deficits in case of clamp-related ischemia. The absence of the cerebroprotective properties of general anesthesia, method-related risks and, most importantly, poor acceptance by patients and surgeons are additional shortcomings of this technique (3, 17).

Somatosensory evoked potentials

During surgery under general anesthesia, the use of somatosensory evoked potentials elicited by median nerve stimulation at the contralateral wrist can identify clamp-related cerebral ischemia as reliably as clinical assessment of the awake patient. Under these circumstances, a loss of the cortical SEP response above the ipsilateral hemisphere after cross-clamping is a reliable index of critical cerebral hypoperfusion (Figure 1). Effective functioning of an intraluminal shunt is also signalled very reliably by instantaneously recovering evoked potentials (Fig. 1). This was the result of our prospective study of 924 carotid operations (Table 1) (6).

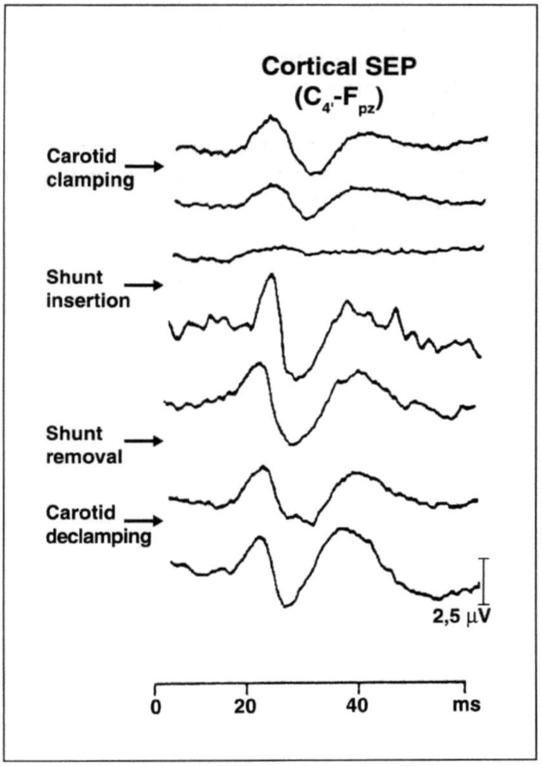

Fig. 1. Example typical of SEP loss that was reversed by use of an intraluminal shunt. The postoperative neurological examination was uneventful.

Table 1. SEP monitoring during carotid artery surgery. Own study comprising 924 consecutive procedures

SEP	Shunt placement	Neurological outcome Unchanged	TIA	Stroke
Identifiable n = 856 (93 %)	no n = 856	n = 853	n = 2	n = 1
Complete loss n = 68 (7 %)	no n = 17	n = 5	n = 11	n = 1
	yes n = 51	n = 37	n = 12	n = 2
Total		n = 895	n = 25	n = 4

According to our analysis, about 7 % of all patients showed insufficient collateral circulation and consecutive SEP loss requiring shunt placement. More than 70 % of the patients with shunt use remained neurologically intact as opposed to 30 % of the patients not receiving a shunt. Two patients suffered a stroke despite the use of a shunt. This was attributable to insufficient shunt blood flow resulting in a permanently erased SEP amplitude in one patient, and to postoperative thrombotic occlusion of the carotid artery in another patient (6).

In our study, apart from patients showing loss of the cortical SEP response, only 3 patients without intraoperative SEP changes revealed postoperative neurological deficits. However, a summarizing assessment of angiographic, computer-tomographic, electrophysiological and surgical findings only allows the conclusion that these neurological deficits were not caused by clamp-related ischemia but by thromboembolisms. As embolic events cannot be prevented but are more likely to be increased by shunt placement, this by no means detracts from the value of SEP monitoring.

Therefore, clinically relevant clamp-related cerebral hypoperfusion is indicated by SEP monitoring with a high sensitivity and specificity. This is born out by our own experience but also particularly by other groups' observations (Table 2) (1, 6, 9, 10, 16, 19). Thus, SEP monitoring not only reliably indicates the necessity of shunt placement, but can also be taken as the gold standard in evaluating the significance of other cerebral monitoring techniques.

Table 2. Sensitivity and specificity of SEP monitoring during carotid artery surgery

Author	Year	Patients (n)	Sensitivity (%)	Specificity (%)
Ruß et al. (19)	1985	106	83	99
Gigli et al. (10)	1987	40	100	83
Lam et al. (16)	1991	64	100	94
Amantini et al. (1)	1992	368	100	100
Fava et al. (9)	1992	151	100	100
Dinkel et al. (6)	1996	924	100	99

Transcranial Doppler sonography

In this respect, the comparison with TCD in our own study showed good correlation between the SEP finding and blood flow velocity in the ipsilateral middle cerebral artery (v-mean MCA). Of 102 patients in whom we were able to perform simultaneous monitoring of SEP and TCD, only those patients who also had a complete disappearance of the Doppler signal showed SEP loss (Table 3) (5). However, this unambiguous result is put in perspective by Thiel's findings. In some 3 patients with pathological SEP response after cross-clamping, he could not find a critical reduction in middle cerebral artery blood flow velocity. On the other hand, he observed critical changes in TCD in 10 patients, 2 of whom even showed a complete loss of signal, without evidence of pathological SEP changes or neurological deficits (21).

It is therefore obviously impossible to make safe predictions about the actual blood flow to functionally relevant areas from measuring blood flow velocity in basal cerebral

Table 3. Somatosensory evoked response and TCD findings during carotid artery cross-clamping

v-mean MCA	Cortical SEP	
	complete loss	identifiable
0 cm/s	n = 5	n = 0
> 0 cm/s	n = 0	n = 97
n = 102		

arteries. The same limitations are true for carotid stump pressure (CSP) measurements (4). Hence it is not surprising that the sufficiency of collateral perfusion cannot be determined reliably by measuring v-mean and that various studies produced dissimilar results when the question of critical values of v-mean MCA indicating cerebral ischemia was investigated (5, 6, 11, 20, 21).

The main disadvantage of TCD, however, is a high rate of primary failure which was about 33 % in our own study (Table 4). In another 10 % of cases, we observed secondary dislocation of the ultrasound probe contributing to the fact that we could not use TCD to monitor cerebral blood flow during cross-clamping in altogether 43 % of patients. The number of patients in whom the MCA could not be identified a priori was especially high among women, old people and patients who experienced SEP loss during the procedure. The observation that TCD can be used successfully in less than 50 % of patients with insufficient collateral circulation raises serious questions about its usefulness as a monitor of ischemia (Table 4) (5).

Table 4. Primary failure of TCD in relation to various disruptive factors

	Number	TCD Failure
Sex		
female	n = 58	n = 30 (51.7 %)**
male	n = 123	n = 29 (23.6 %)
Age		
< 70 years	n = 87	n = 19 (21.8 %)***
> 70 years	n = 94	n = 40 (42.6 %)
Neurological History		
asymptomatic	n = 35	n = 13 (37.4 %)
TIA	n = 102	n = 31 (30.4 %)
stroke	n = 44	n = 15 (34.1 %)
Contralateral Carotid Artery		
not stenotic (< 70 %)	n = 134	n = 45 (33.6 %)
stenotic (> 70 %)	n = 44	n = 14 (31.8 %)
SEP-findings		
identifiable	n = 162	n = 48 (29.6 %)*
complete loss	n = 19	n = 11 (57.9 %)
Total	n = 181	n = 59 (32.6 %)

*$p < 0.05$ **$p < 0.01$ ***$p < 0.001$

This also puts in perspective the fact that by means of TCD there is a chance to identify hyperperfusion states and cerebral embolism as further causes of perioperative strokes. However, clinical interpretation of such TCD findings is in itself difficult. After declamping almost all patients show an overshooting increase in v-mean MCA that normalizes within a few minutes and usually has no clinical consequences (Fig. 2). This reaction probably reflects the process of adaptation of cerebral autoregulation to increased cerebral blood flow after removal of the carotid stenosis (5).

Even high frequency noise signals which are a typical index of cerebral embolism, are seen in almost all patients shortly after release of the cross-clamp (Fig 2). However, we never detected any concomitant neurological deficit. Performing TCD, Jansen registered altogether 75 events of embolism in 55 out of 130 procedures. Of these, only one patient had a neurological deficit that was possibly related to an embolic event (13). The problem with detecting embolism by means of TCD is twofold. On the one hand, it is still impossible to differentiate reliably between artefacts and genuine sources of embolism. On the other hand, quantification of embolic events is problematic and the critical number of embolic events is still unknown.

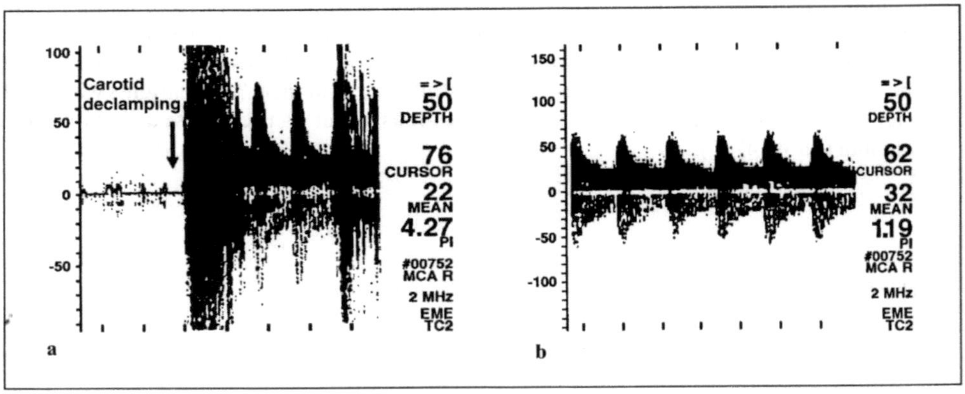

Fig. 2a. Typical hyperperfusion and Doppler signals suspicious of embolism during carotid declamping.
Fig. 2b. 5 min after declamping: normal flow pattern and flow velocity in the middle cerebral artery. Postoperatively, no neurological deficits were observed.

Conclusions

Bearing all this in mind, it emerges that there are clear limitations to a profitable use of TCD during carotid artery surgery. TCD is difficult to perform and prone to failure which might have an adverse effect on the course of surgery. Even more important, however, is the fact that TCD has only limited sensitivity and specificity when it comes to detecting critical cerebral ischemia (Table 5).

In contrast, SEPs fit all the requirements for a suitable neuromonitor. In this respect, SEPs are superior to all clinically available monitoring techniques including EEG and transcranial oximetry (Table 5). Both techniques fail when it comes to reliably detecting critical cerebral hypoperfusion (6). Regarding EEG, there are several reasons for this. EEG is notably susceptible to interference and difficult to interpret and it cannot detect ischemia restricted to subcortical areas. Conversely, the EEG tracing can be pathologically altered even in the situation of prognostically insignificant cortical ischemia, which brings about the limited specificity of EEG (14).

Registration of regional cerebral oxygen saturation (rSO_2) by means of NIRS excels in its uncomplicated use. However, for technical reasons, transcranial oximetry is only possible through the hairless scalp, i.e. over the well-collaterated frontal region of the brain. Therefore, it did not come as a surprise to us that during 83 procedures, we could establish neither a good correlation between rSO_2 and SEP nor a critical rSO_2 value that reflects critical ischemia reliably (6).

Advantages of SEP monitoring

Currently, we consider somatosensory evoked potentials to be the gold standard of monitoring during carotid surgery because they offer various advantages. Due to the high sensitivity of SEPs, ischemic neurological deficits can be prevented reliably. In addition, proper functioning of a temporary shunt is indicated instantaneously by recovering potentials. Due to the high specificity of SEPs, the risks associated with unnecessary shunt use can be minimized. As long as the cortical response can be elicited, there is no need for induced hypertension and cerebral integrity is definitely not put at risk. This facilitates protection of heart and brain. From the surgeon's point of view, SEP monitoring is a valuable aid to perform technically faultless surgery without undue haste, which provides the basis for further improvement of long-term results in carotid surgery. Finally, the underlying mechanisms of neurological deficits are exposed. A postoperative neurological deficit that occurs in the absence of intraoperative SEP loss points towards a source of embolism making surgical revision without further delay imperative.

Table 5. Cerebral neuromonitoring during carotid artery surgery

Requirements	SEP	EEG	CSP	TCD	rSO_2
Easy application	+	O	+	–	+
Low rate of failure	O	–	+	–	+
Continuous monitoring	+	+	–	+	+
Ease of interpretation	+	–	+	+	+
Unimpeded procedure	+	O	O	–	+
No side effects	+	+	+	+	+
Affordable costs	+	+	+	+	O
High sensitivity	+	O	+	O	O
High specificity	+	O	–	O	–

+ requirement fulfilled O requirement partly fulfilled – requirement not fulfilled

References

1. Amantini A, Bartelli M, deScisciolo G, Lombardi M, Macucci M, Rossi R, Pratesi C, Pinto F (1992) Monitoring of somatosensory evoked potentials during carotid endarterectomy. J Neurol 239: 241–247
2. Bishop CCR, Powell S, Insall M, Rutt D (1986) Effect of internal carotid occlusion on middle cerebral artery blood flow at rest and in response to hypercapnia. Lancet 2: 710–712
3. Clark NJ, Stanley TH (1990) Anesthesia for vascular surgery. In: Miller RD, Anesthesia; 3rd Ed., Churchill Livingstone, New York pp. 1693–1730
4. Dinkel M, Schweiger H, Goerlitz P (1992) Monitoring during Carotid Surgery: Somatosensory Evoked Potentials vs. Carotid Stump Pressure. J Neurosurg Anesthesiol 4: 167–175
5. Dinkel M, Langer H, Loerler H, Rügheimer E, Schweiger H (1994) Neuromonitoring in der Karotischirurgie: Möglichkeiten und Grenzen der transkraniellen Doppler-Sonographie. VASA 23: 337–344
6. Dinkel M (1996) Funktionelles, hämodynamisches und metabolisches Neuromonitoring in der Karotischirurgie. Abbott, Wiesbaden
7. European carotid surgery trialists' collaborative group (1991) MRC european carotid surgery trial: interim results for symptomatic patients with severe (70 – 99 %) or with mild (0 – 29 %) carotid stenosis. Lancet 337: 1235–1243
8. Executive Committee for the Asymptomatic Carotid Atherosclerosis Study (1995) Endarterectomy for Asymptomatic Carotid Artery Stenosis. JAMA 273: 1421–1428
9. Fava E, Bortolani E, Ducati A, Schieppati M (1992) Role of SEP in identifying patients requiring temporary shunt during carotid endarterectomy. Electroenceph Clin Neurophysiol 84: 426–432
10. Gigli GL, Caramia M, Marciani MG, Zarola F, Lavaroni F, Rossini PM (1987) Monitoring of subcortical and cortical somatosensory evoked potentials during carotid endarterectomy: comparison with stump pressure levels. Electroenceph Clin Neurophysiol 68: 424–432
11. Halsey JH, McDowell HA, Gelmon S, Morawetz RB (1989) Blood velocity in the middle cerebral artery and regional cerebral blood flow during carotid endarterectomy. Stroke 20: 53–58
12. Hannallah, MS (1995) Anesthetic Management of Patients Undergoing Carotid Endarterectomy. Anesth Clin North Am 3: 147–163
13. Jansen C, Vriens EM, Eikelboom BC, Vermeulen FEE, van Gijn J, Ackerstaff RGA (1993) Carotid Endarterectomy with Transcranial Doppler and Electroencephalographic Monitoring. Stroke 24: 665–669
14. Kearse LA, Brown EN, McPeck K (1992) Somatosensory evoked potentials sensitivity relative to electroencephalography for cerebral ischemia during carotid endarterectomy. Stroke 23: 498–505
15. Kleiser B, Widder B (1992) Course of carotid artery occlusions with impaired cerebrovascular reactivity. Stroke 23: 171–174
16. Lam AM, Manninen PH, Ferguson GG, Nantau W (1991) Monitoring electrophysiologic function during carotid endarterectomy: A comparison of somatosensory evoked potentials and conventional electroencephalogram. Anesthesiology 75: 15–21
17. Mahla ME (1993) Carotid artery surgery: anesthesia and monitoring. ASA Refresher Course 44: 232
18. North American Symptomatic Carotid Endarterectomy Trial Collaborators (1991) Beneficial effect of carotid endarterectomy in symptomatic patients with high-grade carotid stenosis. N Engl J Med 325: 445–453
19. Russ W, Fraedrich G, Hehrlein FW, Hempelmann G (1985) Intraoperative Somatosensory Evoked Potentials as a Prognostic Factor of Neurologic State after Carotid Endarterectomy. Thorac cardiovasc Surgeon 33: 392–396
20. Spencer MP, Thomas GI, Moehring MA (1992) Relation Between Middle Cerebral Artery Blood Flow Velocity and Stump Pressure During Carotid Endarterectomy. Stroke 23: 1439–1445
21. Thiel A, Zickmann B, Stertmann WA, Wyderka T, Hempelmann G (1995) Cerebrovascular Carbon Dioxide Reactivity in Carotid Artery Disease. Anesthesiology 82: 655–661

Author's address:
Priv. Doz. Dr. med. Michael Dinkel
Clinic of Anesthesiology
University of Erlangen Nuremberg
Krankenhausstraße 12
91054 Erlangen
Germany

The choice of method for cerebral protection from ischemia in carotid endarterectomy

P. O. Kazantchian, V. A. Popov, T. V. Rudakova

Department of Vascular Surgery (Head: Prof. P. O. Kazantchian). Moscow Regional Research Clinical Institute (Director: Prof. G. A. Onopriyenko), Moscow, Russia

The outcome of surgical treatment of occlusive diseases of aortic brachiocephalic branches depends not only on irreproachable surgical technique (1), but also upon an adequate intraoperative protection of brain from ischemia (3, 4, 6). In this connection, the major task within the algorithm of examining patients suffering from chronic vascular insufficiency consists of studying intracerebral hemodynamics, the condition and compensatory capacity of collateral circulation, and definition of cerebral tolerance to ischemia. The major goal of the present study includes evaluation of both transcranial Dopplerography (TCD) and electroencephalography (EEG) potentialities to estimate the cerebral tolerance to ischemia and to choose adequate measures to protect it from intraoperative ischemic injuries while reconstructing carotid arteries (2, 5).

Brain tolerance to ischemia was determined using clamping of the common carotid artery (CCA), studying the middle cerebral artery (MCA) circulation, and electroencephalography (EEG). CCA clamping was carried out for 4 min under control of TCD and EEG. The linear blood flow velocity (LBFV) in MCA and EEG data were registered before CCA clamping, at the moment of clamping, and on the 1st, 2nd, 3rd and 4th min after clamping. When performing the above test, the systemic arterial pressure was taken into account and the contact with a patient being supported to reveal complaints and neurologic symptoms. To estimate the results of the test mentioned, we counted the percent MCA circulation speed decrease as compared to its initial level as well as EEG character, which allowed to evaluate both the compensatory capacity of collateral blood circulation and the degree of cerebral tolerance to ischemia.

The foregoing investigations were executed in 113 patients with different degrees of brachiocephalic arteries (BCA) disorders. As an outcome of the study , four degrees of brain tolerance to ischemia has been established (Table 1):

Table 1. Grades of cerebral tolerance from ischemia

Grades of cerebral tolerance	Neurologic symptoms	Decrease of linear blood flow velocities in MCA	Electroencephalography
(I) "HIGH"	Absence	Less than 25 %	Stable
(II) "SATISFACTORY"	Absence	By 25 – 50 %	Stable
(III) "LOW"	Evident neurologic symptoms at 2nd-4th min	By 50 – 70 %	Slowing and lowering of alpha-rhythm amplitude
(IY) "CRITICALLY LOW"	Evident at 10-15 s	By more than 70 %, or low than 20 cm/s	Appearance of irregular slow EEG-waves

1) High, characterized by decrease of circulation speed in MCA by 25 %, absence of both patient complaints and neurologic symptoms; stable EEG.
2) Satisfactory – decrease of MCA circulation speed by 25 – 50 %, absence of both patient complaints and neurologic symptoms; stable EEG.
3) Low – MCA blood flow speed fall by 50 – 75 %, registration of patient complaints and neurologic symptoms at the 2nd – 4th min; slowing down and decrease of EEG a-rhythm amplitude.
4) Critically low – MCA circulation speed fall by more than 75 %, neurologic symptoms registration 10 – 15 s after CCA clamping; slowing, diminishing a-rhythm amplitude, registration of irregular, slow EEG waves.

The adequacy of the results obtained was checked with intraoperative TCD and EEG monitoring in carotid endarterectomy (65 operations) during the period of CCA clamping. In 96 % of cases preoperative monitoring data concurred with intraoperative ones.

The outcome achieved has demonstrated now highly informative the CCA clamping procedure is under control of TCD and EEG to determine the degree of cerebral tolerance to ischemia and to elaborate reliable measures to protect the brain from intraoperative ischemic injuries.

Analyzing ultrasonography, angiography and EEG data, we have come to the conclusion that the degree of cerebral tolerance to ischemia depends on the state of Circulus Willisii (CW) and the degree of BCA injury. In multiple BCA injuries and completely broken CW a critically low brain tolerance to ischemia was noted (3.6 % of patients). In multiple BCA injuries and partially broken CW (frontal connective artery not functioning) a low degree of cerebral tolerance to ischemia was found (7.1 % of cases). Satisfactory brain tolerance to ischemia was demonstrated in patients with multiple BCA impairments and with functioning CW (70.2 %) High degree of cerebral tolerance to ischemia was revealed in patients with isolated disorders of either BCA and functioning CW (19.1 %).

Based on preoperative evaluation of cerebral tolerance to ischemia, the optimal surgical tactics have been elaborated as well as adequate precautions to protect the brain from

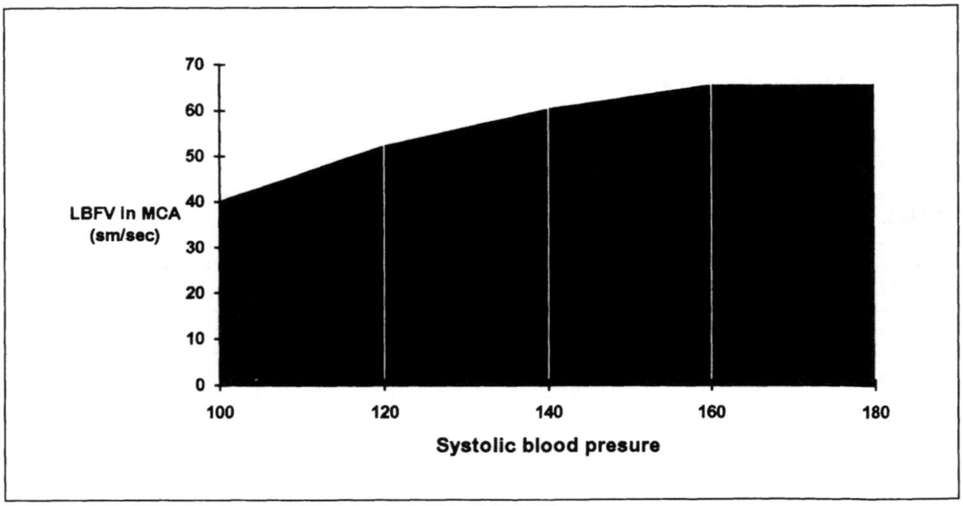

Fig. 1. Changing of linear blood flow velocity in MCA dependent upon systolic arterial blood pressure

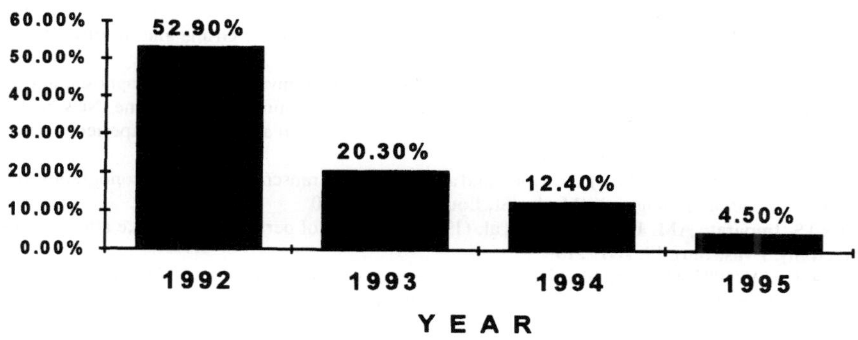

Fig. 2. Use of internal shunt by carotid endarterectomy

ischemia in reconstructive operations on brachiocephalic aortic branches. Thus, in patients with low and critically low brain tolerance to ischemia, while performing carotid endarterectomy, the temporary internal shunting, moderate hypertension and pharmaceutical (dexamethasone, barbiturates) brain protection from ischemia was applied.

Patients with satisfactory cerebral tolerance to ischemia underwent pharmacoprotection and supporting moderate hypertension in patients with high anti-ischemic tolerance special provisions for brain protection were not taken.

Studying indices of MCA circulation velocity in normotension condition and in different levels of artificially created hypertension, we have come to the conclusion that, to some degree, there was a direct dependence between blood pressure rise and enhancement of circulation in MCA. At the same time, artificial increase of blood pressure by more than 30 mm Hg beyond initial readings does not induce further MCA circulation velocity rise (Fig. 1). Therefore, we support creation of moderate hypertension. However, only during operation can we make an exact evaluation of cerebral tolerance to ischemia and reach a final decision about applying an internal shunt. Such an approach allowed us to diminish the frequency of internal shunt usage from 52.9 % at first to 4.5 % at present.

In all reconstructive operations on carotid arteries carried out in terms of pre-determined brain tolerance to ischemia checked with TCD and EEG, no neurologic complications due to intraoperative cerebral ischemic injuries were seen. In two patients acute brain circulation disorder has developed, connected, in the first case, with internal carotid arterial thrombosis, and, in the second case, with embolism of MCA branches.

The experiments performed have shown that application of highly informative methods such as TCD and EEG provides adequate evaluation of intracerebral hemodynamics condition that allows to implement precautions against ischemic injuries of brain and to choose optimal surgical tactics in reconstruction of brachiocephalic branches of aorta.

References

1. Barnes RW (1985) Technical aspects of carotid artery surgery. J Vasc Surg 19: 187–197
2. Callow AD (1985) The value of electroencephalography for cerebral protection. In: Greenhalgh RM, ed. Diagnostic Techniques and Assesment Procedure in Vascular Surgery. Grune and Stratton, London, pp 129–149
3. Hertzer NR (1987) Early complications of carotid endarterectomy: Incidence, diagnosis, and management. In: Moore WS, ed. Surgery for Cerebrovascular Disease. Churchill Livingstone, New York
4. Kirshner LD, O'Brien MS, Ricotta JJ et al. (1989) Risk factors in a community experience with carotid endarterectomy. J Vasc Surg 10: 78–86
5. Otis SM, Ringelstein EB (1993) Principles and applications of transcranial Doppler sonography. In: Bernstein EF, ed. Vascular Diagnosis. Mosby, St. Louse, pp 341–360
6. Riles TS, Imparato AM, Jacowbiz GR et al. (1994) The cause of perioperative stroke after carotid endarterectomy. J Vasc Surg 19: 206–216
7. Schroeder TV (1993) Cerebral blood flow mesurements in carotid artery disease. In: Greenhalgh RM, Hollier LH, eds. Surgery for Stroke. WB Saundrs Company Ltd, London, pp 73–84

Author's address:
Vadim A. Popov, M.D.
Moscow Regional Scientific Research Institute
(MONIKI)
Dpt. Vascular Surgery
Schepkin str. 61/2
129110 Moscow, Russia

SEPs monitoring during carotid surgery: reliability and limitations

M. R. Cirelli, F. Magnoni, L. Pedrini, M. D'Addato

Chair of Vascular Surgery, University of Bologna, Italy

Introduction

Carotid endarterectomy (TEA) remains the treatment of choice for carotid disease characterized by stenosing, hemodynamically significant or embolizing atherosclerotic plaque. One of the greatest risks during surgery is carotid clamping when cerebral ischemia may occur if collateral circulation does not maintain adequate perfusion.

If collateral circulation is insufficient, the brain will suffer varying degrees of ischemic changes leading to functional and/or organic impairment with transient or permanent neurologic deficits apparent on awakening or in the early hours after surgery. The incidence of neurologic postoperative complications in literature reports varies between 0.5 and 4 %; in many cases, neurological deficit is causes by embolism or thrombosis of the endarterectomized segment. Some investigators have elected to prevent brain ischemia during clamping by inserting a vascular shunt in all patients to ensure blood flow to the brain, despite the risks a shunt entails (embolism, dissection, shunt occlusion, intimal changes with early postoperative thrombosis or late ristenosis). Most surgeons prefer to use a shunt selectively and perform intraoperative monitoring to identify patients with poor interhemispheric compensation.

However, all means of technical monitoring present some limitations and are not without problems: the electroencephalogram (EEG) requires specialists to interpret the tracings, Transcranial Doppler (TCD) can only be used in patients with an acoustic window. Somatosensory evoked potentials (SEPs) are easy to monitor, the tracing is straightforward and the wave amplitude is little affected by anesthesia.

This study aimed to find an indicator for brain ischemia during carotid clamping for selective insertion of a vascular shunt.

Materials and methods

We performed a prospective study in a series of 442 patients (328 men and 114 women), average age 71.5 years (range 42.2–84–8 years) who underwent internal carotid endarterectomy (TEA) for hemodynamically significant stenosis. Surgery was performed under general anesthesia in 356 patients and under local anesthesia in 86 (Table 1).

The preoperative work-up in all patients included angiography of the epiaortic vessels and carotid echo color Doppler to determine the percentage of stenosis and plaque characteristics; brain CT scan was performed in symptomatic patients or those presenting occlusion of the controlateral carotid axis.

Table 1. Results in relation to anesthesia, SEPs monitoring and insertion of a vascular shunt

	General anesthesia				Local anesthesia			
SEP	Shunted		Not shunted		Shunted		Not shunted	
	good outcome	TIA stroke	good outcome	TIA stroke	good outcome	TIA stroke	good outcome	TIA stroke
Normal	66	0	230	1	11	0	51	1
Pathologic	35	3	16	5	15	1	7	0

An i.v. bolus of 2500 I.U. heparin was administered to all patients during surgery before clamping, SEPs were monitored throughout and intraoperative angiography performed as a control measure.

Patients presenting thrombosis or embolism following surgery were not included in the study.

SEPs monitoring included the $N_{20}P_{25}$ complex stimulating the controlateral median nerve to the carotid undergoing endarterectomy. Scalp electrodes were positioned at sites C3/F3 of C4/F4 respectively according to the international system 10–20 corresponding to the areas of cortico somatosensory. Basal recordings were made before clamping, for 1 min of test clamping, every 2 min during clamping and 5 and 10 min after clamping.

A vascular shunt was used whenever possible if patients presented a reduced N_{20}-P_{25} amplitude below 50 % and in patients with CT signs of ischemic lesions in the controlateral hemisphere. When a shunt could not be inserted, another bolus of barbiturates and/or vasopressor medication was administered.

Results

Table 2 summarizes clinical outcome in relation to SEPs changes and use of a vascular shunt. Four patients had neurological symptoms on awakening despite the use of a shunt. Of the 11 patients presenting neurological deficits on awakening (9 in GA, 2 in LA), three had an ipsilateral stroke, one a controlateral stroke, 5 a TIA and 2 TIA with minimal residual deficits (TIA-IR). Nine of these 11 patients had presented a pathological fall in SEPs, while SEPs had remained unchanged in the other two.

Analyzing the findings of the latter two patients, they were found to have ischemic lesions in the preoperative CT scan in areas which could not be monitored with SEPs.

The differences between the results in relation to changes in SEPs recordings were statistically significant ($p < 0.0001$ X^2 test). Differences were also statistically significant when only the patients operated without a shunt were considered ($p < 0.0001$ Fischer's exact test).

Table 1 summarizes the results in relation to anesthesia, SEPs monitoring and insertion of a vascular shunt.

Table 2. Clinical outcome in relation to SEPs changes and use of a vascular shunt

	Not shunted		Shunted	
SEP	good outcome	TIA stroke	good outcome	TIA stroke
360 Normal	281 (99.3 %)	2 (0.7 %)	77 (100 %)	0
82 Pathologic	23 (82.1 %)	5 (17.9 %)	50 (92.6 %)	4 (7.4 %)

$p < 0.0001$ X^2 test

Discussion

Improvements in the indications for carotid endarterectomy and major advances in diagnostic and monitoring techniques have led to a reduction in peri- and postoperative complications.

Many surgeons now use SEPs to monitor ischemia during carotid clamping (1, 2). SEPs recording includes monitoring of the N_{20}-P_{25} complex. A fall in SEPs occur with a cerebral blood flow < 18 ml/100 gr/min. Clinical application by many surgeons (4, 2) has suggested as a risk threshold a 50 % fall in the amplitude of the N_{20}-P_{25} complex, i.e., the negative wave recorded about 20 ms, after stimulation and the positive wave recorded in the parietal region after another 5 ms (25 ms after stimulation).

Other investigators propose a prolonged latency (the time taken by stimulation to reach the somatosensory cortex) as an indicative risk limit for clamping ischemia (1, 2).

In our series, four patients had neurological deficits on awakening despite shunt insertion (two with a non-functioning shunt, two with a SEPs fall lasting over 4 min), while no patient with normal SEPs or a shunt inserted within the second minute had postoperative deficits.

Our results confirm that SEPs are an effective method of monitoring functional status and that 4 or more min of attenuation or flattening of the N_{20}-P_{25} complex is an index of permanent neurological deficit.

The limitations of somatosensory evoked potentials are the failure to detect ischemia in the controlateral hemisphere (which can be overcome by positioning and larger number of electrodes and stimulating the two median nerves of each wrist) and the failure to display ischemia in frontal or occipital regions. Contrary to reports using TCD, it is not always possible to detect an embolism during surgery.

Summary

Stroke following carotid clamping is one of the complications of carotid endarterectomy. This prospective study assessed the reliability of monitoring somatosensory evoked potentials (SEPs) during surgery to predict and prevent clamping ischemia. SEPs were recorded in 442 patients undergoing carotid endarterectomy (356 in general anesthesia; 86 in local anesthesia).

On awakening, 11 patients (2.5 %) presented neurological deficits due to carotid clamping; 3 of them had an ipsilateral stroke, 1 a controlateral stroke, 5 TIA and 2 TIA-IR. Nine of them had had a pathological fall in SEPs, whereas 2 patients had a preoperative CT scan displaying ischemic lesions in areas in which SEPs could not be recorded. Of the 11 patients with postoperative deficits, a vascular shunt had been inserted in 4. Seven patients did not receive a shunt as the SEPs attentuation occurred at the end of suture in 5 patients, and SEPs were unchanged in the remaining 2 cases.

Since results could have been affected by shunt insertion and in part by drug administration to those patients not receiving a shunt, reliability of SEPs monitoring was assessed only in patients without shunts. The technique had a reliability of 92 %, a specificity of 92.4 %, and a sensitivity of 72.4 %.

SEPs monitoring is an effective objective method of monitoring cerebral blood flow during carotid surgery in areas perfused by the median cerebral artery.

References

1. Ganji S, Brinkman SD, Morrell RM, Shirley JG, Jacobs LA (1984) Long latency somatosensory evoked potentialis during carotid endarterectomy. In: Evoked Potentialis II, Ed. R. H. Nodar y C. Barber, p 589–593
2. Grundy BL, Nelson PB, Lina A, Heros RC (1982) Monitoring of cortical somatosensory evoked potentialis to determine the safety of sacrificing the anterior cerebral artery. Neurosurgery 11: 64–67
3. Jacobs LA, Brinkman DS, Morrell RM, Shirley JG, Ganji S (1983) Long-latency somatosensory evoked potentials during carotid endarterectomy. Am Surg 49: 338–344
4. Naylor AR, Bell PRF, Ruckley CV (1992) Monitoring and cerebral protection during carotid endarterectomy. Br J Surg 79: 735–741

Author's address:
Maria Rosaria Cirelli
Cattedra di Chirurgia Vascolare
via Massarenti 9
40138 Bologna, Italy

Effect of myocardial revascularization on the blood flow volume in carotid arteries

A. V. Gagaev, A. L. Maximov, I. E. Soboleva, E. V. Chebotar, A. A. Charov, M. V. Riazanov, I. V. Gagaeva

Cardiovascular Surgery Center at Nizhny Novgorod, Russia

A study of blood flow change in carotid arteries (CA) of a patient with combined disease undergoing myocardial revascularization (MR) is reported with the aim to lower the risk of developing perioperative neurological complications.

Material and methods

Between November 1994 and May 1995, a carotid region of 41 patients with coronary artery disease, ages 36 – 69 years, undergoing MR has been examined by ultrasonography with Acuson-128 device. Measurement of blood flow volume (BFV) in common CA was done by Andry Hayes's method (Fig. 1). We divided the patients into three groups: A) with severe carotid stenosis, five patients (12 %); B) with mild carotid stenosis, 13 patients (32 %), and C) stenosis-free, 21 patients (56 %). We performed the measurement of BFV in common CA before carotid endarterectomy (CE), before MR, after 3 weeks and after 3 months in all three groups of patients. *Group A:* We have chosen the policy of two-stage surgery. In case of unilateral lesions, CE is performed before cardiosurgery. In case of bilateral lesions, restoration of blood flow on the more severely diseased side is performed first. Controlateral CA was carried simultaneously with cardiosurgery. As first stage, we performed CA on the side of the more significant stenosis or on the side of manifestations of neurological events. After 2 weeks, we performed MR with simultaneous CA on the opposite side. The well-known technique of CA was used. As second stage CA was exposed simultaneously with the saphenous vein harvest. Then the sternotomy incision was made and preparation for CPB was performed.Then CA was carried out, and MR was done in the usual way. The cervical wound was closed only after heparin had been reversed with protamin sulphate at the end of the entire procedure. In case of unilateral lesions the CA preceded cardiosurgery.

Groups B, C: MR was done with CPB and moderate hypothermia. We constructed the proximal anasthomosis at first with beating heart. Then the distal anasthomosis was performed with cold cardioplegia (average 4.2 ± 1.6 grafts/patients).

Results

Three weeks after MR, decrease of BFV from the base level was seen in all patients (Table 1).

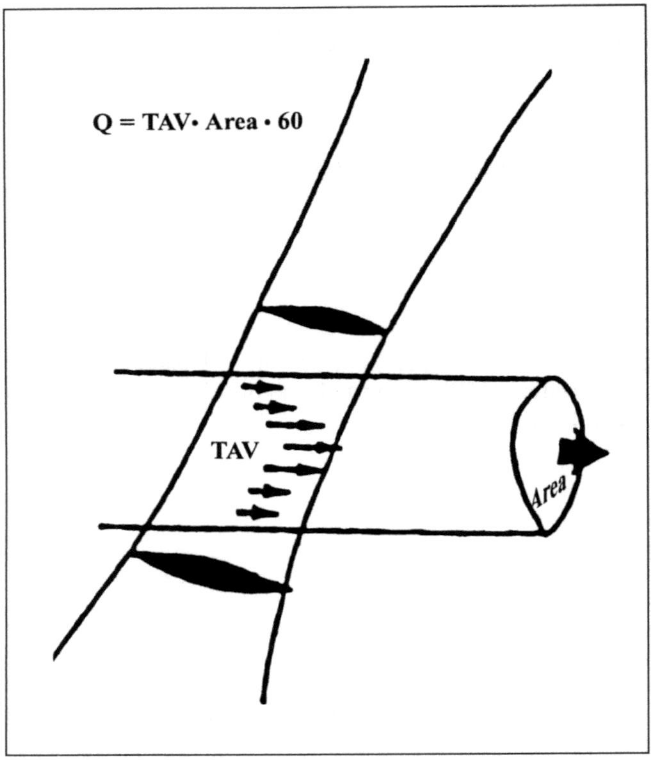

Fig. 1. Hayes' formula for calculating blood flow volume in common carotid artery. Q – blood flow volume; TAV – time average velocity; Area – cross-sectional area of the vessel (mm^2); 60 – coefficient.

Group A: We saw a significant increase of BFV after CA ($p = 0.035$) that was clear and obvious. But in our study BFV has an interesting tendency after cardiac surgery to decrease ($p = 0.037$) throughout 3 weeks (Fig. 2). An average BFV at this stage had no statistically significant difference from base level ($p = 0.291$), but BFV had a statistically significant increase throughout 3 months after MR ($p = 0.049$).

Groups B, C: We obtained equal data for both groups – B and C (Fig. 3) with statistically significant decrease of BFV throughout 3 weeks after MR ($p = 0.044$ for B and $p = 0.050$ for C). After 3 months there was the restoration of BFV with non-significant difference from base preoperative level.

Table 1. Blood flow volume in carotis communis artery (ml/min)

	Before surgery	After CEA, before CABG	3 weeks after CABG	3 months after CABG
W/o carotid disease	994.32±160.95	–	918.84±156.17	1026.35±129.89
Carotid stenosis <60 %	1075.38±180.44	–	960.07±194.22	1170.15±194.98
Carotid stenosis >60 %	718.75±223.64	945.77±98.56	795.81±138.51	815.12±197.54

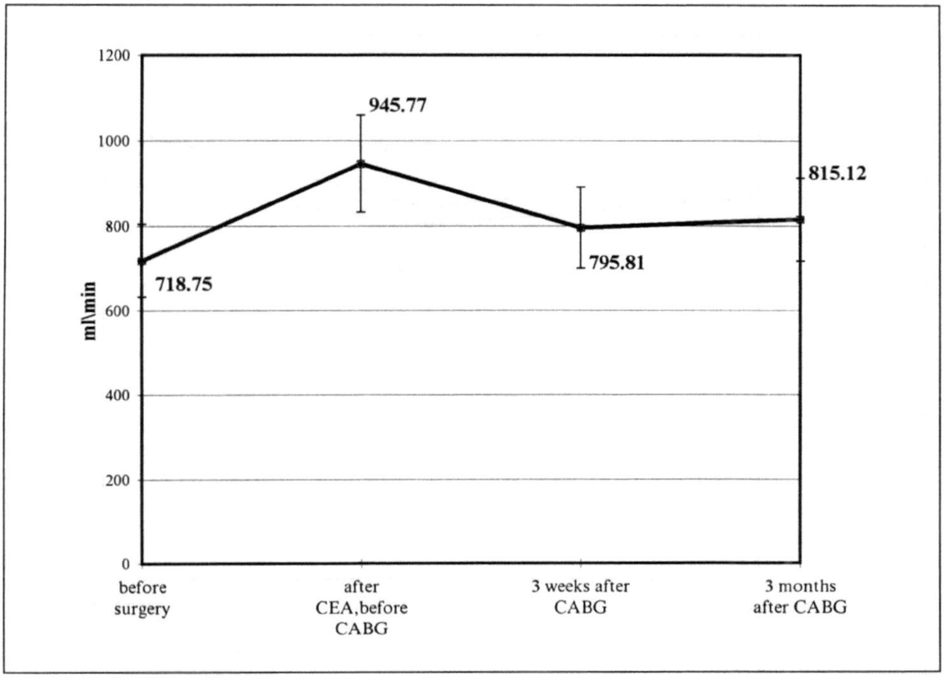

Fig. 2. Change of blood flow volume in common carotid artery in group **A.**

Discussion

The problem of surgical approach to simultaneous coronary and carotid disease has long been unclear. Stroke has been one of the severe complications since the early experience in cardiosurgery and cardiopulmonary bypass (4). Dr. Minami considers that the reasons for stroke are embolization by air, postinfarction left mural thrombus, debris from the ascending aorta during canulation, or ulcerative plaque from the CA (3). Especially important is the low cerebral perfusion through a stenotic extracranial or intracranial artery in the case of hypotension or complete circulatory arrest during the perioperative period. Dr. Faggioli in 1990 showed that stroke occurs not only during surgery, but also during the first postoperative week (1). Reasons for this are unstable hemodynamics, changes in blood viscosity, and platelet adhesion. According to Kertsman's report, acute heart failure is the cause of 80 % postoperative hemispheric events in patients with extracranial carotid disease (2). On the other hand, depressed heart function at short postoperative period may temporarily decrease blood flow to the brain. Our results demonstrate a decrease of BFV in common CA some days after cardiac surgery in all groups of patients. The decrease of BFV in CCA immediately after MR supports the view that the restoration of blood flow in CA is the first priority.

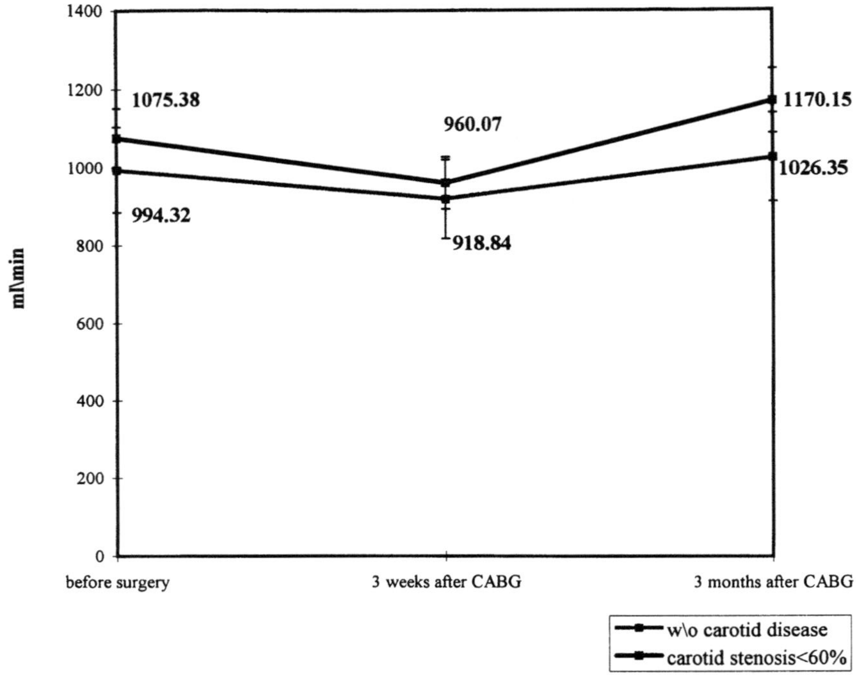

Fig. 3. Change of blood flow volume in common carotid artery in groups **B** and **C**.

References

1. Faggioli GL, Curl GR, Ricotta JJ (1990) The role of carotid screening before coronary artery surgery. J Vasc Surg 12: 724–31
2. Kertsman VP, Kuperberg EB, Serov RA, Bontar YM, Shvarts IP, Bakhutashvili ZV, Karelidis IK (1992) Causes of cerebral complications in patients with coronary heart disease after operations for myocardial revascularization. Thoracic and Cardiovascular Surgery. (Rus., ISSN 0236-2791); 9/10: 26–30
3. Minami K, Sagoo K, Breymann T, Fassbender D, Sewerdt M, Korfer R (1988) Operative strategy in combined coronary and carotid artery disease. J Thorac Cardiovasc Surg 95: 303–9
4. Todd MM, Drammond JC (1983) Cerebral protection during cardiac surgery. In: Kaplan JA (ed) Cardiac Anesthesia. Grune & Stratton, New York; pp 551–577

Author's address:
Dr. Anton L. Maximov
Cardiovascular Surgery Center
Coronary Surgery Division
209, Vaneeva Str.
603136 Nizhny Novgorod
Russia

Cerebral protection during simultaneous cerebrovascular and cardiac surgery using extracorporeal circulation for both procedures

Y. Finkbeiner[1], A. Schiessler[1], J. Ennker[2]

[1] Heart Institute Cottbus, Germany, [2] Heart Institute Lahr/Baden, Germany

Summary

Concomitant significant arteriosclerotic disease of coronary and carotid arteries is a frequent entity and simultaneous surgery appears to be indicated in certain cases.

The time sequence of the two revascularisation procedures, however, has been controversial. Whereas in the past carotid endarterectomy (CEA) was performed before extracorporeal circulation (ecc), we now have routinely applied a concept where the carotid intervention was performed after distal coronary anastomoses, in hypothermia and during ecc.

The results are analysed of 28 patients who underwent this procedure.

Introduction

When patients with a coronary heart disease are assigned to heart surgery for coronary artery bypass grafting (CABG), in a high percentage of cases there are coexistent supra-aortic vessels that are affected by arteriosclerosis, in particular the carotid arteries. This diffuse affect involving at least two major vascular systems presents a challenging management problem, because surgery in one vascular area can lead to severe complications in the other vessel territory. For both vascular systems affected, in 7.3–32.8 % (3, 7, 13, 19, 38, 42, 52, 53, 63, 70), according to the literature, severe neurological deficits occur during heart surgery, whereas myocardial infarction is a feared complication in 7.2–24.5 % (19, 38, 40, 56, 78), when carotid endarterectomy (CEA) is performed alone.

In 1972 Bernhard (6) and Faidutti (24) independantly of each other operated upon a small number of patients using a simultaneous surgical procedure; that is both revascularisating manoeuvres were carried out during the same anaesthesia, whereas carotid desobliteration took place before thoracotomy and institution of extracorporeal circulation (ecc).

The results demonstrated a significant reduction in cardiac deaths as well as in neurological deficits compared to the staged procedure, and simultaneous advance became widespread in many heart-surgical departments (16, 19, 35, 42, 55, 61, 64, 66, 67, 70, 84) during the early 1980s.

Nevertheless valid indications for this kind of simultaneous surgery are still missing: while having reached a large degree of correspondence concerning one stage treatment of patients with high coronary and neurological risk (e.g. left main stem stenosis and symptomatic high-grade carotid stenosis), treatment of neurologically asymptomatic patients remains controversial (18, 35, 39, 42, 43, 50, 52, 54, 58, 59, 77, 83).

In this case, depending on the morphology of carotid stenosis and its lumen reduction and the contralateral affection of the supraaortic vessels as well as the severity of coronary disease, several heart surgical centres developed different protocols: whether to treat these patients one or two staged with coronary revascularisation first or in a second step.

In both heart surgery clinics in Cottbus and in Lahr we favoured the simultaneous approach, using the advantages of ecc. These patients received thoracotomy and institution of cardiopulmonary bypass, after exposing the area of carotid artery only. Only after having performed the distal graft anastomoses, CEA was carried out in hypothermia at 28 °C with the empty beating heart and the additional protective effects of haemodilution and generalised heparinisation by the cardio-pulmonary bypass. According to this strategy, 28 patients were operated from Dec. 1994 to Sept. 1996. This report reviews our experience with the operative treatment of this group of patients.

Patients and Methods

Since the opening of the two new centres for heart surgery in Lahr/Baden and in Cottbus/Brandenburg in Dec. 1994 and in June 1995, in both clinics 3916 open heart surgical procedures were carried out, about 65 % coronary revascularisation operations with ecc. In a total of 28 coronary patients (1.1 %), a simultaneous carotid revascularisation was performed. Table 1 shows the characteristics of these 28 patients.

Table 2 and 3 give the preoperative cardial and neurological symptoms of 28 simultaneously treated patients.

Table 1. Patients' characteristics (n = 28)

Sex distribution	23	Male
	5	Female
Age (mean)	67.4	years
Diabetes (%)	19	67.9 %
Hypertension (%)	18	64.3 %
Obesity	10	35.7 %
Hyperlipoproteinaemia	20	71.4 %
Additional peripheral vascular disease	12	42.9 %

Table 2. Cardial analysis of patients (n = 28)

Preinfarction angina	17	60.7 %
Preoperative myocardial infarction	19	67.9 %
Three vessel disease	21	75 %
Left main stem stenosis	10	35.7 %

Table 3. Neurological analysis of patients (n = 28)

Neurologically asymptomatic	10	35.7 %
Transitory ischaemic attack (TIA)	13	46.4 %
Prolonged reversible ischaemic neurological deficit (PRIND)	3	10.7 %
Complete stroke	1	3.8 %
Contralateral carotid stenosis > 50 % or total occlusion	11	39.3 %

Preoperative diagnosis

In all bypass candidates duplex sonography of supraaortic vessels was performed. In the case of a positive result, showing haemodynamically relevant stenosis, patients received arterial angiography and cranial computer tomography as well as a consultation by a neurologist for accurate preoperative neurological status.

Surgical procedure

Patients received thoracotomy and institution of ecc, after exposing the area of carotid artery only. After thoracotomy, institution of ecc and performing distal coronary bypass graft anastomoses, CEA was carried out in hypothermia at 28 °C. Intraluminar shunting took place only in a few cases.

Figure 1 shows the surgical technique concerning CEA and the onset of ecc.

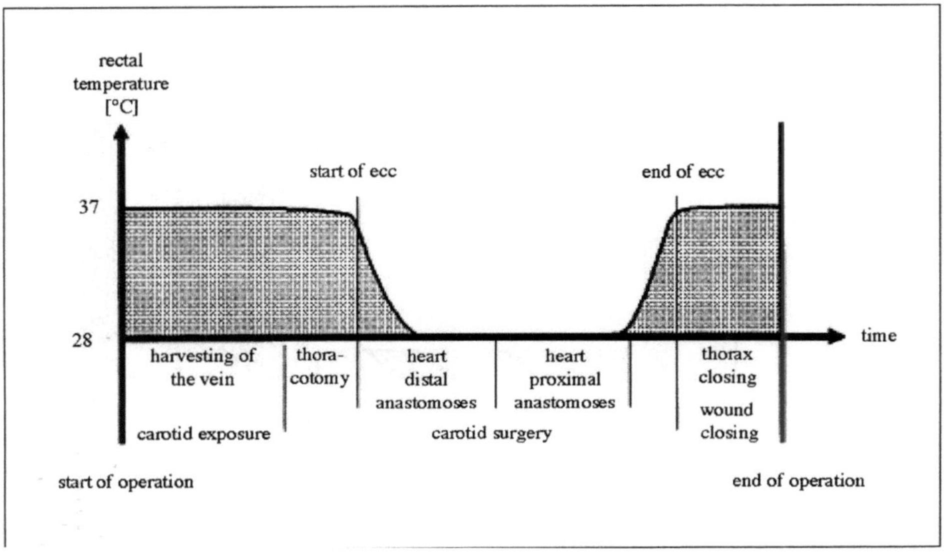

Fig. 1. Simultaneous carotid and coronary surgery. Herzzentrum Cottbus/Herzzentrum Lahr surgical technique

Results

The number of patients with combined surgery using ecc for both procedures was n = 28. During the 30-day postoperative period two major neurological deficits were identified in the 28 patients. Both patients sustained a cerebral infarction ipsilateral to the operated carotid artery. One patient had a contralateral occlusion of the internal carotid artery and had a history of recent transitory ischaemic attack (TIA).

The other patient came to surgery in a neurologically asymptomatic state; the morphology of his carotid stenosis, however, with signs of ulceration in a partially filiformous stenosis, led us to perform simultaneous operation. Intraoperatively vessel tissue was friable and ulcerated so that reconstruction of the bifurcation was only possible by interposing a piece of saphenous vein after excising about 7 cm of native internal carotid artery.

The total neurological complication rate was 7.1 %. There was one death (3.6 %).

This patient came to surgery with an ejection fraction of 24 % and a serious chronical obstructive lung disease; weaning from ecc was only possible after implantation of a balloon pump; this 72-year-old man died from a multi organ failure due to sepsis on the 15th postoperative day. Figure 2 shows the perioperative complications of the 28 simultaneously treated patients.

Discussion

Heart disease and stroke are the two leading causes of cardiovascular death in Europe and the USA. Sharing the same risk factors and similiar pathogenic mechanisms, coronary artery and peripheral vascular atherosclerosis frequently coexist in the same patient. In patients with planned CEA, in up to 49 % (19, 34, 36) a severe coronary heart disease is

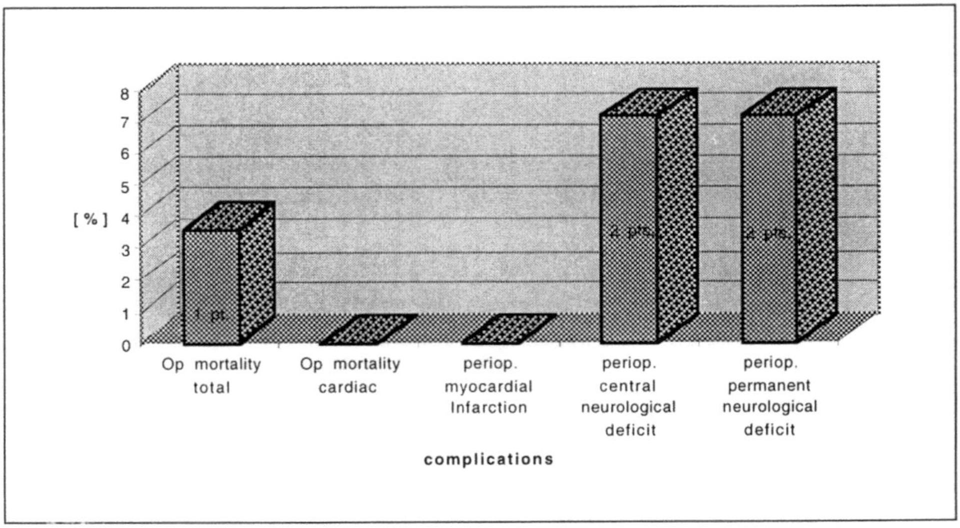

Fig. 2. Perioperative complications

manifest. In 1.5–34 % (3–5, 7, 8, 11, 13, 23, 31, 33, 35, 38, 42, 50, 52–54, 64, 66, 82), depending on the kind of preoperative diagnosis, in patients assigned to heart surgery for CABG, the coexistent carotid stenoses are so severe that also in this vascular area an indication for surgery is seen. In all coronary patients of the two heart surgery centres at Cottbus and Lahr, the incidence for this combined disease was 1.1 %.

This situation poses a therapeutic dilemma, because revascularisation of one vascular lesion alone can lead to detremental effects in the other vessel territory during surgery.

In patients with coexistent severe coronary and supraaortic vessel disease and coronary revascularisation alone, severe perioperative neurological deficits occurred in 7.2–32.8 %. Mortality is reported to be 6.9–16 % (3, 7, 13, 19, 38, 42, 52, 53, 63, 70), whereas neurological complications are between 0.5 and 6 % (1, 7–9, 13, 17, 23, 26, 27, 38, 45, 48, 68, 71) in bypass patients without concomitant carotid stenosis. In coronary patients undergoing carotid desobliteration alone, risk of perioperative myocardial infarction is between 7.2 and 24.5 % with a high mortality (19, 38, 40, 56, 78).

To prevent these complications, Bernhard (6) and Faidutti (24) developed a simultaneous surgical procedure, performing both operations during the same anaesthesia. The results, demonstrating superiority to the staged surgery, were reproducible for other heart-surgical groups (16, 19, 35, 42, 55, 64, 66, 70, 84). Thus, simultaneous carotid and coronary revascularisation became a frequent approach to these seriously ill patients during the early 1980s. Nevertheless, clear indications for the combined procedure are still lacking. Most authors agree to operate simultaneously when the carotid stenosis is symptomatic; in other words, when the patient suffered TIA or prolonged reversible ischaemic neurological deficit (PRIND) within the last 6 months before surgery.

If there are significant supraaortic stenoses in asymptomatic patients, the therapeutic approach varies widely. A large number of reports have been published between 1980 and 1990 by neurologists in particular (49), demanding that the number of neurological complications after a prophylactic surgery must be less than the spontaneous course. Nevertheless concomitant coronary heart disease and additional peripheral vascular disease seemed to allow widening of the indication for surgery, as the spontaneous risk for neurological deficits was estimated to be higher (2, 11, 30, 35). Furthermore, lack of randomised studies in this decade has led to a more restrictive surgical advance and some heart surgical centres stopped performing simultaneous surgery in neurologically asymptomatic patients.

Some other clinics have developed selection protocols, and patients receive either staged or combined surgery according to the severity of the lesion or to the bilateral carotid affect (39, 42, 52, 66, 83). Other centres perform simultaneous carotid and coronary revascularisation independant of neurological symptoms, if a diameter reduction of more than 70 % is present in the carotid artery (43, 50, 54, 58, 77).

These different advances are surely influenced by the controversial discussion about the treatment of patients with extracranial cerebrovaascular disease alone within the last 10 years. After its first description by Cooley and associates (12) in 1956, CEA became one of the most commonly performed vascular surgical procedures in the United States and Europe. In the 1980s, however, concerns were raised regarding the efficacy of carotid endarterectomy in preventing stroke and death compared with that of medical therapy alone for the treatment of extracranial cerebrovascular disease.

Reasons for neurological deficits

Reasons for neurological deficits perioperatively are multiple and differ widely depending on whether CEA alone or in combination with CABG during ecc is performed. Marx (49) by means of CCT and additional neurological and cardiological examinations, tried to conclude from typical brain infarction patterns in CEA-candidates to the aetiology of stroke. About 35 % of neurological deficits are caused by microangiopathy of intraparenchymatous vessels, showing multiple lacunar infarcts in CCT. 40 % are caused by closure of intracerebral territory vessels by emboli of atheromatous plaques of the carotid artery or from atrial or ventricular thrombi (29, 42, 81). Only in an estimated 15 %, haemodynamically relevant carotid stenoses are responsible for cerebral damage.

Simply transferring these data to patients with coexistent coronary disease, who need both vascular systems repaired, and drawing a conclusion concerning indication for two- or one-staged procedures, means negotiating the dangers of ecc itself. Factors to be considered are ecc-specific causes for cerebral dysfunction such as embolisation of air or debris (calcium, fat, microaggregates), embolisation of atherosclerotic debris during cross-clamping the ascending aorta or arterial cannulation, when central onset of ecc is performed as well as inadequate cerebral perfusion. A mean perfusion pressure < 50 mmHg is doubling the risk for cerebral damage after open heart surgery next to further factors like age of patient > 50 years and duration of bypass > 120 min (41).

Moreover, a recent study (85), using serum S100 protein as a marker for cerebral events during ecc, revealed a high correlation between ecc and neuronal damage and increased permeability of the blood-brain barrier. As detected in blood samples of all patients undergoing ecc, highly elevated serum levels of S100 protein, normally found in high concentration in glial and Schwann cells, were linked with severe neurological damage. Conversely, mildly elevated S100 protein levels resulted in no or only subclinical problems, such as cognitive dysfunction or subtle neuropsychological changes.

Similiarly Todd (79) concluded in 1988, taking into account the appearance of primitive reflexes and mild cognitive damage in 60–80 % of patients following CABG, as being suggestive of diffuse brain injury and that hypoperfusion during ecc is an obvious potential mechanism to be blamed.

In this context a recently published study (62) is of high interest, having identified patients with a history of neurological deficit, in particular stroke, to be at a high risk for neurological sequelae. The prospective analysis of 1000 patients undergoing cardiac operations requiring ecc confirmed the vulnerability of the previously injured brain to cardiopulmonary bypass, as evidenced by reappearance or exacerbation of focal deficits in such patients after cardiac surgery. As demonstrated by the characteristics in preoperative patients (Table 2), almost two-third of our patients came to surgery with neurological symptoms.

For the purpose of establishing the efficacy or lack of treatment with CEA, in the late 1980s randomised prospective trials were instituted in both symptomatic and asymptomatic patients. There were three trials concerning symptomatic patients, the North American Symptomatic Carotid Endarterectomy Trial (NASCET; 57), the European Carotid Surgery Trial (ECST; 21), and the Veterans Administration Symptomatic Carotid Stenosis Trial (VAS; 51). All of them demonstrated a clear benefit of CEA in patients with severe (> 70 %) symptomatic carotid stenosis in comparison to only medically treated patients.

Concerning neurologically asymptomatic patients with severe carotid stenosis, three randomised studies have been established: the Asymptomatic Carotid Atherosclerosis Study (ACAS; 22), the Carotid Surgery versus Medical Therapy in Asymptomatic Carotid Stenosis (CASANOVA; 75) study and the Veterans Administrations Asymptomatic Carotid Stenosis Study (VAA; 80). Whereas CASANOVA and VAA showed advantage of surgical versus medical therapy without reaching statistical significance (15), ACAS substantiated clearly that CEA reduces the risk of stroke and its sequelae in asymptomatic patients.

Transferring these data to patients with combined severe coronary and cerebral vascular occlusive disease, it becomes evident that the simultaneous surgical approach even in neurologically asymptomatic patients is a safe way to treat the high-risk group of patients. As demonstrated in Table 1, patients requiring simultaneous surgery were on average 67.4 years old, about 5 years older than the normal coronary patient. Also the higher incidence of risk factors for arteriosclerosis such as diabetes, hypertension, obesity, Hyperlipoproteinaemia and additional peripheral vascular disease demonstrate the clearly higher risk at surgery regarding perioperative complications.

The role of extracorporeal circulation

The results obtained in our series of 28 patients simultaneously treated give support to the logic that improved cerebral protection can be provided by performing the cerebrovascular part of the combined procedure during ecc. Next to generalised heparinisation, haemodilution and safe haemodynamic control by the perfusionist, hypothermia plays a deciding role for cerebral protection during ecc. Hypothermia provides an additional margin of safety during carotid cross-clamping. Henriksen (32), Lundar (46) and Matar et al. (50) reported a marked increase in cerebral blood flow during hypothermic bypass of at least 40 % in the stenosed supraaortic arteries.

Hypothermia induced by moderate systemic blood cooling to c. 28 °C during ecc can be expected to protect the brain by decreasing cerebral oxygen consumption and slowing the accumulation of anoxic metabolites in brain tissue (72, 82).

Cerebroprotection by ecc is common in the repair of the ascending aorta, e.g. in aortic arch aneurysms or in patients with hazardous atherosclerotic debris in the ascending aorta or the transverse arch (14, 20, 47, 69, 74). The repair of supraaortic vessels, in particular the carotid arteries, using ecc for better protecting the brain, however, has yet to reported in more than only a few cases (50, 53, 54, 56, 70). Wickey et al. (86) in 1988 published a case report of a 72-year-old man, who received combined carotid endarterectomy, coronary revascularisation and hypernephroma excision using even hypothermic circulatory arrest.

In 1994 Kouchoukos et al. (44) reported their experiences with hypothermic circulatory arrest during combined carotid and cardiac surgery in 50 patients with severe bilateral carotid artery disease, considered to be at high risk for the development of stroke. There were no early postoperative strokes or ischaemic neurological deficits.

Schwartz and colleagues (70) used the technique of combined carotid and coronary operation under cardiopulmonary bypass in 37 patients and compared it with the standard combined technique, in which the carotid endarterectomy was performed before bypass, in 36 other patients. In their series there was no significant advantage to the performance of the carotid procedure under cardiopulmonary bypass. The overall mortality rate was 10 % and was up to 18.5 % in left main disease. However, flow rates were 2.2 l/m^2 per min, perfusate temperature ranged between 32 and 28 °C, and mean aortic pressure was 50 to 70 mmHg during the carotid cross-clamp time. In our institutions, we followed the recommendations of Matar et al. (50) and Stockard et al. (73) maintaining flow rates between 2.4 and 3 l/m^2 per min, 28 °C, and 60 to 80 mmHg mean aortic pressure.

Minami et al. (53, 54) also perform both surgical procedures during ecc; the difference to our protocol consists in a different time sequence. CEA is carried out immediately after institution of ecc and cooling, trying to maintain a beating heart for pulsatile body perfusion. Nevertheless judgement of pulsatile or non-pulsatile perfusion as brain-protective factors differs widely. Govier et al. (28) saw in 1984 a decrease of regional bloodflow during non-pulsatile ecc, whereas Henriksen (32) and other more recent reports (65, 76) described a clear augmentation of bloodflow, measured by Transcranial Doppler Sonography.

The use of a shunt

The use of a shunt in carotid surgery remains an object of controversial discussion. A general recommendation for using a temporary shunt cannot be maintained, because by the shunt itself severe complications can arise. Mobilising of embolic debris in the distal carotid stump, air emboli and intima dissection next to prolongation of carotid surgery by impeding careful preparation are clear disadvantages (25, 60). On the other hand, using a correctly placed shunt allows, further to the major reason of brain protection against haemodynamically caused ischaemia, free prolongation of carotid-clamping-time and therefore preparation of the occluding plaque without time pressure (10, 37).

In our 28 patients shunt was used only in a very few special cases, e.g. if contralateral carotid occlusion and poor backflow was present and the reconstruction of the carotid artery obviously would last longer than the usual clamping time. In all other cases (92.9 %) no shunt was used.

According to our experiences with shunting during carotid endarterectomy, we believe that shunting with its possible complications can be avoided in carotid desobliteration, when performed during hypothermia on ecc by an experienced surgeon.

In conclusion, the surgical technique with early institution of ecc and CEA in hypothermia during ecc are protecting factors for the brain as well as for the myocardium. Therefore it is a safe way to handle these high-risk patients, who, as our results show, are at the same risk for perioperative complications as bypass candidates alone.

References

1. Astore GW, Meyer BW, Lindesmith GG (1973) Coronary artery disease: surgery in 100 patients 65 years of age and older. Arch Surg 107: 30–33
2. Autret A, Sandeau D, Bertrand P, et al. (1987) Stroke risk in patients with carotid stenosis. Lancet 1: 888–890
3. Barnes RW, Nix ML, Sansonetti D, Turley DG, Goldman MR (1985) Late outcome of untreated asymptomatic carotid disease following cardiovascular operations. J Vasc Surg 2: 843–849
4. Barnes RW, Marszalek PB (1981) Asymptomatic carotid disease in the cardiovascular patient. Is prophylactic endarterectomy necessary? Stroke 12: 497–500
5. Barnes RW, Marszalek PB, Rittger SE (1980) Asymptomatic carotid disease in preoperative patients. Stroke 11: 136–142
6. Bernhard VM, Johnson WD, Petersen JJ (1972) Carotid artery stenosis. Association with surgery for coronary artery disease. Arch Surg 105: 837–840
7. Brener BJ, Brief DK, Alpert J, Goldenkrantz RJ, Parsonnet V (1987) The risk of stroke in patients with asymptomatic carotid stenosis undergoing cardiac surgery. A follow-up study. J Vasc Surg 9: 269–279
8. Breslau PJ, Fell G, Ivery TD, et al. (1981) Carotid arterial disease in patients undergoing coronary bypass operations. J Thorac Cardiovasc Surg 82: 765–767
9. Breuer AC, Hanson MR, Furlan AJ (1981) Central nervous system complications of myocardial revascularization. A prospective analysis of 400 patients. Stroke 11: 1136–1142
10. Browse NL, Ross-Russel R (1984) Carotid endarterectomy and the Javid shunt: the early results of 215 consecutive operations for transient ischemic attacks. Br J Surg 71: 53–57
11. Chambers B, Norris JW (1984) The case against surgery for asymptomatic artery stenosis. Stroke 15: 964–967
12. Cooley DA, Al-Naaman YD, Carton CA (1956) Surgical treatment of arteriosclerotic occlusion of common carotid artery. J Neurosurg 13: 500–506

13. Cosgrove DM, Hertzer NR, Loop FD (1986) Surgical management of synchronous carotid and coronary artery disease. J Vasc Surg 4: 690–694
14. Culliford AT, Colvin SB, Rohrer K, Baumann FG, Spencer FC (1986) The atherosclerotic ascending aorta and transverse arch: a new technique to prevent cerebral injury during bypass; experience with 13 patients. Ann Thorac Surg 41: 27–35
15. Diener HC, Busse O, Hacke W, Hennerici M (1992) Carotis-Endarteriektomie. Eine kritische Analyse aktueller Studien. Dtsch Med Wschr 117: 72–74
16. Duchateau J, Nevelsteen A, Sergeant P, et al. (1989) Combined myocardial and cerebral revascularization. A ten year experience. J Cardiovasc Surg 30: 715–722
17. Dunn EJ (1986) Concomitant cerebral and myocardial revascularization. Surg Clin North Am 66: 385–395
18. Eckel L, et al. (1989) Karotis-plus Koronarstenosen. MMW 31/32: 131 (In: Nachrichten)
19. Ennix CL Jr, Lawrie GM, Morris GC Jr, et al. (1979) Improved results of carotid endarterectomy in patients with symptomatic coronary disease: an analysis of 1546 consecutive caroid operations. Stroke 10: 122
20. Ergin MA, O'Connor J, Guinto R, et al. (1982) Experience with profound hypothermia and circulatory arrest in the treatment of aneurysms of the carotid arch. J Thorac Cardiovasc Surg 84: 649–655
21. European Carotid Surgery Trialists' Collaborative Group (1991) MRC European Carotid Surgery Trial: interim results for symptomatic patients with severe (70–99 %) or with mild (0–29 %) carotid stenosis. Lancet 337 (8752): 1235–1243
22. Executive Committee for the Asymptomatic Carotid Atherosclerosis Study (1995) Endarterectomy for asymptomatic carotid artery stenosis. J Am Med Assoc 273: 1421–1428
23. Faggioli GL, Curl GR, Ricotta JJ (1990) The role of carotid screening before coronary artery bypass. J Vasc Surg 12: 724–731
24. Faidutti B, Steichen FM, Thevoz F, Hahn CJ (1973) Surgical management of coronary artery and associated aortic or major arterial atherosclerosis. J Cardiovasc Surg 13: 157–167
25. Fergusson GG (1982) Intra-operative monitoring and internal shunts: are they necessary in carotid endarterectomy? (Editorial) Stroke 13: 287–289
26. Gardner TJ, Horneffer PJ, Manolio TA, et al. (1986) Major stroke after cornary artery bypass surgery: changing magnitude of the problem. J Vasc Surg 3: 684–687
27. Gonzales-Scarano F, Hurtig HI (1981) Neurologic complications of coronary artery bypass grafting: a case-control study. Neurology 31: 1032–1035
28. Govier AV, Reves JG, Mc Kay RD, et al. (1984) Factors and their influence on regional cerebral blood flow during nonpulsatile cardiopulmonary bypass. Ann Thorac Surg 38: 592
29. Gravlee GL, Cordell AR, Graham JE, et al. (1985) Coronary revascularization in patients witth bilateral internal carotid occlusions. J Thorac Cardiovasc Surg 90: 921–925
30. Hennerici M (1986) Operative Behandlung von asymptomatischen Carotisstenosen. Dtsch Med Wschr 111: 1619–1620
31. Hennerici M, Aurich A, Sandmann W, Freund HJ (1981) Incidence of asymptomatic extracranial artery disease. Stroke 12: 750–758
32. Henriksen L, Hjelms E, Lindeburgh T (1983) Brain hyperperfusion during cardiac operations. J Thorac Cardiovasc Surg 86: 202
33. Hertzer NR, Loop FD, Beven EG, O'Hara PJ, Krajewski LP (1989) Surgical staging for simultaneous coronary and carotid disease. A study including prospective randomization. J Vasc Surg 9: 455–463
34. Hertzer NR (1982) Fatal myocardial infarction following peripheral vascular operations. A study of 951 patients followed 6 to 11 years postoperatively. Clev Clin Q 49: 1–11
35. Hertzer NR, Loop FD, Taylor PC, Beven EG (1983) Combined myocardial revascularization and carotid endarterectomy. J Thorac Cardiovasc Surg 85: 577
36. Hertzer NR, Young JR, Beven EG, et al. (1985) Coronary angiography in 506 patients with extracranial cerbrovascular disease. Arch Intern Med 145: 849–852
37. Hertzer NR, Beven EG (1980) A retrospective comparison of the use for shunts during carotid endarterectomy. Surg Gynecol Obstet 151: 81–84
38. Hertzer NR, Loop FD, Taylor PC, Beven EG (1978) Staged and combined surgical approach to simultaneous carotid and coronary vascular disease. Surg 84: 803–811
39. Jausseran JM, Begeron P, Reggi M, et al. (1989) Single staged carotid and coronary arteries surgery. J Cardiovasc Surg 30: 407–413
40. Javid H, Ostermiller WE, Henges JW, et al. (1970) Carotid endarterectomy for asymptomatic patients. Arch Surg 102: 389–391
41. Javid H, Tufo HM, Najafi H, et al. (1969) Neurological abnormalities following open heart surgery. J Thorac Cardiovasc Surg 58: 502
42. Jones EL, Craver JM, Michalik RA, et al. (1984) Combined carotid and coronary operation: When are they necessary? J Thorac Cardiovasc Surg 87: 7–16

43. Kartchner MM, McRae LP (1982) Carotid occlusive disease as a risk factor in major cardiovascular surgery. Arch Surg 117: 1086
44. Kouchoukos NT, Daily BB, Wareing TH, Murphy SF (1994) Hypothermic circulatory arrest for cerebral protection during combined carotid and cardiac surgery patients with bilateral carotid artery disease. Ann Surg 219: 699–706
45. Lee MC, Geiger J, Nicoloff D (1979) Cerebral vascular complications associated with coronary artery bypass procedure. Stroke 10: 107–110
46. Lundar T, Frøysaker T, Lindegaard K-F, et al. (1985) Some observation on cerebral perfusion during bypass. Ann Thorac Surg 39: 318
47. Mahfood S, Qazi A, Garcia J, et al. (1985) Management of aortic arch aneurysm using profound hypothermia and circulatory arrest. Ann Thorac Surg 39: 412–417
48. Martin WRW, Hashimoto SK (1982) Stroke in coronary bypass surgery. Can J Neurol Sci 9: 21–26
49. Marx P (1989) Karotisendarteriektomie. Ein vertretbares Risiko zur Prophylaxe ischämischer Insulte? Fortschr Med 34: 727–732
50. Matar AF (1986) Concomitant coronary and cerebral revascularization under cardiopulmonary bypass. Ann Thorac Surg 41: 431–435
51. Mayberg MR, Wilson SE, Yatsu F, Weiss DG, Messina L, Hershey LA, et al. (1991) Carotid endarterectomy and prevention of cerebral ischemia in symptomatic carotid stenosis. Veterans Affairs Cooperative Studies Program 309 Trialist Group. J Am Med Assoc 266: 3289–3294
52. Mehigan JT, Buch WS, Pipkin RD, Fogarty TJ (1977) A planned approach to coexistent cerebrovascular disease in coronary artery bypass candidates. Arch Surg 112: 1403–1409
53. Minami K, Gawaz M, Ohlmeier H, Vyska K, Körfer R (1989) Management of concomitant occlusive disease of coronary and carotid arteries using cardiopulmonary bypass for both procedures. J Cardiovasc Surg 30: 723
54. Minami K, Sagoo KS, Breymann T, Fassbender D, Schwerdt M, Körfer R (1988) Operative strategy in combined coronary and carotid artery disease. J Thorac Cardiovasc Surg 95: 303–309
55. Morris GC Jr, Ennis CL Jr, Lawrie GM, et al. (1978) Management of coexistent carotid and coronary artery occlusive atherosclerosis. Clev Clin Q 45: No 1
56. Nishida H, Grooters RK, Yeager AA, et al. (1989) Carotid and aortic arch endarterectomy using hypothermic arrest with coronary bypass. Ann Thorac Surg 48: 865–866
57. North American Symptomatic Carotid Endarterectomy Trial Collaborators (1994) Beneficial effect of carotid endarterectomy in symptomatic patients with high-grade carotid stenosis. N Engl J Med 325: 445–453
58. O'Donnel TF Jr, Callow AD, Willet C, et al. (1983) The impact of coronary artery disease on carotid endarterectomy. Ann Surg 198: 705
59. Okies JE, Macmanus Q, Starr A (1977) Myocardial revascularization and carotid endarterectomy. A combined approach. Ann Thorac Surg 23: 561–564
60. Ott DA, Cooley DA, Chapa L, Coelho A (1980) Carotid endarterectomy without temporary intraluminal shunt: study of 309 consecutive operations. Ann Surg 191: 708–714
61. Palenker J, Hepp W, Bücherl ES (1991) Kombinierte koronare und supraaortale Erkrankung: Ergebnisse des simultanene Vorgehens. In: Aktuelle Herausforderung in der Gefäßchirurgie. Steinkopff Verlag, Darmstadt, pp 49–54
62. Redmond JM, Greene PS, Goldborough MA, et al. (1996) Neurologic injury in cardiac surgical patients with a history of stroke. Ann Thorac Surg 61: 42–47
63. Reul GJ, Morric GC, Howell JF, et al. (1972) Current concepts in coronary artery surgery: a critical analysis of 1287 patients. Ann Thorac Surg 14: 243–257
64. Rice PL, Piffarre R, Sullivan HJ, Montoya A, Bakhos M (1980) Experience with simultaneous myocardial revascularization and carotid endarterectomy. J Thorac Cardiovasc Surg 79: 922–925
65. Ries F, Murday H, Kirchhoff PG (1986) Intraoperatives Monitoring mit der transkraniellen Doppler-Sonographie. Psycho 12: 309
66. Rosenthal D, Candill DR, Lamis PA, et al. (1984) Carotid and coronary arterial disease. A rational approach. Am Surg 50: 233
67. Schiessler A, Hepp W (1984) Zur Problematik operationspflichtiger Koronar-Stenosen bei gleichzeitiger zerebraler Durchblutungsstörung. Klinische Wissenschaft – Herzchirurgie, pp 64–65
68. Schlosser V (1991) Differentialindikation beim gemeinsamen Vorliegen von koronarer Herzkrankheit und Stenosen hirnversorgender Arterien. In: Aktuelle Herausforderung in der Gefäßchirurgie. Steinkopff Verlag Darmstadt, pp 39–47
69. Schmidt CA, Smith DC (1989) Traumatic avulsion of arch vessels in a child: primary repair using hypothermic circulatory arrest. J Trauma 29: 248–250
70. Schwartz RL, Garret JR Kerp RB, et al. (1982) Simultaneous myocardial revascularization and carotid endarterectomy. Circulation 66 (Suppl): 97–101

71. Sergeant P, Flameng W, Suy R (1989) Carotid and aortic arch endarterectomy using hypothermic arrest with coronary bypass. Ann Thorac Surg 48: 865–866
72. Smith AL, Wollmann H (1972) Cerebral blood flow and metabolism: effects of anesthetic drugs and techniques. Anesthesiology 36: 378–384
73. Stockard JJ, Bickford RG, Chir B, Schauble JF (1973) Pressure-dependant cerebral ischemia during cardiopulmonary bypass. Neurology 23: 521
74. Tharion J, Johnson DC, Celemajer JM, et al. (1982) Profound hypothermia with circulatory arrest: nine years' clinical experience. J Thorac Cardiovasc Surg 84: 66–72
75. The CASANOVA Study Group (1994) Carotid surgery versus medical therapy in asymptomatic carotid stenosis. Stroke 22: 1229–1235
76. Thiel A, Russ W, Kaps M, et al. (1990) Transkranielle Doppler-Sonographie während pulsatiler und nicht-pulsatiler extrakorporaler Zirkulation. Anästhesist 39: 30
77. Thompson JE (1983) The developement of carotid surgery. Arch Surg 107: 643
78. Thompson JE, Austin DJ, Patman RD (1970) Carotid endarterectomy for cerebrovascular insufficiency. Long-term results in 592 patients followed up to 13 years. Ann Surg 172: 663–679
79. Todd NV (1988) Cerebral ischemia and surgical practice. Ann Roy Surg Engl 70: 3–7
80. Towne JB, Weiss DG, Hobson RW II (1990) First phase report of cooperative Veterans Administration asymptomatic carotid stenosis study-operative morbidity and mortality. J Vasc Surg 11: 252–259
81. Tufo HM, Ostfeld AM, Shebelle RE (1970) Central nervous system dysfunction following open heart surgery. J Am Med Assoc 212: 1333–1340
82. Turnipseed WD, Berkoff HA, Belzer FO (1980) Postoperative stroke in cardiac and peripheral vascular disease. Ann Surg 192: 365–368
83. Urschel HC, Razzuk MA, Gardner MA (1976) Management of concomitant occlusive disease of the and coronary arteries. J Thorac Cardiovasc Surg 72: 829–834
84. Vermeulen FEE, de Geest R, Pavoordt H.v.D., Eikelboom B (1988) Simultaneous extensive extracranial and coronary revascularization. Long-term-up to 13 years. Eur J Cardio-Thorac Surg 2: 113–123
85. Westaby S, Johnsson P, Parry AJ, et al. (1996) Serum S100 protein: a potential marker for cerebral events during cardiopulmonary bypass. Ann Thorac Surg 61: 88–92
86. Wickey GS, Martin DE, Larach DR, et al. (1988) Combined carotid endarterectomy, coronary revascularization and hypernephroma excision with hypothermic circulatory arrest. Anesth Analg 67: 473–476

Author's address:
Y. F. Finkbeiner, M.D.
Herzzentrum Cottbus
Thiemstr. 111
03048 Cottbus, Germany

Cerebral protection in the pediatric age group

Studies of hypothermic circulatory arrest and low flow bypass as used for congenital heart surgery

R. A. Jonas

Department of Cardiac Surgery, Children's Hospital and Department of Surgery, Harvard Medical School, Boston, MA, USA

Introduction

Following the pioneering studies of hypothermia by Bigelow (4) and the demonstration by Barratt-Boyes (2) that profound hypothermic circulatory arrest could be used to facilitate repair of complex cardiac anomalies in infancy, hypothermic circulatory arrest has been widely applied. The technique has been used in many centers for cardiac procedures in children with congenital heart problems as well as in adults with acquired conditions such as aortic arch aneurysms. Although many studies have attempted to define the risk of brain injury associated with circulatory arrest, they have suffered from a number of study design inadequacies, particularly the heterogeneous nature of the patient population studied. Other limitations have included retrospective study design, nonuniform neuropsychometric testing methods and irrelevance to modern methods of cardiopulmonary bypass such as membrane oxygenators. In fact, refinements in the technique of cardiopulmonary bypass have meant that support modalities other than circulatory arrest such as low flow hypothermic bypass have become increasingly attractive.

Prospective study of circulatory arrest versus low flow bypass

In 1988, we began enrollment of patients under 3 months of age in a prospective randomized study comparing deep hypothermic circulatory arrest with low flow hypothermic bypass. This homogeneous patient population consisted of patients with transposition of the great arteries who were scheduled to undergo an arterial switch procedure. The arterial switch is primarily an extracardiac procedure which can be undertaken equally well under conditions of circulatory arrest or with low flow bypass. In the early 1980s, we had confirmed that this corrective procedure could be undertaken with a very low mortality risk in the first weeks of life (6). In general, these patients were hemodynamically stable in the postoperative period. Thus it seemed likely that intraoperative factors such as the support modality employed would be the primary determinants of neurological and developmental outcome.

Over a 3-year enrollment period up to March 1992, 171 neonates and young infants were enrolled. The mean circulatory arrest duration for those randomized to circulatory arrest was 55 min. The low flow rate employed was 50 cc/kg/min. Perioperative end-points of the study included the incidence of seizures determined clinically and by continuous EEG. EEG monitoring was begun preoperatively and was continued intraoperatively and for 48 h postoperatively. Other endpoints included cumulative release of the brain isoenzyme creatine kinase BB (CK-BB), return of EEG activity, transcranial Doppler assessment of cerebral blood flow velocity, cardiac index, duration of hospitalization as well as complete assessment of fluid and electrolytes, and renal and glucose metabolism. A neurological examination was undertaken at regular intervals. At 1 year of age these same children underwent a brain MRI scan, neurological examination as well as comprehensive developmental assessment of their motor and cognitive function. The neurological and developmental assessments are being repeated currently at 4 years of age.

Perioperative findings

The most important finding of the perioperative studies was that the use of circulatory arrest is associated with a higher risk of seizures determined both by clinical methods as well as by EEG (15). Clinical seizures occurred in 12 % of infants randomized to circulatory arrest while seizures determined by EEG occurred in 26 %. There was a strong correlation between duration of circulatory arrest and the occurrence of seizures ($p = 0.004$) (Fig. 1). No child who had an arrest time less than 35 min had a seizure either clinically or by EEG. Circulatory arrest was also associated with greater release of the brain isoenzyme CK-BB in the first 6 h post-operatively ($p = 0.046$) and longer recovery to first EEG activity ($p < 0.001$). An interesting finding was that the presence of an associated VSD, which was also associated with older age at the time of surgery, had an important

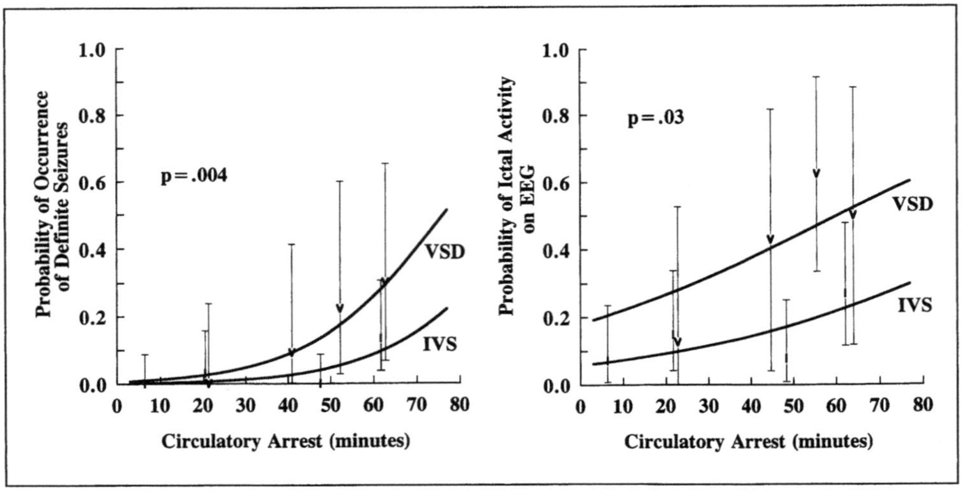

Fig. 1. Results of a prospective randomized study of circulatory arrest (Boston Circulatory Arrest Study): Estimated probabilities of definite seizures in the first week after surgery (panel A) and of ictal activity on continuous video EEG in the first 48 h after surgery (panel B), as a function of the duration of total circulatory arrest. Logistic regression curves are shown for infants with an intact ventricular septum (IVS) and for those with a ventricular septal defect (VSD). In addition, point estimates and exact 95 % confidence intervals for outcome probabilities are plotted for the mean of each quartile of duration of circulatory arest (I and V for the respective groups). The p values shown were calculated by logistic regression for the effect of the duration of circulatory arrest on outcome, with adjustment for diagnosis.

association with risk of seizures. This seemed paradoxical in that the presence of a VSD allows improved mixing of the parallel circulations present in transposition. Therefore these patients are usually less acidotic and less hypoxic than patients with intact ventricular septum and thus are less likely to have suffered a significant preoperative insult.

Findings at 1 year of age

There were 168 survivors of the 171 patients enrolled in the study. Of these, 155 returned at 1 year of age for evaluation (3).

Developmental testing

The Psychomotor Development Index of the Bayley Scale is a measure of fine and gross motor ability in the 1 year old. Scores were significantly lower among children randomized to circulatory arrest by a mean of 6.5 points ($p = 0.01$). Regression analysis revealed an association between longer duration of circulatory arrest and lower score ($p = 0.02$) (Fig. 2). The mean score of the two treatment groups combined was 95.1 (predicted 100).

The Mental Development Index does not accurately predict IQ but is a precursor assessment of cognitive function. The score of the two treatment groups combined was 105.1 with the current norm being 112. Scores tended to be lower among children assigned to circulatory arrest (mean difference 4.1 points, $p = 0.1$) although the scores did not decrease significantly with an increased duration of circulatory arrest. A diagnosis of associated VSD was an independent risk factor for a lower score ($p = 0.004$).

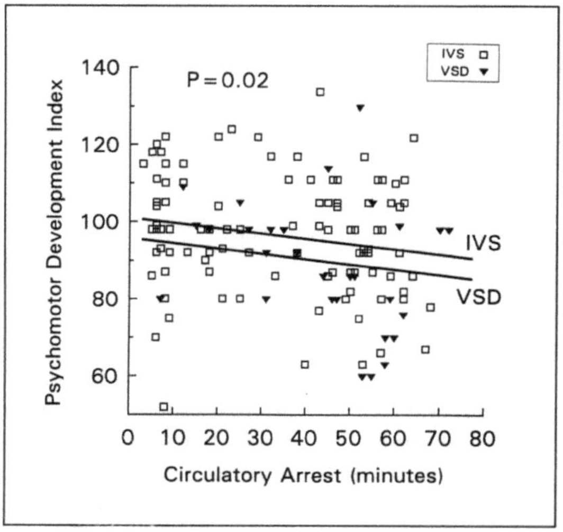

Fig. 2. Boston Circulatory Arrest Study: Score on the psychomotor development index at 1 year as a function of the duration of total circulatory arrest. Regression lines are shown for infants with an intact ventricular septum (IVS) and those with a ventricular septal defect (VSD). The p value shown was calculated by linear regression for the effect of the duration of total circulatory arrest on the score on the psychomotor development index, with adjustment for diagnosis.

Neurologic examination

Thirty-one percent of the 154 children who underwent neurologic examination at 1 year of age had definite abnormalities. All abnormalities were assessed to be mild. Specific abnormalities included hypotonia (18 %), hypertonia (8 %) and cerebral palsy (3 %). Neurologic abnormalities tended to be more common in children randomized to circulatory arrest (41 % versus 28 %, $p = 0.09$). Possible or definite neurologic abnormalities were associated with a longer duration of circulatory arrest ($p = 0.04$).

Magnetic resonance imaging

Fifteen percent of the 142 children who underwent MRI at 1 year of age had definite abnormalities which were mild in 86 %. The prevalence of MRI abnormalities was not related to treatment assignment.

Relation between perioperative seizures and 1 year outcome

As noted above there was a significantly higher incidence of seizures among infants randomized to circulatory arrest compared to those randomized to low flow bypass. In regression analyses with adjustment for the treatment group and the presence or absence of a VSD, the occurrence of EEG seizures in the early postoperative period was associated with a mean reduction of 11.2 points of the Psychomotor Development Index ($p = 0.002$) and with a significantly higher risk of possible or definite abnormalities on MRI scanning ($p < 0.001$). Infants assigned to circulatory arrest also had an increased risk of clinical seizures in the early postoperative period as noted above. Clinical seizures predicted increased risk of possible or definite neurologic abnormalities at 1 year of age ($p = 0.05$).

Findings at 4 years of age

Currently this cohort of children is undergoing neurologic and developmental assessment at 4 years of age. Preliminary analysis suggests a continuing important association between perioperative seizures and outcome, including a correlation with both the cognitive and verbal skills assessments as well as motor skills.

Summary

This unique clinical study raises serious concerns regarding the neurodevelopmental consequences of hypothermic circulatory arrest, particularly when the duration is in excess of 30 to 45 min. Nevertheless, there are many congenital cardiac anomalies in which the technical difficulties of employing continuous cardiopulmonary bypass in the small infant mandate that circulatory arrest be used. Consequently, we have undertaken a number of clinical and laboratory studies that we hope will enable us to reduce the morbidity of the technique.

pH strategy and circulatory arrest

In 1987, Nevin et al. (14) reported that a prebypass pCO2 of less than 35 mm in adult patients undergoing coronary artery surgery was associated with an increased incidence of neuropsychometric deficit. This report stimulated us to review the influence of pCO2 and pH on neurodevelopmental outcome in our infant population undergoing circulatory arrest (10). We were particularly interested to undertake this analysis because in 1985 we had changed our pH strategy for hypothermic cardiopulmonary bypass to a more alkaline strategy, namely "alpha stat", that is maintenance of pH at 7.40 as measured at 37 °C and not corrected to patient temperature. Before 1985, we had used the more acidotic "pH stat" strategy, that is, we had maintained pH at 7.40 corrected to patient temperature. The pH stat strategy is achieved by the addition of carbon dioxide to the oxygenator gas mixture. The resultant respiratory acidosis counteracts the alkaline shift which occurs with hypothermia. Like many other units during the 1980s, our rationale for changing our pH management was based on a number of comparative physiological studies of cold-blooded vertebrates. These reports suggested that animals which remained active when hypothermic tended to employ the alpha stat strategy (16, 17). Intracellular enzyme function is more efficient when the alpha stat strategy is followed. (It is interesting to note however that many hibernating animals which are inactive during hypothermia and are attempting to minimize energy consumption, utilize the pH stat strategy.)

Retrospective clinical study of circulatory arrest and pH strategy

We undertook a retrospective developmental study with a cohort of patients who had undergone surgery for transposition of the great arteries in a time frame which straddled our change in pH strategy (10). Sixteen patients who had undergone Senning procedures under deep hypothermic circulatory arrest between 1983 and 1988 underwent cognitive developmental assessment. Most children scored in the normal range with a median developmental score of 109 (10). The mean duration of circulatory arrest was 43 min ranging from 35 to 60 min. Duration of circulatory arrest was not associated with cognitive outcome. However, a strong positive correlation was found between arterial pCO2 during cooling before circulatory arrest and developmental score (Fig. 3), i.e., children undergoing the alpha stat strategy had a worse developmental outcome. These results must be interpreted cautiously because of the small sample size and the usual limitations of a retrospective study. For example, there were many changes in perfusion technique during this time such as a change from bubble to membrane oxygenators which may have contributed to this result.

Choreoathetosis and pH strategy

Between 1980 and 1984 there were no cases of choreoathetosis at Children's Hospital, Boston. Between 1986 and 1990, following the introduction of the alpha stat strategy in 1985, 19 cases of choreoathetosis were noted (18). Eleven of these were severe with four of the children dying and six having persistent choreoathetosis. As already noted a number of perfusion protocol changes occurred in the mid 1980s which might have contributed to the

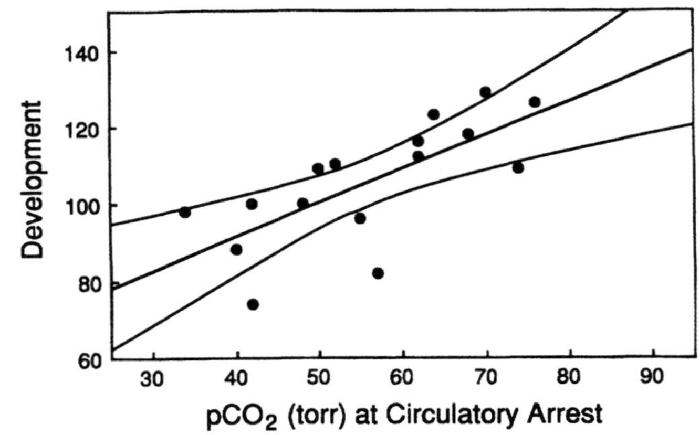

Fig. 3. Association between cognitive function and arterial pCO2 (as measured at 37 °C) before deep hypothermic arrest ($r = 0.71$, $p = 0.002$). (From a small retrospective study of children undergoing circulatory arrest for Senning procedures.)

virtual epidemic of choreoathetosis. At the same time there was an increase in the number of children with complex forms of pulmonary atresia undergoing surgery. In our review of these cases we found the presence of pulmonary atresia and the use of circulatory arrest to be frequently present factors. We were not able to prove that use of a more alkaline pH strategy was associated with choreoathetosis. Nevertheless, it is tempting to speculate that a more alkaline strategy is responsible for a steal of blood from the cerebral to the pulmonary circulation in patients whose pulmonary blood flow is derived from the systemic arterial system because of the opposite effects of alkalosis on cerebral and pulmonary resistance. Decreased cerebral blood flow during cooling may have resulted in inadequate, non-homogeneous brain cooling before circulatory arrest.

Laboratory studies of circulatory arrest

In order to better study the basic mechanisms behind the findings of our clinical studies, we have developed a piglet model of hypothermic circulatory arrest which in many ways replicates the perfusion strategies we use clinically (11).

Four-week-old miniature piglets weighing approximately 3.5 kg are cooled on cardiopulmonary bypass and undergo either circulatory arrest or low flow bypass at 50 cc/kg/min. The animals are rewarmed to normothermia over 45 min and are then maintained at normothermia on partial bypass to ensure maintenance of temperature and cardiac output for 3 more h. Data collected include cerebral magnetic resonance spectroscopy using a 4.7 Tesla horizontal bore magnet, cerebral blood flow by microspheres and electromagnetic flow probe, cerebral metabolism by oxygen and glucose consumption, lactate production and assessment of cerebral edema. More recent studies have included near infra-red spectroscopy (9) and EEG.

Effect of pH strategy on acute recovery of cerebral metabolism after circulatory arrest

In this study all animals underwent 1 h of circulatory arrest (1). However, 14 animals (seven blood flow and metabolism studies, seven magnetic resonance studies) underwent the alpha stat pH strategy during hypothermia and 11 underwent the pH stat strategy (six blood flow and metabolism studies, five magnetic resonance studies).

The pH stat animals had greater cerebral blood flow during core cooling ($p = 0.001$). The intracellular pH during core cooling showed an alkaline shift in both groups but became more alkaline with alpha stat than pH stat at the end of cooling ($p = 0.013$). Recovery of cerebral ATP ($p = 0.046$) and intracellular pH ($p = 0.014$) in the initial 30 min of reperfusion was faster with pH stat. As noted in the previous study, the cerebral intracellular pH became even more acidotic during early reperfusion than it had become during the circulatory arrest period itself with alpha stat, while it showed immediate recovery with reperfusion with pH stat. Brain water content postoperatively was less with pH stat (0.8075) than with alpha stat (0.8124) ($p = 0.05$).

A particularly interesting finding of this study was the redistribution of cerebral blood flow during cooling which was different between the two groups (Fig. 4). Animals undergoing alpha stat had a decrease in the proportion of blood perfusing the basal ganglia in addition to having as expected less total cerebral blood flow than the pH stat animals. Animals undergoing pH stat showed an increase in % distribution to the basal ganglia, cerebellum, pons and medulla oblongata with a decrease in % distribution to the cerebral

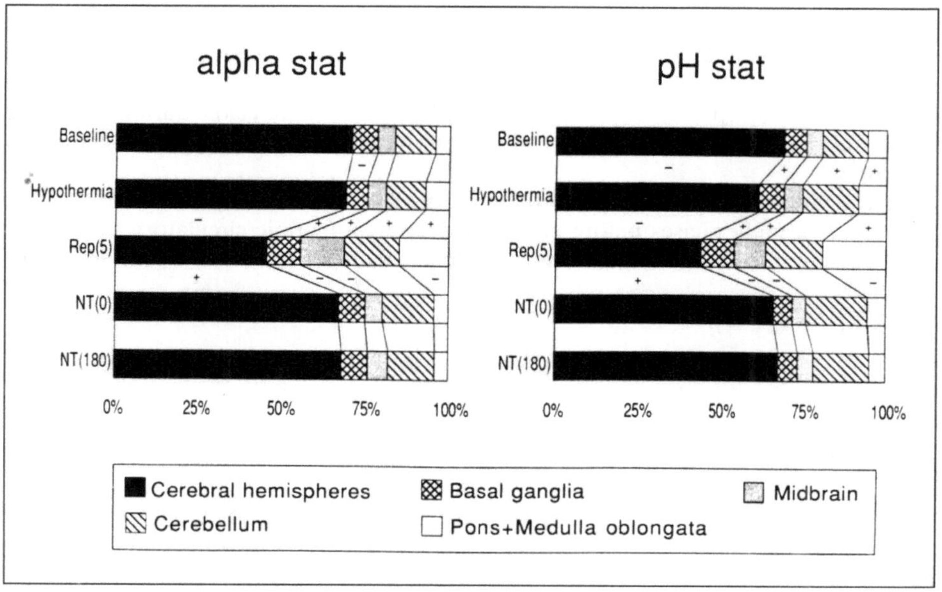

Fig. 4. Intracerebral distribution of blood flow with either alpha stat or pH stat strategy, core cooling and rewarming and 1 h of circulatory arrest NT(O) = after 45 min of rewarming, when normothermia (nasopharyngeal temperature > 35 °C) was achieved, NT (180) = after 180 min of reperfusion at normothermia; REP (5) = 5 min after initiation of reperfusion and rewarming after 1 h of total circulatory arrest; + $p < 0.05$ for the within-group increase by paired *t*-test; $p < 0.05$ for the within group decrease by paired *t*-test.

hemispheres. But even with the shift in distribution, the absolute regional blood flow to the cerebral hemispheres was not less with pH stat than alpha stat.

Although the findings of our initial study of pH strategy were consistent with our retrospective clinical study of pH strategy, further experiments were required to define whether the mechanism of improved protection with pH stat was operative primarily during the cooling or rewarming phase before or after circulatory arrest respectively. We hypothesized that the apparent improved protection with pH stat might be secondary to greater oxygen availability during the cooling phase before circulatory arrest. pH stat causes a rightward shift in oxyhemoglobin dissociation (counteracting the leftward shift induced by hypothermia) as well as increasing cerebral blood flow secondary to the cerebral vasodilation induced by CO2. Alternatively the greater blood flow might be more important in the early reperfusion phase. Furthermore reperfusion after ischemia with a more acidotic reperfusate has been shown in models of both myocardial and cerebral ischemia to be associated with reduced ischemic injury (5, 12). This may be because of competition between calcium and hydrogen ions for intracellular entry with calcium ions causing greater injury than hydrogen ions.

To identify which of these mechanisms was predominant, we studied 49 4-week old piglets undergoing 1 h of deep hypothermic circulatory arrest (8). Four groups were defined according to cooling/rewarming strategy: alpha stat during cooling/alpha stat during rewarming, alpha/pH, pH/alpha and pH/pH.

Once again cerebral blood flow was greater with pH-stat than alpha-stat during cooling ($p < 0.001$). Cytochrome a,a3 measured by near infrared spectroscopy (thought to be a measure of mitochondrial oxygen availability though this has not yet been completely validated) became more reduced during cooling with alpha-stat than pH-stat ($p = 0.049$), similar to findings we have noted in clinical studies (7). Recovery of ATP in the initial 45 min of reperfusion was more rapid in the animals in which pH stat was used both during cooling and rewarming compared with the other groups ($p = 0.029$). Recovery of cerebral intracellular pH in the initial 30 min was faster in the pH/pH group compared with the alpha/alpha group ($p = 0.026$). Intracellular pH became more acidic during early reperfusion only in the alpha/alpha group, whereas it showed continuous recovery in the other groups.

We concluded from this study that there are mechanisms in effect during both the cooling and rewarming phases before and after deep hypothermic circulatory arrest which could contribute to an improved cerebral outcome with pH-stat relative to more alkaline strategies.

Current prospective study of pH strategy

Considerable evidence in the literature supports the continuing use of alpha stat for continuous mildly or moderately hypothermic bypass (13). Because of the limitations of the small retrospective study of pH strategy described above (10), we have not reverted to routine use of the pH stat strategy except with cases where multiple aorto-pulmonary collateral vessels are present. However, beginning in 1992, we embarked on a prospective randomized study comparing alpha stat and pH stat. Patients undergoing deep hypothermia either with circulatory arrest or low flow bypass who are less than 9 months old at the time of surgery and who have not undergone previous surgery are eligible. The same perioperative end points are being examined as were used in the previous randomized comparison of circulatory arrest and low flow bypass including continuous EEG monitoring intraoperatively and for 48 h postoperatively. The children return at 1 year of age for neurological and developmental assessment. Preliminary analysis of the results to date with more than 150 patients enrolled has shown an overall markedly reduced incidence of seizures relative to the previous prospective study, perhaps related to a decreased use of circulatory arrest for durations greater than 30 min.

Conclusion

Current methods of hypothermic circulatory arrest are probably associated with subtle degrees of permanent brain injury when extended beyond 30 to 45 min in neonates and young infants. Nevertheless the technique is unavoidable for a number of congenital repairs. Further studies are required to understand better the mechanisms of injury associated with the method which will allow such injury to be minimized.

References

1. Aoki M, Nomura F, Stromski ME et al. (1993) Effects of pH on brain energetics after hypothermic circulatory arrest. Ann Thorac Surg 55: 1093–1103
2. Barratt-Boyes BG (1973) Complete correction of cardiovascular malformations in the first two years of life using profound hypothermia. In: Barratt-Boyes BG, Neutze JM, Harris EA (eds) Heart Disease in Infancy. Edinburgh, Churchill Livingstone, p 35
3. Bellinger DC, Jonas RA, Rappaport LA (1995) Developmental and neurologic status of children after heart surgery with hypothermic circulatory arrest or low-flow cardiopulmonary bypass. N Engl J Med 332: 549–555
4. Bigelow WG, Lindsay WK, Harrison RC (1950) Oxygen transport and utilization in dogs at low body temperatures. Am J Physiol 160: 125–137
5. Bing OH, Brooks WW, Messer JV (1973) Heart muscle viability following hypoxia: protective effect of acidosis. Science 180: 1297–1298
6. Castaneda AR, Norwood WI, Jonas RA (1984) Transposition of the great arteries and intact ventricular septum: anatomical repair in the neonate. Ann Thorac Surg 38: 438–443
7. du Plessis AJ, Newburger J, Jonas RA et al. (1995) Cerebral oxygen supply and utilization during infant cardiac surgery. Ann Neurol 37: 488–497
8. Hiramatsu T, Miura T, Forbess JM (1995) pH strategy and cerebral energetics before and after circulatory arrest. J Thorac Cardiovasc Surg 109: 948–958
9. Jobsis FF (1977) Non-invasive, infra-red monitoring of cerebral and myocardial oxygen sufficiency and circulatory parameters. Science 198: 1264–1267
10. Jonas RA, Bellinger DC, Rappaport LA et al. (1993) Relation of pH strategy and developmental outcome after hypothermic circulatory arrest. J Thorac Cardiovasc Surg 106: 362–368
11. Kawata H, Fackler JC, Aoki M et al. (1993) Recovery of cerebral blood flow and energy state after hypothermic circulatory arrest versus low flow bypass in piglets. J Thorac Cardiovasc Surg 106: 671–685
12. Matsuda N, Kuroda H, Mori T (1991) Beneficial actions of acidotic initial reperfusate in stunned myocardium of rat hearts. Basic Res Cardiol 86: 317–326
13. Murkin JM, Farrar JK, Tweed WA et al. (1987) Cerebral autoregulation and flow/metabolism coupling during cardiopulmonary bypass. The influence of PaCO2. Anesth Anagl 66: 825–832
14. Nevin M, Colchester AC, Adams S, Pepper JR (1987) Evidence for involvement of hypocapnia and hypoperfusion in aetiology of neurological deficit after cardiopulmonary bypass. Lancet 2: 1493–1495
15. Newburger JW, Jonas RA, Wernovsky G (1993) A comparison of the perioperative neurologic effects of hypothermic circulatory arrest versus low flow cardiopulmonary bypass in infant heart surgery. N Engl J Med 329: 1057–1064

16. Reeves RB (1972) An imidazole alphastat hypothesis for vertebrate acid-base regulation: Tissue carbon dioxide content and body temperature in bullfrogs. Resp Physiol 14: 219–236
17. Swan H (1984) The importance of acid-base management for cardiac and cerebral preservation during open heart operations. Surg Gynecol Obstet 158: 391–414
18. Wong PC, Barlow CF, Hickey PR et al. (1992) Factors associated with choreoathetosis after cardiopulmonary bypass in children with congenital heart disease. Circulation 86 (suppl 2): 118–126

Author's address:
R. A. Jonas, M.D.
Children's Hospital
300 Longwood Avenue
Boston, MA 02115, USA

Alteration of cerebral blood flow velocity (CBFV) in neonates and infants after cardiac surgery. Relation to occurrence of cerebral injury?

H. Abdul-Khaliq[1], A. Gamillscheg[1], F. Uhlemann[1], V. Alexi-Meskishvili[2], Y. Weng[2], R. Hetzer[2], P. E. Lange[1]

Abteilung für Angeborene Herzfehler und Kinderkardiologie[1], und Abteilung für Herz, Thorax- und Gefäßchirurgie[2]. Deutsches Herzzentrum Berlin. Berlin, Germany

Introduction

It has been estimated that 10 – 25 % of all infants undergoing cardiac surgery by means of hypothermic cardiopulmonary bypass with or without circulatory arrest suffer transient or permanent neuropsychologic injury (10, 13, 23, 35, 38, 39, 42).

The etiology of cerebral injury associated with cardiac surgery in neonates and infants is considered as multifactorial and has not been clearly understood (13, 16, 38, 42). In addition to the effects of various physiological extremes during cardiopulmonary bypass (CPB) on cerebral blood flow and oxygenation these infants are subjected to other risk factors before and after surgery. Following CPB hyperventilation, low cardiac output, and variation in intravascular volume during the early postoperative period may also contribute to alteration in cerebral hemodynamics and thereby to the possible development of cerebral injury (15, 42). Bellinger et al. found a strong predictive value of adverse neurologic and developmental outcome at 1 year of age in those with evidence of seizure activity during the first 48 postoperative hours after corrective cardiac surgery (13). Alteration of cerebral and cardiac hemodynamics during this postoperative period could also be a contributing risk factor. Changes in cerebral blood flow velocity (CBFV) determined by the Doppler method have been shown to correlate well with the measurements of volumic cerebral blood flow by other invasive methods such as the microsphere, ^{133}Xenon clearance, and positron emmision tomography in neonatal animals and human infants (17, 18, 36).

The objective of this study was to investigate by ultrasonography the relationship between the alteration of cerebrovascular hemodynamics and subsequent occurrence of visible cerebral complications such as intraventricular hemorrhage (IVH) in a homogenous group of term newborn infants with d-transposition of the great arteries (d-TGA) before and after cardiac surgery involving full flow cardiopulmonary bypass.

Methods

Between January 1994 and September 1995, 58 infants below the age of 8 months were consecutively studied by serial cranial ultrasound and cerebral Doppler sonography before and after surgery at the German Heart Centre in Berlin. This paper will be focused on the 27 infants with d-TGA undergoing cardiac surgery of primary and two-stage arterial switch operation. Cerebral blood flow patterns and cardiac hemodynamic parameters in those infants with and without neurological complication such as IVH were compared.

The inclusion criteria for the enrollment of infants with d-TGA in this study group were: term newborn infants with appropriate weight for age, diagnosis of d-TGA with or without ventricular septum defects, and primary arterial switch operation by means of full flow cardiopulmonary bypass (CPB) without circulatory arrest. The exclusion criteria were: preoperatively diagnosed IVH or seizures, the presence of hemodynamically effective residual aortic valve regutation after corrective surgery, and arrythmia with variation in cardiac ejection. Infants undergoing two-stage arterial switch operation for d-TGA beyond the neonatal period because of previous palliative cardiac surgery of associated other heart defects such as coarctation of the aorta, aortopulmonary shunt and pulmonary arterial banding, were included in a separate group.

Full flow cardiopulmonary bypass (120 – 150 ml/kg/min) and moderate hypothermia (20 – 25 °C) were used. The management of the acid base status during CPB was used according to the alpha-stat method. Primary open sternotomy was used to avoid pericardial tamponade and low cardiac output after operation (6).

Serial measurements of cerebral blood flow velocity (CBFV) in the anterior cerebral artery (ACA) and internal carotid artery (ICA) were performed using color Doppler sonography 24 h before surgery, immediately after surgery and thereafter at the intervals, 30 min, 1, 2, 4, 8, and 24 h, and then daily for 6 days. The Doppler measurements in the anterior cerebral artery and the internal carotid artery were carried out using 5 MHz Doppler probe in a standardized localization in the isonated vessels. Using color flow system the vessels were visualized to ensure accurate reproducible placement of the sample volume which was set at 4 mm. Wall filter setting was kept to a minimum of 200 Hz to appreciate low enddiastolic flow signal.

Cerebral blood flow velocity was measured in the internal carotid artery immediately beneath the lateral edge of the sella turcica, in the anterior cerebral artery directly anterior to the third ventricle beneath the lower edge of corpus callosum (3). The Doppler signal was recorded when the sharpest visual and highest audible signals were obtained. In each postoperative examination two consecutive measurements in each infant were performed. The mean of the maximal, the enddiastolic, the flow velocity integral of the area under the flow signal, and the acceleration time of systolic peak flow in three equal heart cycles were documented for further statistical calculation. The resistance index (RI) was calculated according to the formel maximal systolic flow velocity-enddiastolic flow velocity/maximal systolic flow velocity. The flow signal in the left ventricular outflow tract was imaged by color Doppler in subcostal plane, the sample volume was placed immediately over the aortic valve to measure flow velocity integral and acceleration time.

Prior to each Doppler examination, ultrasonography of the brain in standardized planes was performed to assess the presence or absence of intra- and periventricular hemorrhage or other structural abnormalities. Determination of the presence of blood in the germinal matrix and in the lateral ventricle was made by coronal and parasagittal ultrasound scan. The severity of the intraventricular hemorrhage was graded according to the classification by Volpe (45).

Results

From 21 newborn infants with d-TGA who underwent primary arterial switch operation in the neonatal period below the age of 20 days after birth, moderate IVH was detected in 9 newborn infants. All IVH were diagnosed during the first 24 h postoperatively. The severity of hemorrhage was moderate (6/9): 2 infants with IVH grade I, 4 infants with grade II, and 3 with grade III. No IVH was detected in older infants undergoing cardiac surgery beyond the neonatal period (1, 2).

Two infants with IVH grade III developed internal hydrocephalus during the postoperative period and required later ventriculoperiteneal shunts. After 2 weeks the structural changes in the germinal matrix were not more detectable in the the majority of infants.

There was no significant difference in gestational age, birth weight and minimal temperature during CPB between the infants with and without hemorrhage (Table 1). Infants with hemorrhage had a significant longer bypass time ($p < 0.01$) (Table 1). Infants with the two-stage switch operation were nearly 3 months of age at time of operation. In this group, 2 infants had clinical seizure activity, and in 1 infant cerebral infarction in the left middle artery area was diagnosed by cranial tomography. In both groups of newborn infants with and without hemorrhage no significant difference in mean arterial blood pressure and arterial carbon dioxide tension were found (Fig. 4).

In comparison to the preoperative values, cerebral blood flow velocities and FVI decreased significantly following cardiac surgery in all infants during the early postoperative hours (Fig. 2). The preoperative values of RI in newborn infants, who underwent primary switch operation, were significantly higher due to hemodynamically effective patent ductus arteriosus (Fig. 1). In those 9 newborn infants with hemorrhage, the enddiastolic flow velocity was increased, resulting in a significantly lower RI prior to the occurrence of IVH ($p < 0.01$). After surgery, the RI was still significantly higher in the other newborn infants without hemorrhage and increased significantly during the 24 – 72 postoperative hours ($p < 0.01$) in infants with two-stage switch operation (Fig. 1). After the development of IVH, the RI increased significantly for a period of 24 to 48 h (Fig. 1).

Figure 3 shows the flow signal in the anterior cerebral artery immediately after switch operation. Four hours later the enddiastolic flow velocity was markedly increased resulting in lower calculated resistance index. Subsequent ultrasonography scans of the brain showed an intraventricular hemorrhage grade III in the lateral ventricle.

Table 1. Clinical data of the 3 group of infants with d-TGA (mean ± SD). * $p < 0.01$

	Age (day)	Weight (g)	Bypass time (min)	Min. Temp. during CPB (°C)
prim. switch with IVH (n = 9)	10.3 ± 4	3234 ± 317	196 ± 39*	21.7 ± 5
prim. switch without IVH (n = 12)	6.3 ± 1.2	3416 ± 312	161 ± 23	24.8 ± 5.6
two-stage switch-op (n = 7)	85 ± 35	4054 ± 630	159 ± 25	23 ± 5

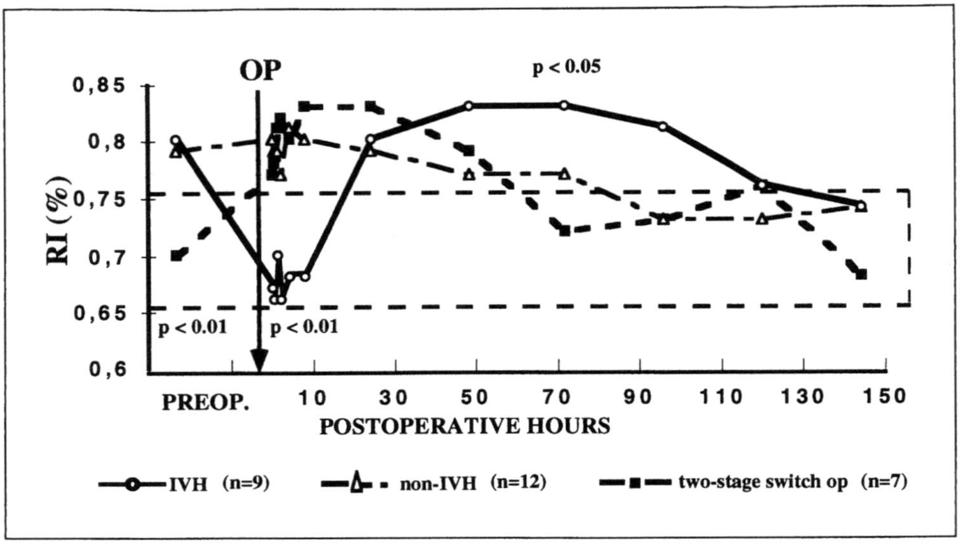

Fig. 1. Mean of resistance index (RI) in the anterior cerebral artery in infants with and without intraventricular hemorrage (IVH) 24 h before and after switch-op. In comparison to older infants with two-stage switch operation the preoperative values of RI in newborn infants who underwent primary switch operation were significantly higher due to hemodynamically effective patent ductus arteriosus ($p < 0.01$). The decreased RI during the early postoperative period in infants with IVH ($p < 0.01$) may indicate higher cerebral perfusion and lower cerebrovascular resistance. The RI increased significantly 48 h after occurrence of IVH ($p < 0.05$).

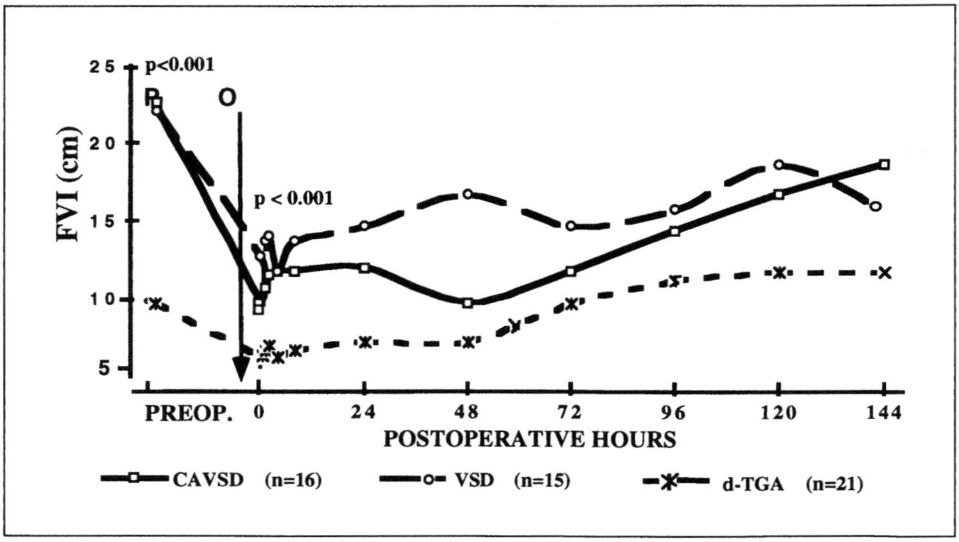

Fig. 2. Mean of flow velocity integral (FVI) in the anterior cerebral artery 24 h before and after surgery in infants with complete atrioventricular septum defect (CAVSD), ventricular septum defect (VSD) and d-transposition of great arteries (d-TGA). There was a significant difference in the preoperative values of FVI between the newborn infants with d-TGA and both groups of older infants with CAVSD and VSD. The immediate fall in FVI values in the early postoperative period in all infants may indicate decreased cerebral perfusion, which is most distinct in infants with CAVSD.

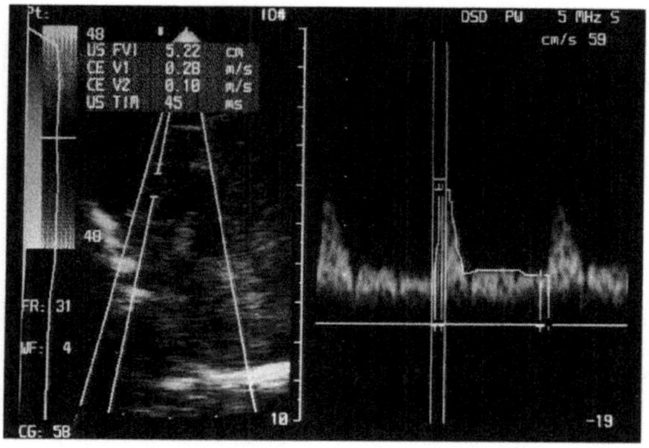

Immediately after surgery

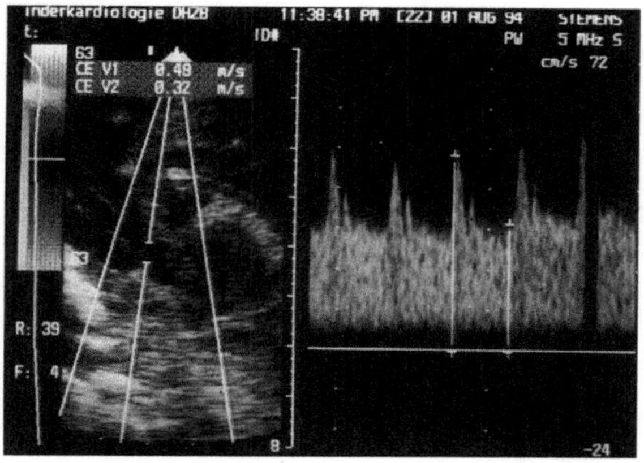

5 hours after surgery

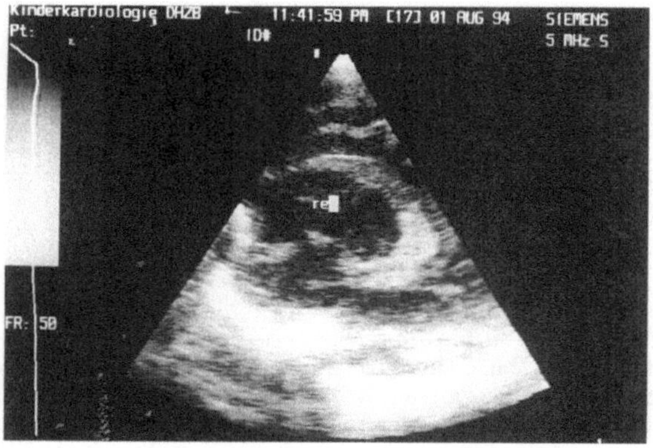

IVH grade III

Fig. 3. Cerebral blood flow velocity patterns in an infant with intraventricular hemorrhage (IVH) after switch operation for transposition of great arteries. Increased enddiastolic flow velocity indicating vasodilation and impaired autoregulation was found prior to the subsequent detection of IVH.

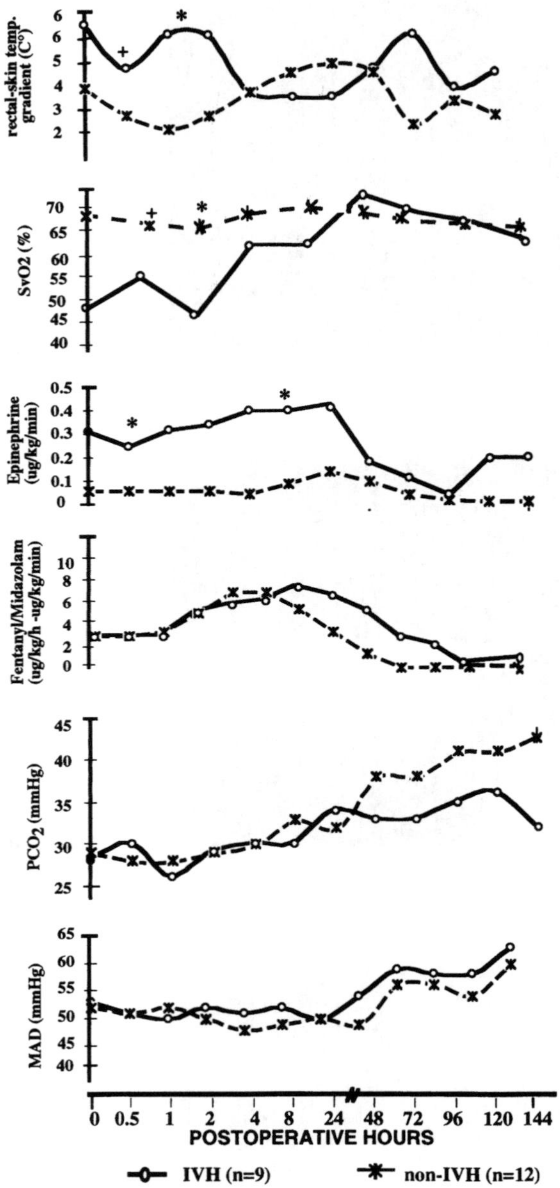

Fig. 4. Sequential measurements (mean) of rectal skin temperature gradient, central venous blood saturation (SvO2), Epinephrine infusion rate, Fentanyl/Midazolam infusion rate, arterial carbon dioxide tension (pCO2) and mean arterial blood pressure (MAD) in infants with intraventricular (IVH) and without intraventricular hemorrhage (non-IVH) after switch operation of transposition of great arteries. Significant differences were found particulary during the first 24 postoperative hours. The change of these hemodynamic parameters may indicate low cardic output and delayed left ventricular adaptation in those infants with IVH particularly during the early postoperative hours.
$+ p < 0.05$. $* p < 0.01$.

The mean values of the flow velocity integral in the left ventricular outflow, which correlates with cardiac output, was significantly lower in the first 4 h postoperatively in the group of infants with hemorrhage.

The sequential measurements of other hemodynamic parameters are summarized in figure 4. The simultaneously measured mean arterial blood pressure and arterial carbon dioxide tension were not significantly different between IVH and non-IVH groups. Rectal-toe-skin temperature gradient was significantly higher in those infants with hemorrhage. Central venous blood saturation during the early postoperative period was significantly lower in those infants who subsequently developed intraventricular hemorrhage. Epinephrine infusion rate was significantly higher in those infants with hemorrhage. The infusion rate of other inotrop and vasodilatative agents were not significantly different. In both groups the infusion rate of Fentanyl and Midazolam during the first 24 postoperative hours was not different. However, infants with hemorrhage were ventilated longer and needed sedation and analgesation for a longer time.

Discussion

The occurrence of intraventricular hemorrhage (IVH) in a homogeneous group of term newborn infants following a uniform procedure of cardiac surgery such as the switch operation has not been studied. Although IVH is still an important neurological complication of premature infants below the 32nd week of gestational age, it is not as common in term infants (20, 22, 35, 45). However, the fact that all detected intracerebral hemorrhages in our studied infants after switch operation occurred in the germinal matrix may indicate similar pathogenesis as in premature infants. The significantly higher enddiastolic flow velocity resulting in lower calculated resistance index (RI) and thereby in a possible higher cerebral perfusion, which was found in the IVH group during the first postoperative hours (Fig. 1) may indicate vasodilation and possible impairment of cerebral autoregulation (8, 33, 43, 44). This interpretation is supported by the association of vasoparalysis and abolished autoregulation with cerebral damage in asphyxiated term infants (32) and following hypoxia in an experimental newborn lamb model (41). Increased enddiastolic flow velocity indicating hyperperfusion was also observed in similar Doppler studies in term newborn infants following birth asphyxia (8, 43, 44), during seizures (33), and in premature infants prior to subsequent onset of IVH (4, 8, 21, 43).

The distinctive localization of the hemorrhage within the choriod plexus and germinal matrix, the oldest phyogenetic brain region with rich capillary network (24), may be an expression of the functional (83) and structural (30, 40) vulnerability of this cerebrovascular region not only in the premature but also in the term infants. Similar to the premature infants the choroid plexus and germinal matrix vessels also remain extremely vulnerable to hypotension in term infants (29, 38). Low capability of autoregulation in the germinal matrix was also demonstrated in newborn beagle puppies (29). In infants undergoing cardiac surgery by means of hypothermic CPB, impairment of the metabolism of endothelial vasoactive substances , which play an important role in the regulation of cerebrovascular tone (12, 19, 24, 25), could not be excluded. In an experimental animal model, the combination of hypoxia with variations in cerebral intravascular pressure was the most effective method to produce hemorrhage in the geminal matrix (7, 14, 26, 29). Similar cardiovascular and cerebrovascular hemodynamic reactions which include variation in perfusion pressure of non-pulsative CPB followed by reperfusion may predispose to cerebral vascular injury and IVH in this vulnerable area of the brian (9, 14, 26, 27, 29).

Furthermore, during the early postoperative period following switch operation myocardial dysfunction and delayed left ventricular adaptation may also play an additive etiological role. However, the same perfusion pressure in both groups of our studied infants (Fig. 4) may not reflect equal cardiac output, since there was a significant difference in those hemodynamic parameters, which pointed at altered left ventricular function and low cardiac output in the infants with IVH, such as mixed venous blood saturation, rectal peripheral skin temperature gradient (5) and epinephrine infusion rate during the first 24 postoperative hours (Fig. 4). The intra- and postoperative course in the infants with IVH was more complicated than those without hemorrhage, being longer ventilated and needing significantly more epinephrine. These cardiovascular hemodynamic results (Fig. 4) and the corresponding change in cerebral blood flow velocity patterns in infants with IVH (Fig. 2) may be in accordance with other Doppler studies, which demonstrated an increase in cerebral enddiastolic flow velocity as a result of loss of cerebral autoregulation in infants with myocardial dysfunction following birth asphyxia (44).

Although other cerebral and hemodynamic changes before cardiac surgery may also act as contributing factors, we did not find any relationships between the preoperative change in CBVF patterns and the occurrence of IVH after surgery (Fig. 1). All newborn infants with and without postoperative IVH had a hemodynamically effective patent ductus resulting in decreased values of flow velocity integral (FVI) (Fig. 2) and increased RI (Fig. 1) (43, 46). The magnitude and duration of postnatal hypoxia and low oxygenation prior to the diagnosis of the cyanotic heart defect and the start of prostaglandine therapy was difficult to evaluate because our infants were admitted from external neonatal units. Silent hypoxic cerebral events in our studied infants during this period coud not be excluded. The perinatal clinical data in both groups were not significantly different. Seizure activity and IVH grade I–II was diagnosed preoperatively in 2 infants who were excluded from this cohort.

We suggest that altered cerebral hemodynamics may be a contributing factor inducing cerebral injury after cardiac surgery in hemodynamically unstable newborn infants. Serial determinations of cerebral blood flow velocity in these infants by Doppler sonography may provide an additional method to identify those at increased risk. The immediate postoperative period following CPB should be considered as a vulnerable critical phase. The prognostic neurological value of these observations will be determined in folllow-up studies.

References

1. Abdul-Khaliq H, Gamillscheg A, Berger F, Uhlemann F, Alexi-Meskishvili V, Weng Y, Hetzer R, Lange PE (1995) Cerebral blood flow velocities (CBFV) in neonates and infants before and after corrective repair of congenital heart defects by means of cardiopulmonary bypass (CPB). Pediatric Res 37: A229
2. Abdul-Khaliq H, Gammelscheg A, Uhlemann F, Berger F, Alexi-Meskishvili V, Weng Y, Hetzer R, Lange PE (1995) Cerebral blood flow velocity (CBFV) in relation to occurrence of intraventricular hemorrhage (IVH) in newborn infants following corrective surgery of transposition of great arteries (d-TGA) by means of cardiopulmonary bypass (CPB). J Neuroimaging 5 (suppl. 2): A33
3. Abdul-Khaliq H, Segerer H, Luck W, Obladen M (1993) Increased cerebral blood flow velocity in newborn infants of smoking mothers. Eur J Pediatrics 152: 232–235
4. Ahmann PA, Dykes FD, Lazzara A, Holt PJ, Giddens DP, Carrigan T (1983) Relationship between pressure passivity and subepenymal/intraventricular hemorrhage as assessed by pulsed Doppler ultrasound. Pediatrics 72: 665–669

5. Alexi-Meskishvili V, Popov SA, Nikoljuk AP (1984) Evaluation of hemodynamics in infants and small babies after heart surgery. Thorac Cardiovasc Surgeon 32: 4–9
6. Alexi-Meskishvili V, Weng Y, Uhlemann F, Lange PE, Hetzer R (1996) Prolonged open-heart sternotomy after pediatric open heart operation: experience with 113 patients. Ann thorac Surg (in press)
7. Ashwal S, Dale PS, Longo LD (1984) Regional cerebral blood flow: studies in the fetal lamb during hypoxia, hypercapnia, acidosis, hypotension. Pediatric Res 18: 1309–1316
8. Bada HS, Hajjar W, Chue C, Summner DS (1979) Noninvasive diagnosis of neonatal asphyxia and intraventricular hemorrhage by Doppler ultrasound. J Pediatr 95: 775–779
9. Bada HS, Korones SB, Perry E et al. (1990) Mean arterial blood pressure changes in premature infants and those at risk for intraventricular hemorrhage. J Pediatr 117: 607–14
10. Bellinger DC, Jonas RA, Rapport LA et al. (1995) Developmental and neurologic status of children after heart surgery with hypothermic circulatory arrest of low-flow cardiopulmonary bypass. N Engl J Med 332: 549–55
11. Brent WA, Martin CG, Alexander BJ, Chen T, Fleming LR (1991) Autoregulation of brain blood flow during hypotension and hypertension in infant lamb. Pediatric Res 29: 110–115
12. Edmunds LH (1993) Vasoactive substances released during CPB. Pathophysiology and techniques of cardiopulmonary bypass. 14th annual San Diego Cardiothoracic Surgery Symposium: 60–66
13. Ferry PC (1990) Neurologic sequelae of open-heart surgery in children. AJDC 144: 369–373
14. Goddard-Finegold J, Michael LH (1984) Cerebral blood flow and experimental intraventricular hemorrhage. Pediatr Res 18: 7–11
15. Greeley WJ, Ungerleider RM, Kern FH, Brusino FG, Smith R, Revers JG (1989) Effects of cardiopulmonary bypass on cerebral blood flow in neonates, infants, and children. Circulation 80 (Suppl. I) I: 209–215
16. Greeley WJ, Kern FH, Mault JR, Ungerleider R (1993) Mechanism of injury and methods of protection, during cardiac surgery in neonates and infants. Cardiol Young 3: 317–330
17. Greisen G, Johansen K, Ellison PH, Fredriksen PS, Mali J, Friis-Hansen B (1984) Cerebral blood flow in the newborn infants: Comparison of Doppler ultrasound and 133 Xenon clearance. J Pediatr 104: 411–418
18. Hansen NB, Stonestreet BS, Rosenkrantz TS, Oh W (1983) Validity of Doppler measurements of anterior cerebral artery blood flow velocity: Correlation with brain blood flow in piglets. Pediatrics 27: 526–531
19. Heros RC, Zervas NT, Varsos V (1983) Cerebral vasospasm after subarachnoid hemorrhage: An Update. Ann Neurol 14: 599–608
20. Hill A, Volpe JJ (1985) Pathogenesis and management of hypoxic-ischemic encephalopathy in the term newborn. Neurologic Clinics 3 (1): 31–46
21. Hill A, Perlman JM, Volpe JJ (1982) Relation of pneumothorax to occurrence of intraventricular hemorrhage in the premature newborn. Pediatrics 69: 144–149
22. Hayden CK, Shattuck KE, Richardsen CJ, Ahrendt DK, House R, Swischuk LE (1985) Subependymal germinal matrix hemorrhage in full-term neonates. Pediatrics 75: 714–718
23. Keck EW, Kimm E, Grävinghoff L, Sieg K, Lagenstein I, Kühne D (1981) Neurologische Veränderung und zerebrale Läsionen bei Kindern mit Transposition der großen Arterien (TGA). Monatsschr Kinderheilkd 129: 45–47
24. Longo LD, Pearce WJ (1991) Fetal and newborn cerebral vascular response and adaptations to hypoxia. Sem Perinatol 15: 49–57
25. Leuschen MP, Ehrenfried JA, Willet LD et al. (1991) Prostaglandin F1æ levels during and after extracorporeal membrane oxygenation. J Thorac Cardiovasc Surg 101: 148–152
26. Ment LR, Stewart WB, Duncan CC, Lambrecht R (1982) Beagle puppy model of intraventricular hemorrhage. J Neurosurg 57: 219–223
27. Merhabani D, Gowen CW, Kopelman AE (1991) Association of pneumothorax and hypotension with intraventricular hemorrhage. Arch Dis Child 66: 48–51
28. Newburger JW, Jonas RA, Wernowsky G et al. (1993) A comparison of the perioperative neurologic effects of hypothermic circulatory arrest versus low flow cardiopulmonary bypass in infant heart surgery. N Engl J Med 329: 1057–64
29. Pasternak JF, Groothuis DR, Fisher JM, Fisher DP (1983) Regional cerebral blood flow in the beagle puppy model of neonatal intraventricular hemorrhage: studies during systemic hypertension. Neurology 33: 559–566
30. Pearce WJ, Ashwal S (1987) Developmental changes in thickness, contractility, and hypoxic sensitivity of newborn lamb cerebral arteries. Pediatric Res 22: 192–196
31. Pyrds O (1991) Control of cerebral circulation in the high-risk neonate. Ann neurol 30: 321–329
32. Pyrds O, Greisen G, Lou H, Friis-Hansen B (1990) Vasoparalysis associated with brain damage in asphyxiated term infants. J Pediatr 117: 119–125
33. Raju TNK (1991) Cerebral Doppler studies in the fetus and newborn infants. J Pediatr 119: 165–174
34. Rogers BT, Msall ME, Buck GM, Lyon NR, Norris MK, Roland JMA, Gingell RL, Cleveland DC, Pieroni DR (1995) Neurodevelopmental outcome of infants with hypoplastic left heart syndrome. J Pediatr 126: 496–498

35. Ronald EH, Flodmark O, Hill A (1990) Thalamic hemorrhage with intraventricular hemorrhage in the full-term newborn. Pediatrics 85: 737–742
36. Rosenberg AA, Narayanan V, Jones MD (1985) Comparison of anterior cerebral blood flow velocity and cerebral blood flow during hypoxia. Pediatr Res 19: 67–70
37. Swain JA (1995) Cardiac surgery and the brain. N Eng J Med 329: 1119–1118
38. Szymonowicz W, Walker AM, YU VYH, Stewart ML, Cannata J, Cussen L (1990) Regional cerebral blood flow after hemorrhagic hypotension in the preterm, near-term, and newborn lamb. Pediatric Res 28: 361–366
39. Tam VKH, Cameron DE (1993) Cerebral blood flow following hypothermic circulatory arrest. Cardiol Young 3: 281–286
40. Trommer BL, Groothuis DR, Pasternak (1987) Quantitative analysis of cerebral vessels in the newborn puppy: the structure of germinal matrix vessels may predispose to hemorrhage. Pediatric Res 22: 23–28
41. Tweed A, Cote J, Lou H, Gregory G, Wade J (1986) Impairment of cerebral blood flow autoregulation in the newborn lamb by hypoxia. Pediatric Res 20: 516–519
42. Ungerleider RM (1994) Cerebral response to CPB in neonates and infants. Pathophysiology and techniques of cardiopulmonary bypass. 14th annual San Diego Cardiothoracic Surgery Symposium: 88–98
43. Van Bel F, Van der Bor M, Stijinsen T, Baan J, Ruys JH (1987) Aetiological role of cerebral blood flow alterations in development and extension of peri-intraventricular haemorrhage. Dev Med Child Neurol 29: 601–614
44. Van Bel F, Walther FJ (1990) Myocardial dysfunction and cerebral blood flow velocity following birth asphyxia. Acta Paediatr Scand 179: 756–762
45. Volpe JJ (1995) Intracranial hemorrhage: subdural, primary subarachnoid, intracerebellar, intraventricular (term infant), and miscellaneous. Volpe JJ, ed. Neurology of the Newborn. 3rd ed. Philadelphia: W. B. Saunders: 211–463
46. Wright LL, Baker KR, Hollander DI, Wright JN, Nagy DA (1988) Cerebral blood flow velocity in term newborn infants: changes associated with ductal flow. J Peditr 112: 768–73

Author's address:
H. Abdul-Khaliq M.D.
Abteilung für Angeborene Herzfehler und Kinderkardiologie
Deutsches Herzzentrum Berlin
Augustenburgerplatz 1
13353 Berlin, Germany

Change of regional cerebral hemoglobin saturation (rSO_2) in children undergoing corrective cardiac surgery of congenital heart disease by means of high-flow cardiopulmonary bypass (CPB)

H. Abdul-Khaliq[1], T. Weipert[1], V. Alexi-Meskishvili[2], Y. Weng[2], R. Hetzer[2], P. E. Lange[1]

Abteilung für Angeborene Herzfehler und Kinderkardiologie[1],
und Abteilung für Herz-Thorax- und Gefäßchirurgie[2]. Deutsches Herzzentrum Berlin. Berlin, Germany

Introduction

Neuropsychological morbidity following cardiac surgery of congenital heart disease (CHD) – considered to be most likely due to alterations of cerebral oxygenation and hemodynamics – could possibly be in part prevented by early detection by means of continuous non-invasive monitoring during and after cardiac surgery (8, 11, 12). However, determination of capillary blood saturation is limited during non-pulsatile CPB. Continuous monitoring of regional cerebral blood saturation (rSO_2) by near infrared spectroscopy (NIRS) may provide qualitative information on cerebral oxygen supply and consumption, since a significant correlation was found between the spectroscopic measurement of rSO_2 and the invasive (1) and noninvasive (14) determination of cerebral venous blood saturation in the jugular bulb. The aim of this study therefore was to investigate the relationship between the change in rSO_2 and other hemodynamic parameters during the different stages of CPB in a heterogeneous group of infants and children undergoing corrective and palliative cardiac surgery by means of high flow CPB.

Methods

In 32 children and infants (15 children with cyanotic CHD, age 1 week-9 years, median 3 years, and 17 children with non-cyanotic CHD, age 2–16 years, median 6 years) undergoing surgical correction by means of high flow cardiopulmonary bypass (CPB) (120–150 ml/Kg/BW) with moderate hypothermia (30 ± 3 °C) were studied. Total circulatory arrest was used only in three infants. Continuous measurement of rSO_2 was performed using a two channel cerebral oximeter (INVOS 3100A, Somanitics, USA). The sensor with a light source and superficial and deep receiver was placed in standardized localization at the left temporal head side (Fig. 1). The alpha stat method for management of acid base status was used. Conventional hemodynamic parameters were simultaneously documented. The mean of three representative 5-min periods of spectroscopic measurements for each of the following periods were compared. A: before CPB, B: begin of CPB, C: clamp of the aorta,

D: minimum of rSO_2 during CPB, E: after rewarning/reperfusion, F: stop of CPB, G: closure of the Thorax (Fig. 2).

Results

Before CPB the mean values of rSO_2 in children with cynotic congenital heart disease (CHD) were significantly lower ($p = 0.002$) than those with non-cyanotic CHD (Fig. 2). After the onset of cardiopulmonary bypass (CPB) there was a continuous fall in the regional cerebral hemoglobin saturation (rSO_2), which reached minimal values within 15–40 min ($p < 0.01$) (Fig. 2).

During and after CPB rSO_2 was nearly 8–10 % lower but not significantly different (Fig. 2). An abrupt decrease in mean arterial blood pressure (MAD), hemoglobin concentration (Hb) and central venous pressure (CVP) which were associated with the aortic cannulation and hemodilution did not have a significant abrupt effect on the alterations of rSO_2, which fell gradully (Fig. 2). During CPB the MAD was kept in a range between 40 and 50 mmHg. After the end of CPB nearly pre-CPB values were observed. After rewarming and

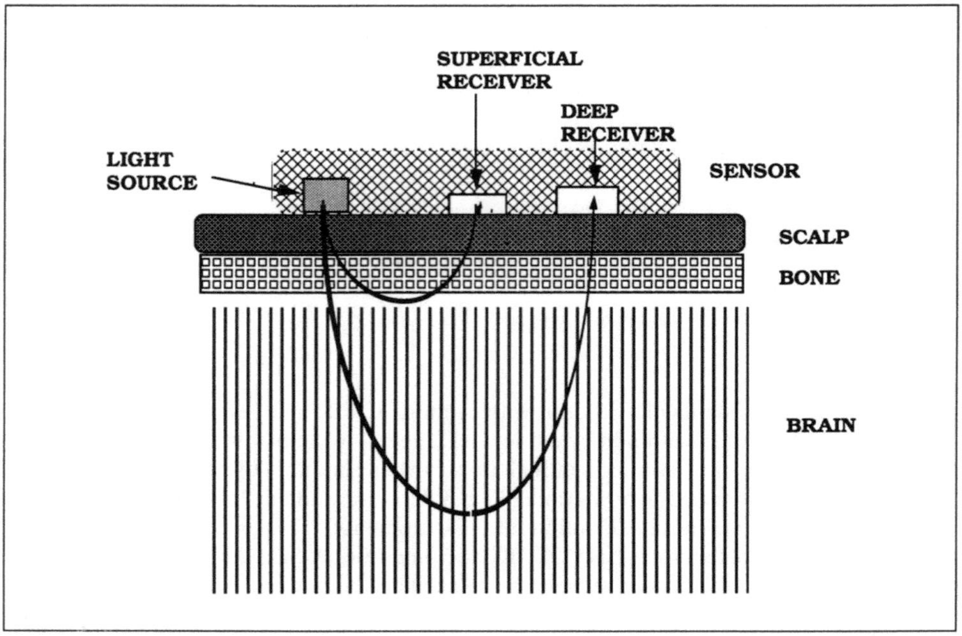

Fig. 1. The sensor with a light source and superficial and deep receivers was placed in standardized localization at the left temporal head side. The reflected signal from the superficial vessels in scalp and bone is substracted from the displayed calculated value of regional cerebral hemoglobin saturation (rSO_2).

cessation of CPB rSO_2 decreased up to 15 % in individual patients, especially in young infants. Before, during and after CPB a significant decrease in arterial pO_2 or perfusion pressure was associated with prompt decrease in rSO_2 (Fig. 2). There was no significant correlation between the change in rSO_2 and MAD, CVP, Hb and body temperature in all infants during the period of monitoring.

Figure 3 demonstrates the orginal monitor values of rSO_2 in a cyanotic infant for a period of 10 h during palliative surgery of a complex pulmonary atresia by means of high

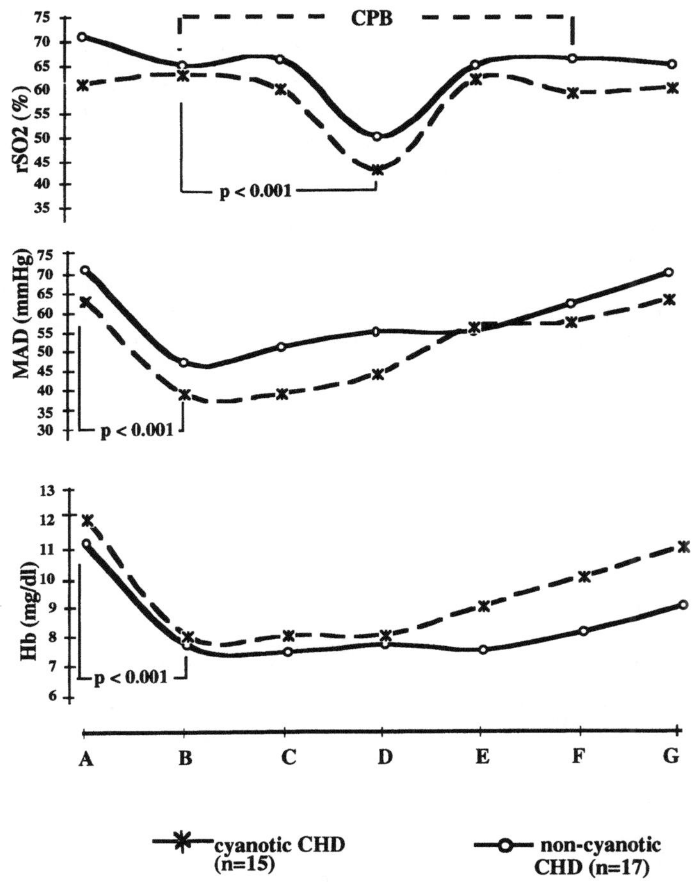

Fig. 2. Mean values of sequential measurement of regional cerebral hemoglobin saturation (rSO_2), mean arterial blood pressure (MAD) and hemoglobin concentration (Hb) during corrective cardiac surgery of cyanotic and non-cynotic congenital heart disease (CHD) by means of full flow cardiopulmonary bypass (CPB). A = before CPB, B = begin of CPB, C = clamp of the aorta, D = minimum of rSO_2 during CPB, E = after reperfusion, F = end of CPB, G = thorax closure. Aortic cannulation and initiation of CPB was associated with abrupt fall in MAD and Hb, where rSO_2 decreased gradually and reached minimal values after 15–40 min of CPB.

flow CPB and total circulatory arrest (TCA). After the start of CPB rSO_2 increased. Cooling resulted in an initial increase in rSO_2 up to 30 %. However, there was a continuous fall in rSO_2 during total circulatory arrest with prompt rise after reperfusion (Fig. 3).

Discussion

Because intracranial blood has been estimated to be 70 % venous (13), determination of cerebral hemoglobin oxygen saturation (rSO_2) by near-infrared spectroscopy (NIRS) may reflect mainly venous blood saturation. We have recently validated this method invasively and found a good correlation ($r = 0.95$, $p = 0.001$) between the spectroscopic measurement of rSO_2 by NIRS and oxymetric measurement of venous blood oxygen saturation in the jugular bulb, as determined during routine diagnostic cardiac catheterization by manipulating the catheter into the jugular bulb in 30 infants and children (1). Thus, it seems possible that continuous non-invasive monitoring of regional cerebral blood saturation during the different stages of hypothermic cardiopulmonary bypass (CPB) (Figs. 1 and 2) may provide qualitative information on change in global cerebral oxygen consumption (7, 8, 10).

During hypothermic CPB the cerebral metabolic rate for oxygen was found to be reduced due to decreased cerebral flow and cross brain oxygen extraction as determined by invasive methods (3, 6, 7). If the arterial oxygen supply and delivery during hypothermic high flow cardiopulmonary bypass is assumed to be constant, rSO_2 – correlating with

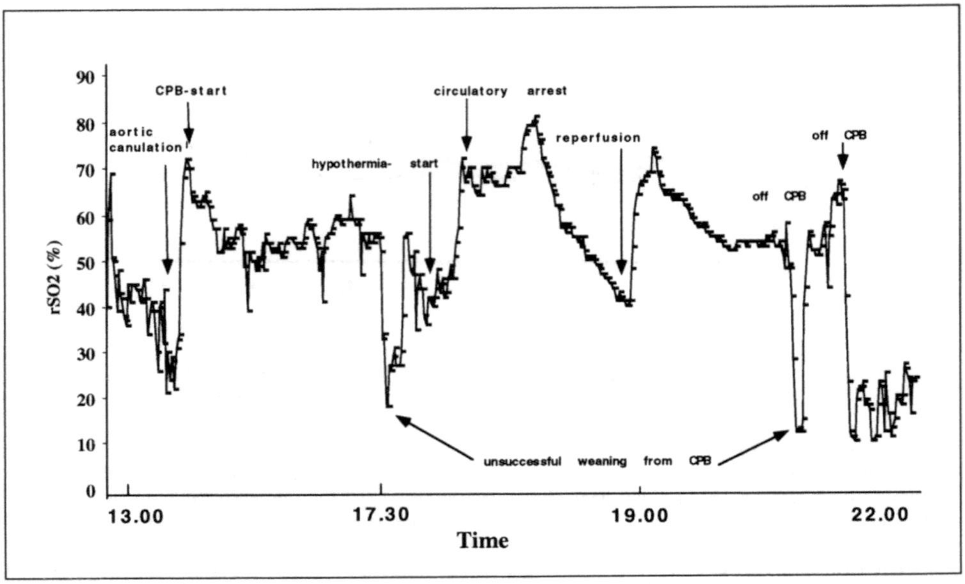

Fig. 3. Original $rSaO_2$ values in a 3-month-old cyanotic infant during cardiac surgery by means of high flow CPB and total circulatory arrest in deep hypothermia (16 °C).

cerebral venous blood saturation – should be increased due to lower brain oxygen consumption. However, we found a significant gradual decrease in rSO_2 after the begin of CPB and moderate cooling indicating either a possible decrease of cerebral blood flow or decrease of cross-brain oxygen extraction during non-pulsatile hypothermic CPB. Insufficient delivery of oxygen or alteration of the affinity and diffusion of hemoglobin for oxygen during hypothermic cardiopulmonary bypass however cannot be excluded. Increased cerebrovascular resistance associated with non-pulsatile flow or the alkaline pH stat strategy (11) which was demonstrated during and after non-pulsatile CPB (12) in previous studies, may also probably play an additional role in the alteration of cerebral oxygenation.

In those patients who underwent cardiac surgery in deep hypothermia (temp < 20 °C), rSO_2 increased initially after cooling probably reflecting lower brain oxygen consumption and thereby possible higher cross-brain oxygen extraction than those with moderate hypothermia (Fig. 3) (5, 9). However, during total circulatory arrest rSO_2 decreased gradually, indicating active cerebral metabolism and oxygen utilization in absence of blood supply. After the renewed institution of CPB, rSO_2 increased abruptly reflecting improvement of cerebral oxygen delivery (Fig. 3).

In addition, age, weight and kind of congenital heart disease itself may contribute to the alterations and pattern of changes in rSO_2 before and during CPB (Fig. 2). The rSO_2 values in cyanotic infants were significantly lower ($p < 0.01$) than those with non-cyanotic congenital heart disease before CPB (Fig. 2). In addition, the lowest minimal values of rSO_2 during and after CPB were found in preoperatively cyanotic infants. Other conventional registered hemodynamic data such as mean arterial blood pressure, arterial oxygen saturation and carbon dioxide tension seem to have no statistical influence on the change of rSO_2 during moderate hypothermic high flow CPB.

The statistically not significant correlation which was found between the change in rSO_2 and mean arterial blood pressure may support the suggestion of Kern et al. (1995) that there is an intact cerebral perfusion pressure-flow autoregulation during the moderate hypothermic CPB (11, 12). A contributing effect of hemodilution which occurred abruptly following aortic cannulation (Fig. 2) can be expected, but could not be proved, since no significant correlation was found between the change in rSO_2 and hemoglobin concentration during the different stages of CPB.

The determination of rSO_2 by NIRS may reflect only a change in intravascular hemoglobin oxygenation. A discrepancy between the change in the intravascular and intracellular oxygen metabolism was found during reperfusion and rewarming following cardiac surgery involving deep hypothermic CPB with total circulatory arrest in newborn and infants (4, 7). Other studies have previously demonstrated a corresponding change in the concentration of oxygenated hemoglobin and intracellular oxycytochrom during moderate hypothermic low flow CPB (2, 5, 7).

In conclusion, the change of cerebral oxygenation independent of the change in conventional hemodynamic parameters and arterial blood oxygenation confirm the necessity of separate monitoring of cerebral oxygenation and hemodynamics during and after cardiac surgery in infants and children. The rewarming and total circulatory arrest should be considered as a vulnerable phase for alteration of cerebral oxygenation and possible development of cerebral injury, particularly in young infants. Further follow-up studies are necessary to evaluate the neurological significance of the magnitude and duration of the decreased change in rSO_2 during and after CPB.

References

1. Abdul-Khaliq H, Berger F, Dähnert I, Nürnberg J, Lange PE (1996) Relationship between regional cerebral hemoglobin saturation (rSO_2) and jugular venous oxygen saturation ($SjVO_2$) in infants and children (in preparation)
2. Abdul-Khaliq H, Uhlemann, Nürnberg J, Berger F, Weng Y, Alexi-Meskishvili V, Hetzer R, Lange PE (1995) Monitoring of cerebral oxygenation during extracorporeal circulation (ECC) in children undergoing cardiac surgery. (Pilot study). Intensive Care Med 21 (Suppl 1): 30
3. Cook DJ, Anderson RE, Michenfelder JD, Oliver WC, Orszulak TA, Daly RC, Bryce RD (1995) Cerebral blood flow during cardiac operations: Comparison of Kety-Schmidt and Xenon-133 Clearance methods. Ann Thorac Surg 59: 614–620
4. Du Plessis AJ, Newburger J, Jonas RA, Hickey P, Naruse H, Tsuji M, Walsh A, Walter G, Wypij D, Volpe JJ (1995) Cerebral oxygen supply and utilization during infant cardiac surgery. Ann Neurology 37: 488–497
5. Fallon P, Roberts I, Kirkham FJ, Elliot MJ, Lloyd-Thomas, Maynard R, Edwards AD (1993) Cerebral hemodynamics during cardiopulmonary bypass in children using near-infrared spectroscopy. Ann Thorac Surg 56: 1473–1477
6. Frewen T, Kisson N, Kronick J, Fov M, Lee R, Bradwin N, Chance G (1991) Cerebral blood flow, cross-brain oxygen extraction, and fontanelle pressure after hypoxic-ischemic injury in newborn infants. J Pediatr 118: 265–271
7. Greeley WJ, Bracey VA, Ungerleider RM, Greibel JA, Kern FH, Boyed JL, Reves JG, Piantadosi CA (1991) Recovery of cerebral metabolism and mitochondrial oxidation state is delayed after hypothermic circulatory arrest. Circulation 84 (suppl III): III-400–III-406
8. Greeley WJ, Ungerleider RM (1991) Assessing the effect of cardiopulmonary bypass on the brain. Ann Thorac Surg 52: 417–419
9. Groughwell N, Smith LR, Quill T, Neuman M, Greeley W, Kern F, Lu J, Rves JG (1992) The effect of temperature on cerebral metabolism and blood flow in adults during cardiopulmonary bypass. J Thoracic Cardiovasc Surg 103: 549–554
10. Gruz J, Raps EC, Hoffstad, OJ, Jaggi JL, Gennarelli TA (1993) Cerebral oxygenation monitoring (Review). Critical Care Medicine 21: 1242–1246
11. Kern FH, Hickey PR (1994) The effect of cardiopulmonary bypass on the brain. In: Jonas RA and Elliott MJ (eds) Cardiopulmonary Bypass in Neonates, Infants and Young children, 1st. ed. Oxford, Butterworth-Heinemann, pp 263–281
12. Kern FH, Greeley WJ, Ungerleider RM (1995) Cardiopulmonary bypass. In: Nichols DG (eds) Critical Heart Disease in Infants and Children, 1st. ed. St. Louis, Missouri, Mosby, pp 496–529
13. McCormick PW, Stewart M, Goetting MG, Dujovny M, Lewis G, Ausman JI (1991) Noninvasive cerebral optical spectroscopy for monitoring cerebral oxygen delivery and hemodynamics. Critical Care Medicine 19: 89–97
14. Wickramasinghe YABD, Livera LN, Spencer SA, Roffe P, Thorniley MS (1992) Plethysmographic validation of near infrared spectroscopic monitoring of cerebral blood volume. Arch Dis Child 67: 407–411

Authors' address:
H. Abdul-Khaliq M.D.
Abteilung für Angeborene Herzfehler und Kinderkardiologie
Deutsches Herzzentrum Berlin
Augustenburger Platz 1
13353 Berlin, Germany

The relation between arterial oxygen tension and cerebral blood flow during cardiopulmonary bypass

G. Chow[1], I. G. Roberts[2], P. Fallon[1], M. Onoe[1], A. Lloyd-Thomas[1], M. J. Elliott[1], A. D. Edwards[2], F. J. Kirkham[1]

[1] Great Ormond Street Hospital for Children, London, England
[2] Department of Paediatrics and Neonatal Medicine, Royal Postgraduate Medical School, London, England

Introduction

Neurological impairment occurs in up to 25 % of all infants and children undergoing hypothermic cardiopulmonary bypass (CPB) (3). In our unit, a recent survey found a 6 % incidence of acute neurological disturbance (2).

The normal range of arterial oxygen tension (PaO_2) in humans varies from about 9 – 14 kPa, but during CPB, PaO_2 may range from 10 kPa to above 40 kPa. There is evidence from studies in animals that an elevated PaO_2 causes vasoconstriction under normal conditions (1). If this occurs during CPB in addition to CBF reduction via other mechanisms, CBF might be reduced to low enough levels to cause ischaemic brain damage. A previous study in adults undergoing CPB showed a vasoconstrictor effect of high PaO_2 (4). During CPB, arterial oxygen tension can vary widely and may rise very high because of the efficiency of the blood gas delivery system. Little is known about the effect of high oxygen tension on CBF in children under these circumstances, when other changes may be occurring, for example in pump flow or temperature.

Near infrared spectroscopy

Biological tissues are relatively transparent to light in the near infrared spectrum (700 – 1000 nm), as first described by Jobsis in 1977 (5). Within the brain the two main absorbers of near infrared light (chromophores) are oxyhaemoglobin (HbO_2) and deoxyhaemoglobin (Hb). Changes in concentration of these chromophores can be calculated from measured changes in light absorption at the wavelengths used. CBF can be estimated using a modification of the Fick principle which employs indocyanine green (ICG) as an intravascular and non-diffusible tracer (6).

Aims

Our hypothesis was that increasing PaO_2 during CPB decreases CBF. We have used near infrared spectroscopy (NIRS) to test this hypothesis through the range of oxygen tensions used in normal clinical practice.

Patients and methods

Patients

Fifteen patients, median age 1 year, 6 months (range 1 month to 10 years, 11 months), undergoing open surgical correction of congenital heart defects, were studied.

Cardiopulmonary bypass management

CPB was conducted using hypothermic haemodilution techniques using a non-pulsatile roller pump (Stöckert, Munich, Germany) and membrane oxygenator (701 or 702, Dideco, Mirandola, Italy). The alpha-stat method of arterial blood gas management was used. Measurements were made during steady-state hypothermic bypass (14.9° to 34.6 °C).

Experimental protocol

A commercial spectrophotometer (NIRO 500, Hamamatsu, Hamamatsu City, Japan) was used. Light at four wavelengths (776, 819, 843 and 913 nm) was conveyed to the child's head via a flexible fibre optic bundle which terminated in an optode that was applied to the frontoparietal region of the child's head after induction of anaesthesia. Transmitted light emerging was collected via another optode and fibre optic bundle leading to the photon detector in the spectrophotometer. Measurements were displayed instantaneously and stored on computer disc for subsequent analysis.

The arterial concentration of tracer was optically quantified by using a fibreoptic probe and dye densitometer (Pulsion Medizintechnik, Munich, Germany) with the probe placed in the arterial line of the CPB circuit at its junction to the aorta. ICG (0.1 $mg \cdot kg^{-1}$) was injected upstream to this probe (Fig. 1).

CPB conditions were considered to have reached steady-state when the PaO_2 and the temperature were stable. The oxygen saturation was kept at > 99 %.

The PaO_2 was altered in temperature uncorrected increments from 10 kPa to up to 60 kPa. Ten minutes after each increment of approximately 10 kPa, two successive measurements of CBF were made in rapid succession, with each change of oxygen tension at approximately 15 minute intervals.

Results

Cerebral blood flow measurements

A total of 168 measurements were made during stable hypothermia in the 15 patients. Multivariate analysis shows that pump flow is the only variable with a significant relation to CBF.

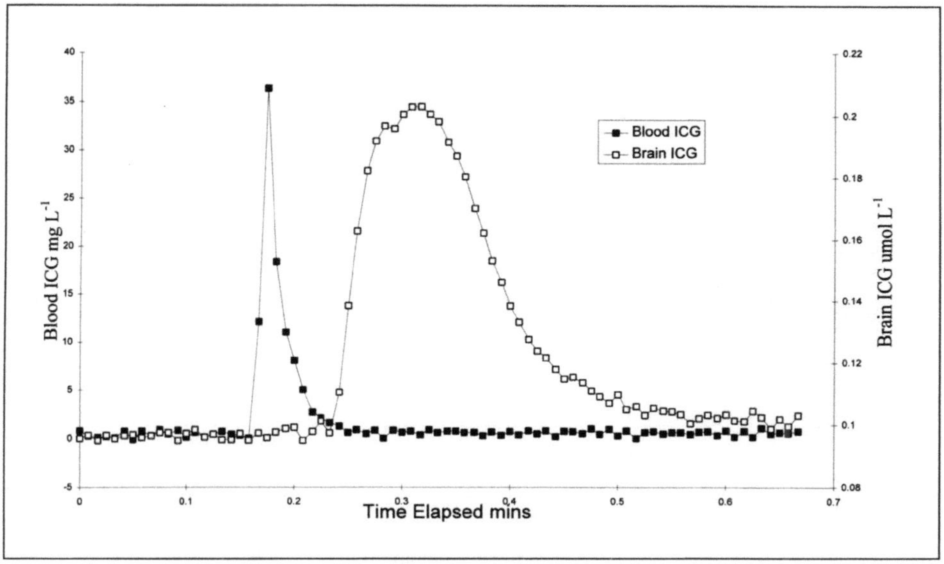

Fig. 1. Blood and brain concentrations of indocyanine green after injection of dye into the cardiopulmonary bypass circuit.

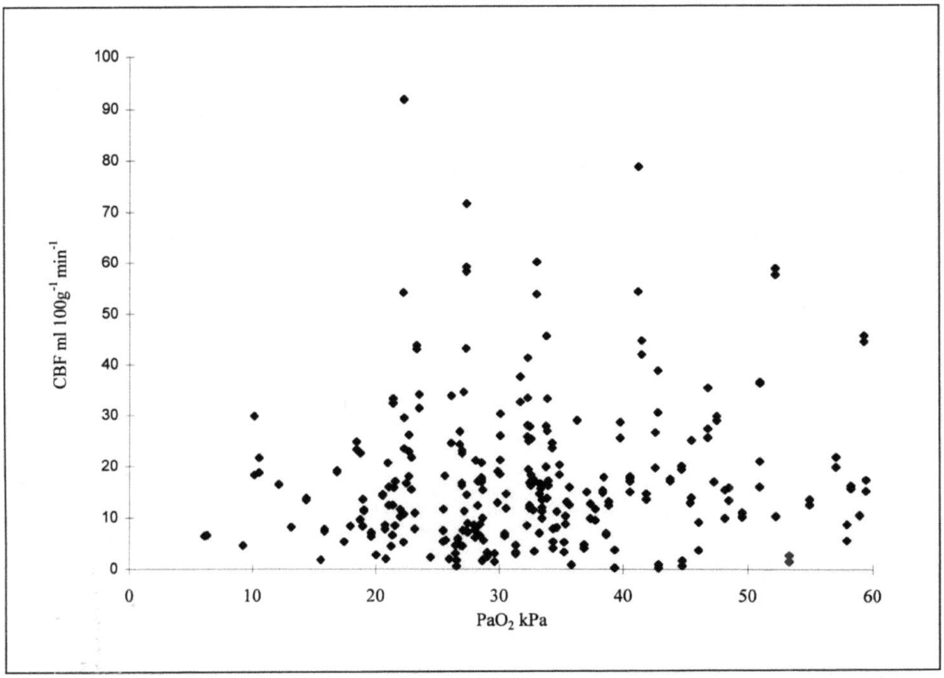

Fig. 2. Graph showing the relation of cerebral blood flow and arterial oxygen tension. Each symbol represents a diffferent patient.

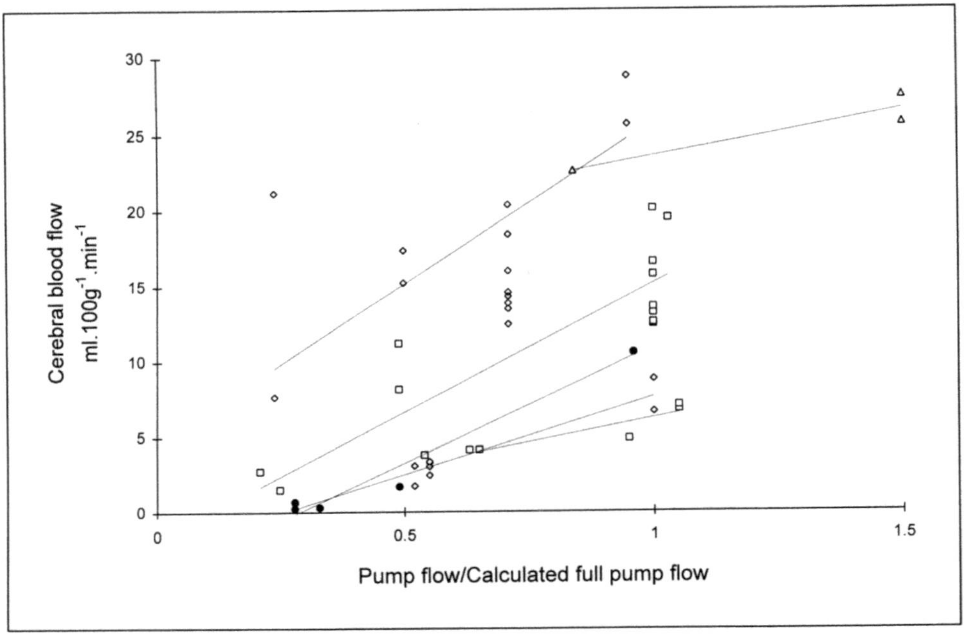

Fig. 3. Graph showing the relation of cerebral blood flow to pump flow rate, expressed as a fraction of full pump flow rate (2.4 $L.m^{-2} \cdot min^{-1}$). Each symbol represents a different patient. In these six patients, CBF decreases by 5.6 – 31.9 $ml \cdot 100\,g^{-1} \cdot min^{-1}$ (mean 18.7 $ml \cdot 100\,g^{-1} \cdot min^{-1}$) for each $L.min^{-1}$ decrease in pump flow rate.

Table 1. The results of multivariate analysis showing the relation of CBF with variables and their confidence limits

Independant variable:	Slope	SD	p value	% change in CBF	95 % confidence limits
Uncorrected arterial oxygen tension	N.R.	N.R.	0.170	N.R.	N.R.
Temperature corrected arterial oxygen tension	N.R.	N.R.	0.699	N.R.	N.R.
Pump flow	21.8 ml $100\,g^{-1} \cdot L^{-1}$	4.72	<0.00001	4.2 % $L^{-1} \cdot m^{-2} \cdot min^{-1}$ change in pump flow rate	+7.4, +12.6
Nasopharyngeal temperature	2.02 $ml \cdot 100\,g^{-1} \cdot min^{-1} \cdot °C^{-1}$	0.26	<0.00001	1 % per °C	−2.0, +3.0
Arterial carbon dioxide tension	2.54 $ml \cdot 100\,g^{-1} \cdot min^{-1} \cdot kPa^{-1}$	0.84	0.003	1 % per kPa	−1.0, +3.2
Mean arterial pressure	N.R.	N.R.	0.117	N.R.	N.R.
Haematocrit	N.R.	N.R.	0.597	N.R.	N.R.

N.R. – No Relation
SD – Standard Deviation

Conclusions

This study failed to show any direct relationship between CBF and PaO_2 in the range of PaO_2 greater than 10.5 kPa (Fig. 2) and there was no evidence of any vasoconstriction up to a PaO_2 of 59.4 kPa.

There was a significant relationship between CBF and pump flow rate (Fig. 3). CBF decreased by 4.2 % $L^{-1} \cdot m^{-2} \cdot min^{-1}$ decrease of pump flow rate (Table 1).

Our data suggests that there is no need to change current practice with regards to management of PaO_2. However, the change in CBF associated with a decrease in pump flow rate requires further study.

References

1. Busija DW, Orr JA, Rankin JHG, Liang HK, Wagerle LC (1980) Cerebral blood flow during normocapnic hyperoxia in the unanesthetized pony. J Appl Physiol 48: 10–15
2. Fallon P, Aparicio JM, Elliott MJ, Kirkham FJ (1995) Incidence of neurological complications of surgery for congenital heart disease. Arch Dis Child 72: 418–422
3. Ferry PC (1990) Neurological sequelae of open-heart surgery in children. Am J Dis Child 144: 369–373
4. Henriksen L (1986) Brain luxury perfusion during cardiopulmonary bypass in humans. A study of the cerebral blood flow response to changes in CO2, O2 and blood pressure. J Cereb Blood Flow Metab 6: 366–78
5. Jobsis FF (1977) Noninvasive infrared monitoring of cerebral and myocardial oxygen sufficiency and circulatory parameters. Science 198: 1264–7
6. Roberts I, Fallon P, Kirkham FJ, Lloyd-Thomas A et al. (1993) Estimation of cerebral blood flow with near infrared spectroscopy and indocyanine green. Lancet 342: 1425

Authors' address:
Dr. G. Chow
Research Fellow
Department of Cardiothoracic Surgery
Great Ormond Street
London WC1N 3JH
England

Cerebral perfusion during low-flow cardiopulmonary bypass with circulatory arrest in rabbits – An experimental study for CPB in neonates

D. Troitzsch, S. Vogt[1], A. Peukert[2]

University of Leipzig, Clinic for Neurosurgery, [1]Transplant Surgery and [2]Veterinary Surgery, Germany

Introduction

Cardiopulmonary bypass may be associated with multiorgan damage, resulting in either immediate or long-term effects (1, 2, 5). This damage may occasionally be related to inadequate regional tissue oxygen delivery. Several clinical and experimental studies have clearly shown the precise and close correlation among electrical cerebral activity (EEG), cerebral blood flow (CBF), intracranial pressure (ICP), and metabolic activity ($CMRO_2$). The purpose of our study is to assess the cerebral perfusion in neonates by evaluating differences in CBF and $CMRO_2$-metabolism during low-flow CPB with circulatory arrest in deep hypothermic temperatures in an experimental model for heart- and heart-lung-transplantation in rabbits.

Materials and methods

After review and approval of the protocol by the Animal Care Committee, 10 New Zealand white rabbits, weighing 2.5 – 3 kg, undergoing experimental surgical procedures with deep hypothermia cardiopulmonary bypass technique (alpha-stat pH-management, non-pulsatile) and circulatory arrest in deep hypothermic temperatures (below 18 °C rectal) were monitored in a pilot study.

Anesthesia

Animals were anesthetized with fentanyl, midazolam and pancuronium. An ear vein was cannulated and the trachea was intubated with a cuffed tracheal tube. Pancuronium was given intravenously and the lungs were mechanically ventilated. Catheters were surgically inserted into both of the abdominal aorta and inferior vena cava via the femoral vessels. Therefore, a continuous monitoring of mean arterial and central venous pressure (MAP and CVP) was permitted.

Physiological Monitoring included ECG, direct arterial pressure, esophageal and rectal temperature, urine output, and continuous neurophysiological monitoring. Furthermore, the CBF was monitored with an invasive method: H_2-clearance method and with a noninvasive method: Transcranial Doppler Sonography (TCD) of the middle cerebral artery (MCA) (3).

The animals were turned prone and the head fixed in a stereotaxic frame. After infiltration with bupivacaine the scalp was incised in the midline and reflected. Using a drill, the bone was then removed from the area around the occipital protuberance and the confluence of venous sinuses was exposed in the midline. A 20-gauge spinal needle catheter was introduced into the confluence with the bevel of the needle facing anteriorly. The distal 0.5 mm tip of a 300 micrometer diameter platinum-iridium needle electrode was introduced into the venous confluence. The electrode and the sampling needle catheter were both fixed at place with cyanoacrylate adhesive glue. Finally, a Ag/AgCl reference electrode was applied to an area of shaved skin on the animal's back. For ICP-monitoring a special catheter was stereotactically inserted into the right lateral brain ventricle.

The Cerebral Perfusion Pressure (CPP) was calculated as the difference between mean arterial pressure (MAP) and intracranial pressure (ICP). A standard CPB-technique for human infants was used. Before cannulation, animals were anticoagulated with heparin 3 mg/kgBW. The bypass circuit consisted of an infant oxygenator and a centrifugal pump (Biomedicus BP-50) primed with 300 ml of fresh heparinized blood from two crossmatch compatible rabbits and lactated Ringer's solution to achieve a PCV of 25 %. There were no differences in Hct, MAP, PFR and $paCO_2$ among animals at the measurement intervals. A circulatory arrest was induced. After 60 min, the rewarming of the animals was started and anticoagulation was reversed with protamine.

Forebrain CBF was measured using the hydrogen-clearance technique with flow calculated by the $T_{1/2}$ method. To determine $CMRO_2$, ~1 ml samples of arterial and cerebral venous blood were drawn simultaneously. Withdrawal was completed immediately prior to beginning the H_2 washout period.

The PO_2, PCO_2, pH and hematocrit (Hct) were determined for each sample and these values were then used to determine arterial and venous blood oxygen content. The $CMRO_2$ was calculated as the product of CBF and the arterial-sagittal sinus O_2 content difference.

TCD-monitoring for CBF

Using a Medasonics 2 MHz pulsed TCD-probe the CBF was monitored in the middle cerebral artery (MCA) on the right and left temporal window.

EEG-analysis

Bitemporal multichannel EEG were recorded with a filter window of 1 – 60 Hz in 4-s sampling epoch. The signal was simultaneously passed to an IBM-computer, the signal was than subjected to a fast-Fourier analysis and the resultant power spectrum was used to calculate total EEG-power.

Somatosensory evoked potentials (SSEP) were recorded using the Nicolet Pathfinder (Nicolet Biomedical Instruments) with the following stimulation and recording parameters: rectangular constant current pulses delivered to the median nerve or to the posterior tibial nerve. The stimulus lasted 200 ms; 256 stimuli were delivered at a rate of 5.9/s and averaged. High-amplitude electrical artifacts were automatically rejected by the computer-aided system. Cerebral abnormalities were preoperatively excluded on FFT-EEG, Computertomography, SPECT and SSEP.

Results

All animals showed decrease in $CMRO_2$ during deep hypothermic temperatures (below 18 °C). With rewarming $CMRO_2$ returned to pre-cooling values (see Fig. 2). Cerebral blood flow during CPB was not significantly different from pre-CPB levels. With cooling, below 28 °C, the CBF decreased with the reduction of pump flow (Fig. 1). CVR values increased and the CPP decreased with reduction of temperatures (see Figs. 3, 4).

Table 1. Measurement points

I	– baseline value	III	– rectal temperature below 18 °C
II	– after anesthesia induction	IV	– OP-end

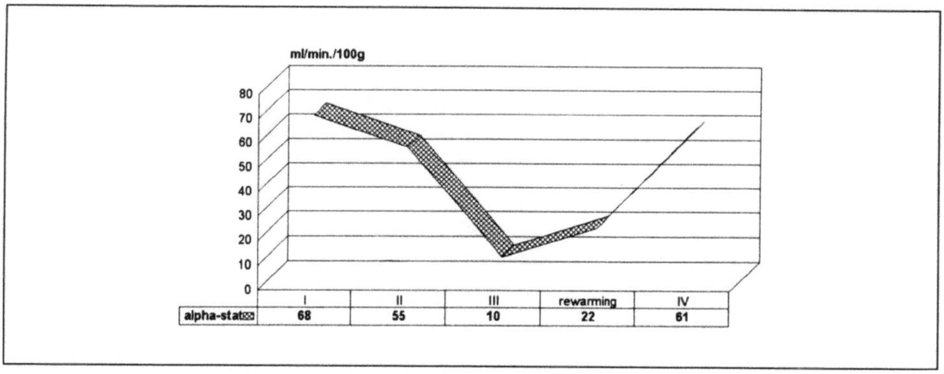

Fig. 1. Cerebral blood flow versus measurement points

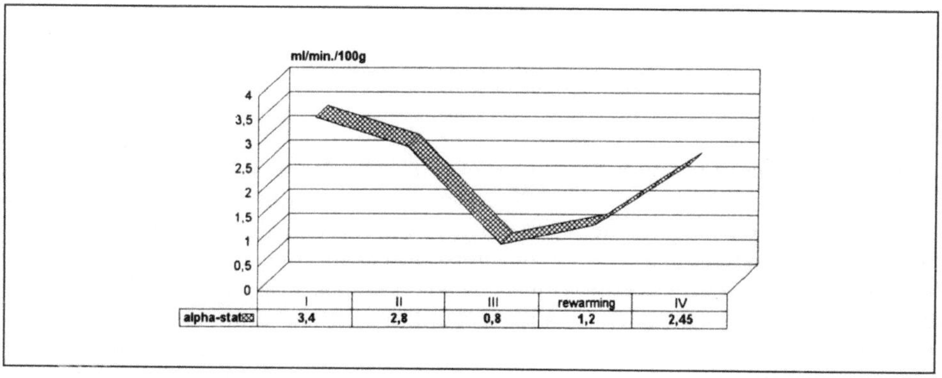

Fig. 2. $CMRO_2$ versus measurement points

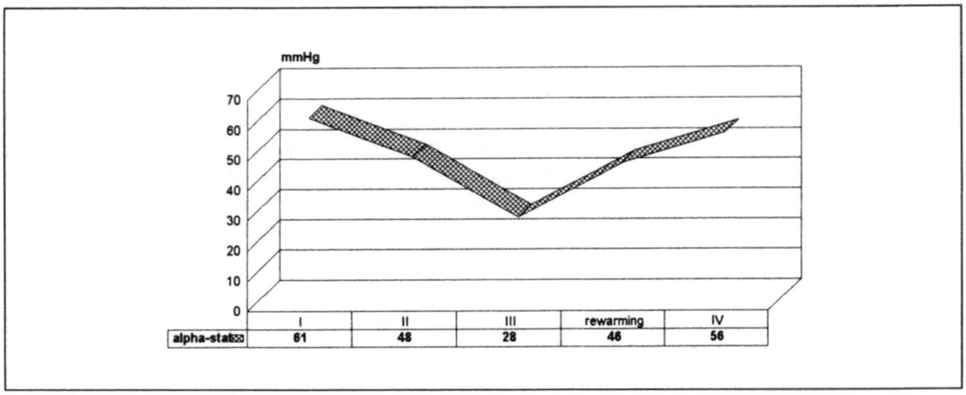

Fig. 3. Cerebral perfusion pressure versus measurement points

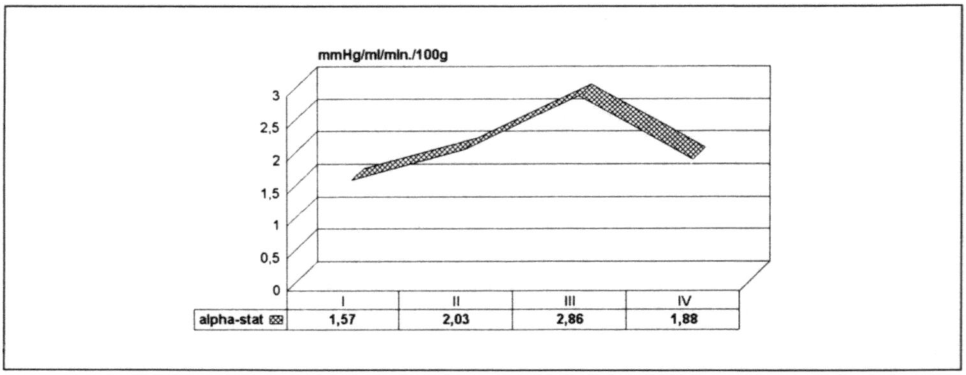

Fig. 4. Cerebral vascular resistance versus measurement points

Discussion

In any discussions of the pathophysiology of cerebral ischemia it is important to differentiate between global and regional ischemia, low-flow ischemia, absolute (no-flow) ischemia, and the cerebral ischemia that occurs as a consequence of a full body failure of the circulation (cardiac arrest). CBF and metabolism allow the integrated functions of the central nervous system to be performed on a continuous basis (4). Prevention of organ damage associated with deep hypothermic CPB with and without circulatory arrest remains one of the goals of pediatric cardiac surgeons in the near future. Cerebral damage has been well documented in neonates and children (6). The reasons for these alterations are inadequate perfusion and micro- and macroembolism. As the body temperature is reduced, a progressive reduction in cerebral metabolic requirement for oxygen enhances the brain tolerance to ischemia. Disadvantages include longer bypass time and increased peripheral vasoconstriction.

Conclusion

Finally, examination of the relationship between CBF and $CMRO_2$ suggests that most of the CBF changes are probably coupled to changes in metabolic demand. Deep hypothermic temperatures below 18 °C are associated with a persistent decrease in $CMRO_2$ and with an indefinite episode of reduced cerebral perfusion during rewarming. More clinical research and basic investigative work in appropriate experimental models will enable the development of better techniques for directly dealing with the critical cerebral ischemic damage and will provide more accurate assessment of the efficacy of these various interventions in the setting of cerebral ischemia during deep hypothermic cardiopulmonary bypass with and without circulatory arrest in neonates. The potential for effective neurocellular protection as a clinical reality appears bright.

References

1. Thomas SJ, Kramer JL (eds) (1993) Manual of Cardiac Anesthesia. 2nd Edition, Churchill Livingstone, New York Edinburgh London Madrid Melbourne Tokyo
2. Jonas RA, Elliott MJ (1994) Cardiopulmonary Bypass in Neonates, Infants and Young Children. Butterworth-Heinemann Ltd., Oxford
3. Scremin OU, Sonnenschein RR, Rubinstein EH (1982) Cerebrovascular anatomy and blood flow measurements in the rabbits. J Cereb Blood Flow Metab 2: 55–66
4. Kuschinsky W (1982) Coupling between functional activity, metabolism and blood flow in the brain: state of the art. Microcirculation 2: 357–78
5. Govier AV (1989) Central nervous system complications after cardiopulmonary bypass. In: Tinker JH (ed) Cardiopulmonary Bypass: Current Concepts and Controversies. W. B. Saunders, Philadelphia, pp 41–68
6. Haka-Ikse B, Blackwood MJ, Steward DJ (1978) Psychomotor development of infants and children after profound hypothermia during surgery for congenital heart disease. Developmental Medicine & Child Neurology 20: 62–70

Authors' address:
D. Troitzsch
Ruhrstraße 38
06846 Dessau
Germany

Neurophysiology, monitoring, cardiopulmonary bypass technique

Cerebral protection in surgery of the aortic arch: The place of neurophysiologic monitoring

B. Zickmann, K. Wulf, F. Dapper[1], G. Hempelmann

Department of Anesthesiology and Intensive Care Medicine, [1]Department of Cardiac and Vascular Surgery, Justus-Liebig University, Giessen, Germany

The aortic arch is the origin of the brachiocephalic arteries. Surgical interventions in this area bear the risk of impairment of cerebral perfusion and are associated with a relatively high rate of adverse cerebral outcome (10, 18). Aside from specific hemodynamic monitoring and anesthesia in aortic root surgery cerebral protection is one of the major challenges to the anesthetist. Several techniques have been suggested to protect the brain during the period of cerebral circulatory arrest. Temporary tube bypasses, temporary or permanent bypass grafts, cardiopulmonary bypass with selective perfusion of one ore even more cerebral arteries, retrograde cerebral perfusion and deep hypothermic cardiocirculatory arrest (DHCA) have been recommended to protect brain function during these operations (1, 9, 21, 22). All concepts of cerebral protection are based on a close cooperation of the surgical and anesthesiological team. New monitoring technologies have been introduced into clinical practice within the last years. And last not least, the combination of innovative surgical techniques and new monitoring technologies has lead to new options to perform cardiopulmonary bypass in patients with aortic arch disease without the continuous fear of a cerebral disaster.

Cerebral outcome in aortic arch surgery: Influence of surgical techniques

At present *deep hypothermic cardiocirculatory* arrest (DHCA) is the most common surgical technique in aortic arch replacement (6, 8). The patient is placed on cardiopulmonary bypass after arterial (femoral artery) and venous cannulation and is cooled down. Controlled hypothermia diminishes oxygen consumption and thus increases the viability of tissues under ischemic conditions. Depending on the degree of cooling of the patient this method provides a limited time of cerebral tolerance to circulatory arrest (11, 20, 25). The safe duration of DHCA is derived from empirical data. At body core temperatures of 18–20° DHCA up to 60 minutes is considered to be "safe". However, these data are empirically derived and can differ in a given patient. There are no means to measure cerebral function during DHCA period (flat-line EEG, evoked potentials suppressed) and to provide the surgeon with sufficient information on the safety of this procedure in the individual patient. The incidence of neurologic complications after DHCA depends on the method of evaluation (8, 9, 23). Most of the undesired effects of DHCA are caused by reperfusion. The extent of reperfusion injury in the individual patient is unpredictable. DHCA is associated with additional problems: Coagulation disorders, particularly platelet dysfunction, are observed more frequent than in operations with only moderate hypothermia.

Liver and kidney dysfunction are more frequent and the immunosuppressive effect of cardiopulmonary bypass is more pronounced after DHCA as well, resulting in a higher risk of infectious complications. If prolonged time of DHCA is mandatory in a specific patient, the frequency of complications, particularly cerebral ones, is increasing rapidly.

Selective cannulation of the innominate artery (truncus brachiocephalicus) is an alternative surgical technique in many cases additionally to femoral artery cannulation. In the period, when the distal part of the aorta and the cerebral vessels are clamped, the perfusion of the innominate artery supplies blood to the cerebral circulation and to the right arm. Blood supply to the brain is sufficient with this method on the condition, that the circle of Willis is intact and blood is supplied to any part of the brain by collateral blood flow. This assumption is not met in all patients. In the development of the cerebral circulation malformations are not uncommon. Insufficient collateral circulation after cannulation of the innominate artery can be expected in up to 7 % of the population. Therefore cannulation of cerebral vessels on both sides and the perfusion of the cerebral circulation with a separate pump have been recommended, with number of arteries cannulated and the exact cannulation sites dependent on the extent of the lesion of the aortic arch (3, 7).

The cannulation of several cerebral vessels has the disadvantages of being time and, even more important, space consuming. The use of an additional pump for the cerebral perfusion can be avoided by division of the flow of the routine arterial pump to the femoral artery and the cerebral circulation. Under conditions of selective cerebral perfusion no ischemia of the brain is necessary. The time of operation on the structures of the aortic arch can be extended without a strict time limit. The operation can be performed at moderate hypothermia (28–30 °C body core temperature) and thus the negative effects of hypothermia on organ function can be avoided or at least diminished. Selective cerebral perfusion techniques have been reported by several groups (2, 3, 14, 19, 24). The methods differ in cannulation sites, cerebral blood flow, separate versus standard arterial pump for brain perfusion, core temperature of the patient and other factors. However, encouraging results regarding the incidence of cerebral complications were observed (13–15). The incidence of cerebral complications ranged from 1.3 % to 15 % and thus seems to be probably even lower than after DHCA. Unfortunately it is not possible to distinguish between the neurologic complications attributable to the pathway of brain perfusion per se and those caused by technical problems associated with cannulation of the supraaortic vessels. Additionally the risk of thromboembolic events, particularly of air embolism into the cerebral circulation is probably higher than in routine cardiac surgery, though comparable data can not be obtained. At present quantification of air bubbles embolized into the cerebral circulation is not possible, though transcranial Doppler sonography provides a tool for measurement.

Selective cerebral perfusion in our institution

In our institution the blood flow from the heart-lung machine to the femoral cannula and the one in the innominate artery is realized by an "Y"-connector. Though the total flow of the ECC to the patient is well known, the amount flowing to the cerebrum remains uncertain. The supply of blood to the cerebral arteries depends on the resistance of the vascular system of the lower body (flow via the femoral cannula) and the distribution of the flow via the truncus cannula to brain and arm. Thus the exact blood flow to the brain is unknown.

This may cause periods of hypo- as well as hyperperfusion of the brain. Therefore cerebral monitoring should be available to detect the effects of each of these perfusion disturbances on cerebral function. Additionally dislocations of the innominate artery cannula should be easily detectable, if cerebral perfusion is compromised.

Because the exact blood flow to the brain during selective perfusion remains unknown some precautions have to be considered. It is necessary to have an arterial pressure monitoring in the area, which is perfused by a special cannula. This is preferably the right radial artery pressure. If we are not sure, whether the perfusion of the right arm is adequate, for instance in cases of aortic dissection which might involve the right arm's perfusion even distally to the cannulation site, blood pressure monitoring in the carotid artery is recommended. Blood pressure values obtained at the level of the heart-lung-machine or from the arterial line are not sufficient. Ideally blood pressure in the cerebral circulation (and the right arm, respectively) remains at the same level as before selective perfusion. We aim at perfusion pressures of 50–100 mmHg. Particular attention has to be paid to the moment of aortic clamping. If blood pressure increases above this limit, the flow of the arterial pump has to be reduced to avoid brain edema or even hemorrhage.

With increasing experience with this perfusion method we today recommend to perform a test-clamping period prior to definitive clamping of the distal aorta. After initiation of CPB the patient is perfused via both cannula and via his own circulation (beating heart). Moderate hypothermia is initiated. If the temperature aimed at is achieved, the supra-aortic vessels are closed by snares or clamps and selective perfusion of the brain is initiated for a period of 5 to 10 minutes. The topographic EEG changes (as described below) as well as hemodynamic changes are observed with respect to the situation prior to clamping. According to our experience with this method in TEA of carotid arteries a 10-minutes period should be long enough to detect changes in cerebral function caused by malperfusion. If changes in cerebral function are detected the surgical concept has to be modified. In situations indicating insufficient collateralisation either additional cannulation sites have to be used to ensure cerebral perfusion of non collateralized areas or the concept has to be changed to the use of DHCA in this patient. In cases indicating hyperperfusion of the preferentially perfused hemisphere the flow of the arterial pump has to be decreased or the size of the cannula in the innominate artery has to be reduced. If global cerebral hypoperfusion is suspected, the position of the selective cannula has to be checked. This test period allows return to routine cerebral perfusion within seconds and provides decision making without being pressed for time.

Demands on the ideal cerebral function monitor

As mentioned above, anomalies of the cerebral collateral circulation are common. In some patients parts of the brain are not supplied by collateral perfusion. Therefore the requirements for an ideal monitoring device are detection of:

- global cerebral hypoperfusion
- global cerebral hyperperfusion (development of edema, risk of intracranial bleeding)
- regional perfusion deficits
- and more important: The impact of these changes on cerebral function
- monitoring of cortical and subcortical structures

- continuous on-line monitoring in real-time
- high sensitivity
- high specificity

A measurement of global or even regional cerebral blood flow is neither sufficient nor feasible under conditions of the intraoperative situation. Of crucial importance is the effect of this flow on the function of the brain's cells and the integrity of the intracerebral functional network.

Therefore the optimal device should provide a parameter for global as well as for local cerebral function, which is easy to handle and provides this information on-line and in real time to the anesthetist.

Modalities of cerebral monitoring

Several investigations focused on the impact of intraoperative neurophysiologic monitoring on outcome after cardiac operations or in aortic arch surgery (4, 5, 17, 18).

The electroencephalogram is the oldest of these monitoring modalities. In the setting of aortic arch surgery it seems to be the only modality, which can provide topographic information on virtually any point of the cortex on-line and in real time. On the other hand information on the electrophysiologic situation in the deeper (older) parts of the brain is limited. Though these structures influence cerebral cortical activity, and the surface-EEG is regarded (at least in part) as a projection of the activity of these deeper structures a direct monitoring of subcortical structures is not possible.

Evoked potentials seem to provide more information on the afferent pathway of sensory information from the point of a stimulus to the cortical receptive areas. In the situation of aortic arch surgery the different modalities of evoked potentials (somatosensory, acoustical, visual) do not provide a topographic information yet. The marketing of topographic systems has begun recently, and the place of these systems in intraoperative monitoring has to be determined in the next years. In our opinion evoked potentials are not optimal for the demands of aortic arch surgery at present.

Transcranial Doppler sonography provides information on blood flow velocity in the basal cerebral arteries. It is of minor value in aortic arch surgery, because is gives only limited information on the intracerebral collateralisation. A measurement of blood flow velocity does not even provide quantitative information on cerebral blood supply.

Near infrared spectroscopy claims to measure oxygen saturation within the brain tissue. Though these devices can be used at different points over the cortex and thus could provide topographic information, the interpretation of changes in regional cerebral oxygen saturation remains cumbersome. Changes in oxygen saturation can be caused by changes in blood flow to the respective cerebral area, but can be associated also with changes in venous run off, with cerebral ischemia or brain edema, without the possibility to differentiate between the underlying pathophysiologic situations. Further data have to be obtained to evaluate the place of this modality in intraoperative monitoring.

Measurements of global and regional cerebral blood flow by washout characteristics of inert gases or radioactive substances are the gold standard to assess cerebral perfusion. These measurements are time-consuming, expensive and are not practicable during a typical situation of an emergency operation of aortic arch structures. Additionally these methods give specific information on blood flow, not on brain function.

Quantitative topographic electroencephalometry

At present the topographic monitoring of the electroencephalogram (EEG) is the monitoring modality of choice in our hands and therefore will be described in detail.

We use "computer-aided topographical electro-encephalo-metry" (CATEEM®, MediSyst, Linden, FRG). The EEG is continuously recorded at 16 points on the scalp according to the international 10-20-system (12), using Cz as the physical reference. The 16 analog-signals are amplified and digitized (512 Hz, 12 bit) close to the patients head and transferred to the processor-unit by optic fibers. The EEG-amplifier and the analog-digital converting subunit are accumulator powered, to make the system independent of line power and all electrical paraphernalia. The high input resistance of the amplifier (> 20 MΩ) ensures a sufficient signal/noise-difference in cases of alteration of the individual electrode-resistances between 1 Ω and 100 Ω. The common average reference (16) is calculated from these 16 analogous signals, and a transformation of the bipolar (16 signal-channels) to the unipolar relationship of this virtual reference (17 signal-channels) was performed. The raw EEG is digitized with 512 Hz; by averaging 4 consecutive data points an effective sampling rate of 128 Hz is achieved. For each recording point a frequency analysis is performed, using a Hanning-window followed by a fast-fourier-transformation on epochs of 4 seconds each, continuously. The power spectrum is calculated with a spectral resolution of 0.25 Hz. This power spectrum (1.25–35 Hz) is devised into 6 frequency bands (see table 1). The absolute power densities ($\mu V^2/Hz$) of each frequency-band and each recording point are used as a quantitative measure of cerebral activity.

In patients with stable hemodynamics monitoring is begun prior to induction of anesthesia and continued until the end of the operation. In the remaining patients, monitoring started as soon as possible after induction of anesthesia but in any case before clamping of supraaortic vessels. The topographic electrophysiologic situation directly prior to clamping is used for comparison with results during the period of selective cerebral perfusion.

Results

Quantitative topographic electroencephalometry (CATEEM) has been performed in 18 patients, who required surgery of the aortic arch and who were perfused with the selective cannulation technique. None of the patients so far showed signs of impaired collateralisation perfusion, neither in the test period, nor during the reconstruction phase. In three

Table 1. Frequency bands of CATEEM

frequency band	range
delta	1.25 Hz – 4.50 Hz
theta	4.75 Hz – 6.75 Hz
alpha-1	7.00 Hz – 9.50 Hz
alpha-2	9.75 Hz – 12.50 Hz
beta-1	12.75 Hz – 18.50 Hz
beta-2	18.75 Hz – 35.00 Hz

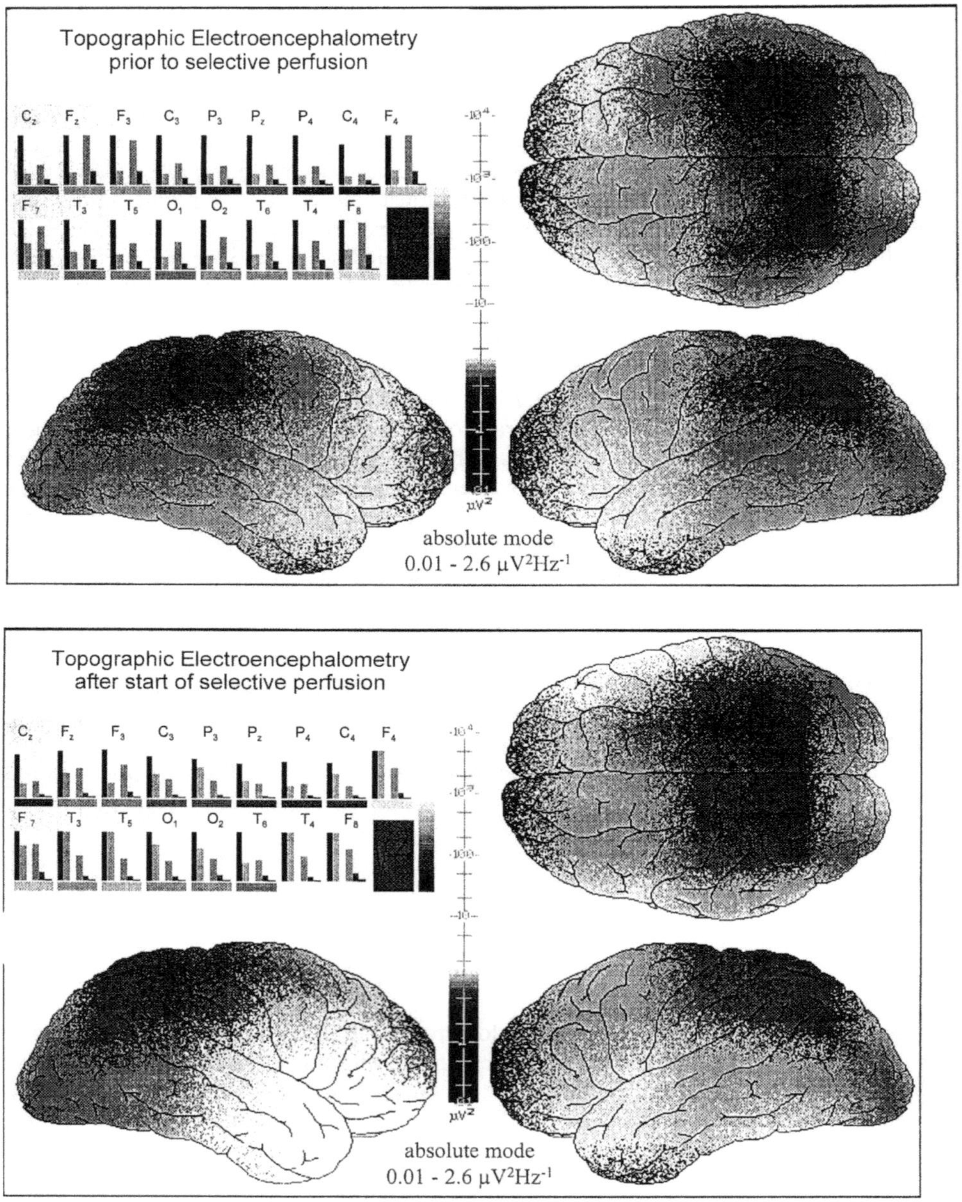

Fig. 1. Topographic electroencephalometry in selective cerebral perfusion. Cerebral electrical power in each frequency-band and at each electrode position prior (figure 1a) and shortly after start of selective cerebral perfusion (figure 1b). In the left upper quadrant of each figure the absolute power in each of the frequency bands is displayed with the bars representing (from left to right) the power in the delta, theta, alpha-1, alpha-2, beta-1 and beta-2 power band. The spectral content of power at each physical recording point and additional 82 intermediate points (calculated from amplitude, frequency and phase delay of the measured data) is displayed on topographic maps of the brain as sighted from left and right side and from above. Clamping of the supraaortic vessels resulted in increases in theta- and alpha-1 cerebral power in the right hemisphere (mainly temporally) and was suspected to indicate hyperperfusion. Cerebral activity above the left hemisphere remained constant, thus collateral perfusion was assumed to be sufficient. With reduction of blood flow to the selective cannula cerebral power above the right hemisphere returned to pre-clamping values within minutes.

patients lateralisation of cerebral activity was noticed. In these cases cerebral power at electrodes of the right (predominantly perfused) hemisphere increased particularly in the alpha-bands, with the power at the electrodes of the left hemisphere (perfusion depending on collateralisation) remaining constant. This observation was suspected to represent the electrophysiologic correlate of hyperperfusion of the right hemisphere and regarded as a sign of edema formation. With this hypothesis it was decided to reduce the flow through the selective cannula in these cases and the EEG-changes disappeared within minutes. To support the hypothesis of a correlation between flow through the selective cannula and changes in ipsilateral cerebral function the flow was increased again after disappearance of the EEG changes. In two out of three patients these EEG changes were reproducible, supporting strongly our hypothesis.

Anesthesia

Anesthesia was induced and maintained with fentanyl or sufentanil as the analgesic, midazolam as the hypnotic and pancuronium. Dosages were adapted to the actual hemodynamic situation and demands of the patients. With this combination of anesthetics cerebral electrical activity decreases continuously with cooling of the patient, but is still present and can be adequately monitored at moderate hypothermia (28–30° body core temperature). Flat line EEG or burst suppression patterns, which are well known from anesthesia with volatile anesthetics (isoflurane, enflurane), barbiturates or propofol were not seen at these temperature levels with opioid plus benzodiazepine anesthesia. Thus this kind of anesthesia ensures sufficient recording conditions for quantitative topographic electroencephalometry. Normocarbic artificial ventilation was performed with an inspired oxygen fraction of 1.0 until start of the extracorporeal circulation. ECC was performed using non-pulsatile flow (2.4 $l/m^2/min$) and membrane oxygenators; α-stat principles were applied.

Pharmacological methods

The discussion about a prophylactic use of steroids and barbiturates is still controversial and depends on the preferences of the anesthetist. We use steroids (dexamethasone 1 mg/kg or prednisolone 10 mg/kg) with the start of ECC. Mannitol is added to the ECC prime (3 ml/kg) to increase intravascular colloidosmotic pressure and by this preventing brain edema. Barbiturates are given in patients, when deep hypothermic cardiac arrest is necessary. They are not used, if selective cannulation is performed, because the depression of cerebral activity down to burst-suppression-EEG or flat-line EEG is well known. These phenomena are on the one side associated with a maximum suppression of cerebral metabolism, which would be beneficial. On the other, quantitative topographic EEG-monitoring is not possible under these conditions.

Conclusion

Surgery of the aortic arch is still associated with a relatively high risk of permanent or transient neurologic dysfunction. The risk of neurologic or psychopathologic sequelae seems to depend on the method of cerebral protection used. The surgical technique determines procedures of cerebral protection available for the individual patient. In operations under deep hypothermic cardiac arrest unspecific methods of prevention of cerebral edema should be used, though the value of steroids, barbiturates, calcium channel blocker and other pharmacological approaches is still matter of debate. Neurophysiologic monitoring is only of minor importance under these circumstances. Flat-line and burst-suppression EEG indicate the degree of suppression of cerebral metabolic function, but at the temperatures aimed at for DHCA (18–20 °C) cerebral electric activity will have come to arrest in virtually any patient. In this setting neurophysiologic monitoring does not help to improve the patients' safety or neurologic outcome.

If selective perfusion techniques of the cerebral circulation are chosen, the situation is completely different. Disadvantages of deep hypothermic cardiac arrest with respect to organ or platelet function or to duration of extracorporeal circulation can be diminished. On the other hand global or regional malperfusion of the brain in these patients would result in neurologic sequelae without delay. In this situation cerebral monitoring is strongly recommended, if not even required. At moderate hypothermia and under conditions of anesthesia as described above, the quantitative topographic EEG is a promising and in our hands already an established tool in monitoring of the cerebral status. In this situation the concept of brain protection is controlled and changed if necessary by continuous monitoring of cerebral function. Computerized data acquisition, processing and presentation are necessary to establish a "stand-by" device to the anesthetist. The relatively high prevalence of patients with malformations of their cerebral collateral circulation makes topographic neurologic monitoring desirable.

References

1. Antunes MJ, Colsen PR, Kinsley RH (1983) Hypothermia and circulatory arrest for surgical resection of aortic arch aneurysms. J Thorac Cardiovasc Surg 86: 576–581
2. Aoyagi S, Akashi H, Kubota Y et al. (1992) Partial brachiocephalic perfusion under hypothermic cardiopulmonary bypass. An experimental study. Eur J Cardiothorac Surg 6: 508–513
3. Aoyagi S, Akashi H, Kubota Y et al. (1993) Surgical treatment of aneurysms of the aortic arch using a simplified selective cerebral perfusion technique. Thorac Cardiovasc Surg 42: 279–284
4. Arom KV, Cohen DE, Strobl FT (1989) Effect of intraoperative intervention on neurological outcome based on electroencephalographic monitoring during cardiopulmonary bypass. Ann Thorac Surg 48: 476–483
5. Bashein G, Nessly ML, Bledsoe SW et al. (1992) Electroencephalography during surgery with cardiopulmonary bypass and hypothermia. Anesthesiology 76: 878–891
6. Crawford ES, Saleh SA (1981) Transverse aortic arch aneurysms. Ann Surg 194: 180–188
7. Crawford ES, Snyder DM (1983) Treatment of aneurysms of the aortic arch. A progress report. J Thorac Cardiovasc Surg 85: 237–246
8. Ergin MA, O'Connor J, Guinto R, Griepp RB (1982) Experience with profound hypothermia and circulatory arrest in the treatment of aneurysms of the aortic arch. Aortic arch replacement for acute arch dissections. J Thorac Cardiovasc Surg 84: 649–655
9. Galloway AC, Colvin SB, LaMendola CL et al. (1989) Ten-year operative experience with 165 aneurysms of the ascending aorta and aortic arch. Circulation 80: I249– I256

10. Govier AV (1989) Central nervous system complications after cardiopulmonary bypass. In: Tinker JH, Cardiopulmonary bypass: Current concepts and controversies. W. B. Saunders, Philadelphia: 41–68
11. Greeley WJ, Kern FH, Ungerleider RM et al. (1991) The effect of hypothermic cardiopulmonary bypass and total circulatory arrest on cerebral metabolism in neonates, infants, and children. J Thorac Cardiovasc Surg 101: 783–794
12. Jaspers HH (1958) The ten twenty system of the international federation. Electroencephalogr Clin Neurophysiol 10: 371–375
13. Kazui T, Kimura N, Komatsu S (1995) Surgical treatment of aortic arch aneurysms using selective cerebral perfusion. Eur J Cardio-thorac Surg 9: 491–495
14. Kazui T, Kimura N, Yamada O, Komatsu S (1994) Surgical outcome of aortic arch aneurysms using selective cerebral perfusion. Ann Thorac Surg 57: 904–911
15. Kuwabara M, Nakajiama N, Andou M et al. (1988) A study on the methods of selective cerebral perfusion on aortic arch replacement. J Jpn Assoc Thorac Surg 36: 466–471
16. Lehmann D (1987) Principles of spatial analysis. In: Gevins AS, Remond A, eds. Methods of analysis of brain electrical and magnetic signals, EEG Handbook Vol.1. Elsevier Science Publishers, 309–354
17. Levy WJ (1992) Monitoring of the electroencephalogram during cardiopulmonary bypass. Know when to say when. Anesthesiology 76: 876–877
18. Levy WL (1987) Central nervous system monitoring. In: Kaplan JA, ed. Cardiac anesthesia. W. B. Saunders Company, Philadelphia: 319–338
19. Matsuda H, Nakano S, Shirakura R et al. (1989) Surgery for aortic arch aneurysm with selective cerebral perfusion and hypothermic cardiopulmonary bypass. Circulation 80: I243–I248
20. Mizrahi EM, Patel VM, Crawford ES, Coselli JS, Hess KR (1989) Hypothermic-induced electrocerebral silence, prolonged circulatory arrest, and cerebral protection during cardiovascular surgery. Electroencephalogr Clin Neurophysiol 72: 81–85
21. Murase M, Maeda M, Koyama T et al. (1993) Continuous retrograde cerebral perfusion for protection of the brain during aortic arch surgery. Eur J Cardiothorac Surg 7: 597–600
22. Ott DA, Frazier OH, Cooley DA (1978) Resection of the aortic arch using deep hypothermia and temporary circulatory arrest. Circulation 58, Suppl 1: I-227–I-231
23. Svensson LG, Crawford ES, Hess KR (1993) Deep hypothermia with circulatory arrest: determinants of stroke and early mortality. J Thorac Cardiovasc Surg 106: 19–31
24. Tabayashi K, Ohmi M, Togo T et al. (1994) Aortic arch aneurysm repair using selective cerebral perfusion. Ann Thorac Surg 57: 1305–1310
25. Treasure T, Naftel DC, Conger KA, Garcia JH, Kirklin JW, Blackstone EH (1983) The effect of hypothermic circulatory arrest time on cerebral function, morphology, and biochemistry. J Thorac Cardiovasc Surg 86: 761–770

Authors' address:
Dr. Bernfried Zickmann
Department of Anesthesiology and Intensive Care Medicine
Justus-Liebig University
Rudolf-Buchheim-Str. 7
35385 Giessen, FRG

Neurophysiological consequences of circulatory arrest with hypothermia

T. Treasure

Department of Cardiothoracic Surgery, London, England

In 1925, Henry Souttar, a surgeon in The London Hospital performed his first and only heart operation, a mitral valvotomy. In his paper describing this operation he wrote:

> In animals ... the circulation has been clamped for as long as two minutes. This, however, would never be justified in a human being in view of the extreme danger to the brain from even the shortest check to its blood supply. Any manipulations which are carried out must therefore be executed in the full flow of the blood stream, and they must not perceptibly interfere with the contractions of the heart. (15)

Written 70 years ago, Souttar's paper reveals a stark appreciation of the problems that had to be overcome before cardiac surgery could be safely performed, and although he could not have foreseen the use of cardiopulmonary bypass to support the circulation, and hypothermia to protect the brain, his preoccupation with the vulnerability of the human brain is shared by the modern cardiovascular surgeon.

The use of a planned period of circulatory arrest has played an important part in the operative strategy in three quite separate types of surgery.

1) Before bypass was developed and refined, moderate hypothermia to about 30 °C, induced by surface cooling, was used to provide a few minutes of protection, just long enough to suture a fossa ovalis atrial septal defect. This is no longer applied clinically but is of considerable historical interest (19).
2) The repair of complex congenital heart disease in tiny hearts is made much easier if the heart is still and empty and the operative field is uncluttered by suckers and cannulae. This remains an important application of the technique. The emphasis on recent research has been to define safe limits and to see if these can be extended by periods of low flow (11), intermittent flow, or pharmacological interventions (7).
3) Our own most frequent use of circulatory arrest is in surgery of the aorta, particularly where the arch itself is involved and the blood supply to the brain must be interrupted (17). Here again the duration of arrest that is tolerated without permanent damage must be known. The means of extending the time beyond this limit include selective cannulation of arch vessels, and retrograde perfusion through the venous system. In the future, we may also use pharmacological adjuncts to modify the tolerance of the brain, or some form of "cerebroplegia".

The consequences of cerebral ischaemia

The neurophysiological consequences of circulatory arrest can be expressed quite simply. The brain has no reserve of oxygen and the high energy phosphates are lost rapidly. Cell death follows soon. In a recent study in dogs (13) the most vulnerable regions were the cortex, followed by the cerebellum, then the basal ganglia and the hippocampus.

An important distinction which should be made at this point is between "stroke" and diffuse brain injury. Stroke is a non-technical term, from common English usage, for sudden incapacity including paralysis or loss of speech, or both. In the sense in which we use the word, the deficit is typically a consequence of a discrete brain injury due to ischaemia and is usually embolic. Studies of circulatory arrest which rely on retrospective analysis of clinical notes in which stroke has been recorded will both underestimate the true incidence of brain injury and wrongly attribute neurological events of other aetiology to the use of circulatory arrest. Furthermore, the ability of our patients, particularly children, to make a good recovery in spite of a diffuse brain injury, leads us to overestimate the safe duration of circulatory arrest, by underestimating the incidence of brain damage, unless we specifically look for it. We will return to this question of semantics later.

The most valuable method to protect the brain, and the one used uniformly, is hypothermia. For reasons that are lost in time, and are almost certainly more dependent on logistics than science, the commonest temperature employed is 18 °C. When I embarked on my studies of circulatory arrest it was widely taught that at 18 °C, an hour of circulatory arrest was safe for the brain. The sum of clinical and experimental evidence already available at the time, if reviewed critically, indicated that this was a substantial overestimate (18, 19).

What is the time limit?

In 1981, we embarked upon a series of experiments in the University of Alabama with the specific objective of defining the earliest time at which irretrievable damage was evident in the mammalian brain. We used the Mongolian gerbil because in this creature the circle of Willis is deficient. Occlusion of the carotid arteries renders the cerebrum ischaemic while permitting the animal to maintain its vital functions because the rest of the body, including the brain stem, is perfused. Matched animals were either killed after reperfusion or allowed to recover. The animals killed early were rapidly frozen so that the brain chemistry could be studied. Those which were allowed to recover were assessed daily for neurological function over the ensuing week and then the brains were fixed by perfusion to study the histology (20).

The method was not without flaws. Because the animals relied on their own cardiovascular system while being surface cooled to 18 °C, and during rewarming, they were almost certainly exposed to a progressively lower cardiac output during that time. Some have reasonably questioned the reliability of a neurological examination in the gerbil, and one is always left with uncertainties in applying animal experiments to humans. Nevertheless, there was an internal consistency in the results and consistency with data obtained in other ways.

The conclusion of this study was that by 35–40 minutes there was a 10% risk of brain damage (20). This correlated with a number of other animal experiments and clinical studies that had been performed at the time (19).

Since then we have always tried to plan operations so that the period of arrest is less than 30 min and have felt confident that if we stay within that time, we have done our best to minimise the risk of brain damage. Times beyond that have been associated with good outcome but cause us increasing anxiety.

Another study published relatively recently (5) re-explores these issues in neonatal pigs at 15 °C subjected to 70 to 120 min of arrest. No histological changes were demonstrable at 70 min but they were evident by 90 min. My own view is that the conclusion "the maximum time of circulatory arrest without histopathological and neuropsychological sequelae should not exceed 70 min" is bold. It implies that there is safety up to that time. The statement is out of line with other evidence and is based on a limited study in an immature animal. The conclusion is not transferrable to clinical practice.

Most recent animal studies have looked at methods to ameliorate damage and the authors have used a period of ischaemia which is presumably deliberately chosen to be damaging. An hour (9, 14, 21) or even 2 h (3, 8, 13) have been used in studies designed to explore methods of reducing damage.

Clinical evidence of "safe duration" of circulatory arrest

A very recent review of a practice of circulatory arrest in 114 children undergoing planned circulatory arrest showed that the IQ measured 9–10 years later was negatively correlated with circulatory arrest time ranging from 10 to 70 min (12). This concurs with much of the findings in the older surgical literature previously reviewed (19).

It would be interesting to find further clinical validation of our estimates of the time at which damage begins to occur. The best clinical study of clinical use of planned circulatory arrest is from the group at Boston's Children's Hospital (7, 11). Babies, all under 3 months of age, having repair of transposition of the great vessels by arterial switch, were randomised to planned arrest or low flow strategies. For the circulatory arrest group the median was 53 min with an interquartile range of 45–59 min, providing a good sample of data in the range of interest. The indices of brain damage were the occurrence of clinically evident seizures and ictal activity on the EEG monitored continuously for 48 h. The authors point to these as close correlates with the concept of excitatory transmitters as mediators of neuronal damage. No child with arrest less than 35 min had seizures. There was a clear relationship between the duration of arrest and the probability of seizures (Fig. 1). The probability of EEG detected ictal activity was also time related.

This practice of circulatory arrest in babies is very different to our own application which is in adult, and often elderly patients, having aortic surgery. There may be some differences between the immature brain and the mature brain, and for that matter between the adult brain and the "old" brain and its possibly deteriorating vascular system.

The report from the late Stanley Crawford's colleagues and associates provides valuable clinical data about patients undergoing major aortic surgery at a median age of 64 over a 12 year period from 1979 to 1991 (16). Here we come across the difficulties alluded to earlier, both that the study is retrospective and that "stroke" may not be the best clinical indicator of damage due to global ischaemia. In this report a "broad definition" of stroke was used:

> This definition included all transient or permanent deficits, either global or focal. Any patients who had not recovered neurologically from the operation within 48 hours; who were comatose, semicomatose, or disorientated; or who had obvious neuropsychiatric changes were included in the broad definition of stroke.

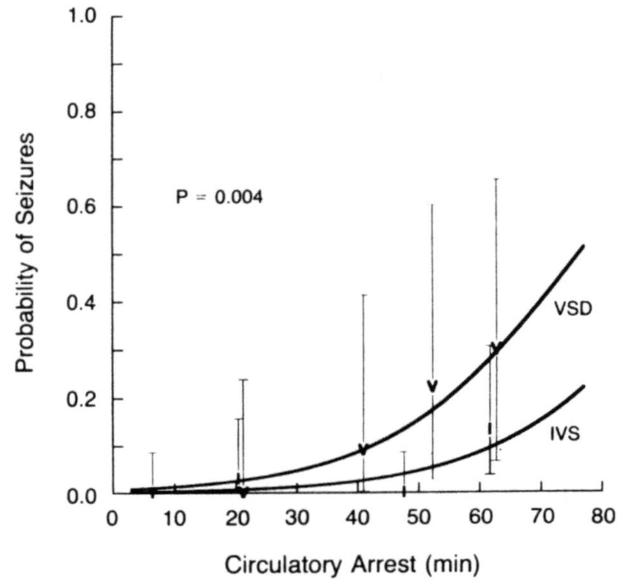

Fig. 1. The risk of seizures increases with the duration of circulatory arrest and reaches 10 % before 40 min of arrest in infants with TGA and VSD at 15–18 °C even with the additional protection of barbiturates (ref. Newburger et al. 1992).

The authors are well aware of the shortcomings of a retrospective study depending largely on recorded clinical observations in detecting all examples of neurological injury, nevertheless, it is clear that there was a high level of awareness of possible brain injury in this practice. The definition is indeed "broad" but comprehensively defined.

The risk of "stroke" as defined was clearly time related and they concluded that the risk of "stroke" began increasing after 40 min of arrest (Table 1).

Temperature

The temperature chosen for circulatory arrest of 18 °C seems to have been arrived at more or less by chance. There is clearly some variation but the publications from Crawford (16) and Jonas (11) indicate that a temperature of 18 °C is usual. Is there any further advantage in cooling further? Animal data in a publication from Mount Sinai (9) indicate that there is indeed further reduction in oxygen consumption of the dog's brain at lower temperature and that the oxygen consumption which had fallen from 34 % of baseline by 18 °C, fell further to 20 % of baseline with a further 5 °C reduction to 13 °C. The EEG that was present at 18 °C became silent at lower temperatures (Table 2). The loss of EEG may be important in the additional prolongation of circulatory arrest at very low temperatures (10).

Table 1. Time related incidence of "stroke" (16)

Arrest time minutes	number	% "stroke" (95 % confidence limits)
7– 29	298	4 % (2– 7)
30– 44	201	8 % (4–12)
45– 59	84	11 % (5–19)
60–120	48	15 % (6–28)

Table 2. Circulatory arrest in dogs (9)

Arrest temperature	18 °C	13 °C	8 °C
EEG	present	absent	absent
O_2 consumption	34 %	20 %	5 %

Other animal studies have used 20 °C (21) 18 °C (8, 13, 14) or 15 °C (3, 5) introducing some uncertainty in the equivalence of one study to another in addition to doubts about the applicability of data to humans.

The brain during ischaemia

If we are to extend the period of arrest we first need to know what are the changes in the cold ischaemic brain that are usually tolerated up to 30 min but are not tolerated beyond 45 min.

Usui and colleagues (21) explored the changes in cerebral tissue oxygen and carbon dioxide, oxygen consumption, ATP, and lactate: pyruvate ratio during an hour at 18 °C in the dog either with arrest or with retrograde perfusion. The cerebral tissue oxygen fell from about 50 mmHg (with a wide range) to 10 mmHg (Fig. 2) and carbon dioxide climbed from 30 mmHg to 140 mmHg (Fig. 3). Tissue oxygen reached a nadir by 15 min. ATP fell from 0.75 mmol/g to 0.2 by about 30 min and then fell no further (Fig. 4) following a similar but inverse pattern to carbon dioxide (Fig. 3) and lactate (Fig. 5). Metabolism is still occurring between 15 and 30 min and after that there is not much further change in these indices of metabolism.

In these dogs retrograde flow of 20 mls/100 g/min maintained a tissue oxygen of 30 mmHg (Fig. 6), ameliorated the rise in carbon dioxide and the fall in ATP. They both continued to change in the second 30 min and were still short of the 30 min state associated with total circulatory arrest.

Our current practice is to use retrograde arterial perfusion through a cannula in the superior vena cava, in any operation where the planned period of arrest is likely to exceed 25–30 min, a practice supported by these data. This is extremely simple to employ but has certain imprecisions. For example, how much goes to the brain and how much to other parts of the upper body we cannot say. Typically we run 500–700 mls per minute, achieve a pressure of 25 to 35 mmHg in the superior vena cava, and see a steady flow of very dark, desaturated blood flowing freely from the arch vessels.

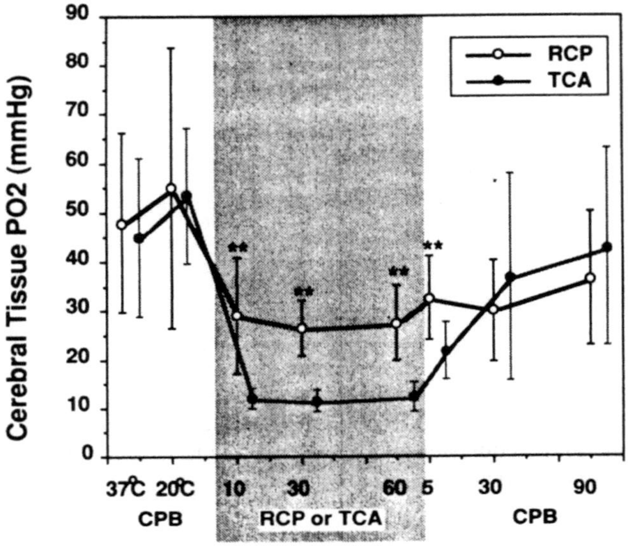

Cerebral Tissue PO2 (mmHg)
90
80
70
60
50
40
30
20
10
0
RCP
TCA
**
**
**
**
37°C 20°C 10 30 60 5 30 90
CPB
RCP or TCA
CPB

Fig. 2

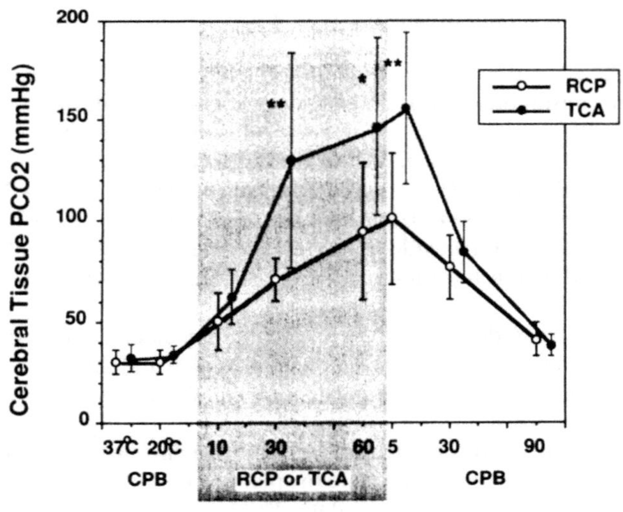

Cerebral Tissue PCO2 (mmHg)
200
150
100
50
0
RCP
TCA
**
*
**
37°C 20°C 10 30 60 5 30 90
CPB
RCP or TCA
CPB

Fig. 3

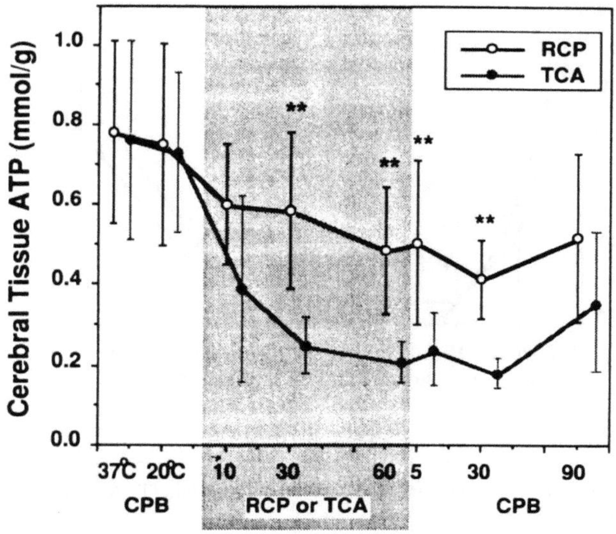
Cerebral Tissue ATP (mmol/g)
1.0
0.8
0.6
0.4
0.2
0.0
RCP
TCA
**
**
**
**
37°C 20°C 10 30 60 5 30 90
CPB
RCP or TCA
CPB

Fig. 4

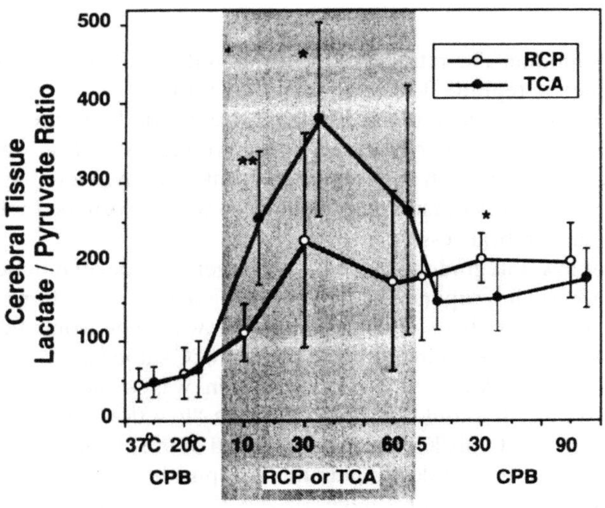
Cerebral Tissue
Lactate / Pyruvate Ratio
500
400
300
200
100
0
RCP
TCA
**
*
37°C 20°C 10 30 60 5 30 90
CPB
RCP or TCA
CPB

Fig. 5

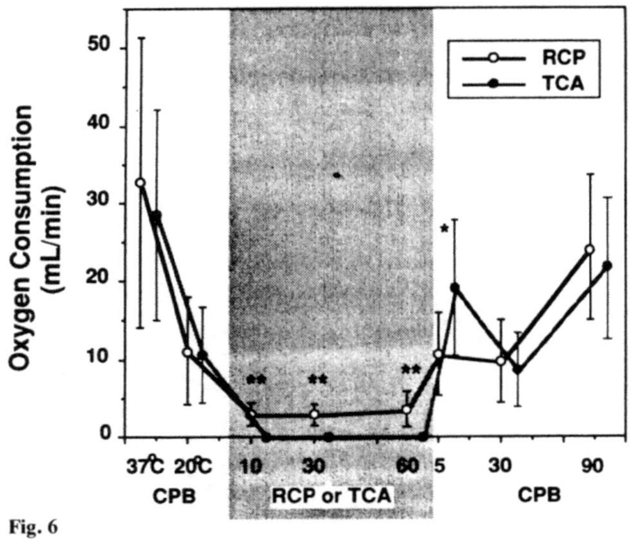

Fig. 6

Figs. 2, 3, 4, 5, 6. Experimental data in dogs with arrested circulation for 60 min (TCA) compared with those with retrograde cerebral perfusion (RCP).
The figures show cerebral tissue oxygen (2) tissue PCO2 (3) ATP (4) lactate/pyruvate ration (5) and oxygen consumption (6) (ref. Usui et al. 1994).

There is a bonus to this technique. The retrograde perfusion reduces the risk of embolisation of air and particles when antegrade flow is reestablished (16).

We have used antegrade cerebral perfusion through cannulae inserted into the orifices of the arch vessels during aortic arch surgery if a very extensive reconstruction was predicted. It is much more difficult to establish and carries inherent risks. We were happy to give this up when we learned about retrograde perfusion which we, and others, first used as a means of flushing air from cerebral vessels.

The alternative strategy of low antegrade flow for aortic surgery can be abandoned for the same reasons in aortic surgery; it is superseded. However, it is a practical option in congenital surgery (11). There has always been a worry that low flow may be worse than no flow. There is some evidence for that belief in a study in pigs at 18 °C subjected for an hour to full flow, 10 % flow, or arrest. Low flow at 10 % (10 mls/Kg/min) was considerably worse than no flow at all (Table 3) (14). It should be noted that the "low flow" group in the Boston Children's study was about 50 mls/Kg/min, about a third of the normal flow (11).

Another approach is to use intermittent flow. Again this is applicable to the situation in congenital heart disease, but has all the disadvantages of selective vessel cannulation and antegrade flow in aortic surgery. It has been studied in dogs at 18 °C where 120 min of arrest has been interrupted at 20-min intervals by 10 min of flow (8). The study is complicated but merits close attention. It suggests that by about 20 min the brain is anaerobic and reperfusion for 10 min restores tissue oxygen. It seems to be consistent with the observations I have made above on Usui's study (21).

Table 3. Pigs at 18 °C under circulatory arrest for 60 min EEG isoelectric (14)

	Golgi morphology disturbance		
	None	Mild	Severe
Normal flow	49 %	31 %	20 %
Circulatory arrest	29 %	42 %	29 %
Low flow (10 %)	13 %	23 %	64 %

Drugs

Barbiturates

The debate about the use of barbiturates to protect the brain has run for a long time and the issue remains unresolved (23). An intravenous bolus of thiopentone does halt EEG activity and slow the cerebral metabolic rate. It is a sustainable argument that this will prolong the tolerance to circulatory arrest and reduce damage due to excitatory neurotransmittors. However, in routine cardiopulmonary bypass for low risk elective cases, the prolonged ventilation required after its use is sufficient reason to eschew barbiturates.

In the special case of planned circulatory arrest, the balance of risks and benefits is different. My own experiments in gerbils convinced me that neurological recovery was better (18) but there was sufficient doubt in our minds about confounding factors in some of the control animals that we did not publish the work formally at the time. The accumulation of knowledge from other sources has led me to use thiopentone prophylaxis in our clinical practice of circulatory arrest (17).

Jonas' group included 10 mg/Kg thiopentone just prior to circulatory arrest (11). Crawford's practice was also to use thiopentone (50 mg/Kg) prior to arrest (16). We too used to give a bolus at this stage (17) but have changed our practice to giving the same total dose but by infusion during the period of cooling on bypass. We believe that this gives time for the drug to be distributed in the fat, a process which probably occurs more efficiently while the patient is still warm. The cerebral benefit is thus considered to be possibly enhanced while the complicating effects on the cardiovascular system are, if anything, reduced.

Nimodipine

Part of the sequence of events in neuronal death is an influx of calcium. It has been suggested that nimodipine may be useful in this respect and it has been found to reduce death and degree of damage in stroke (6) and an earlier study suggested a small benefit in subarachnoid haemorrhage, presumed to be due to a reduction in vasospasm (2). Although other calcium antagonists are used in the treatment of angina and hypertension, nimodipine is only listed in the Association of the British Pharmaceutical Industry (ABPI) Data Sheet Compendium for the treatment or prophylaxis of neurological ischaemia (1).

The great opportunity for the cardiovascular surgeon, denied to the neurologist, is that we have the opportunity to pretreat the patient, before the ischaemic event whether this is due to the imperfections of cardiopulmonary bypass, or the abrupt cessation of flow in planned circulatory arrest. In a randomised controlled trial in valve replacement surgery, patients were given nimodipine or placebo from 12 h before to 5 days after surgery. There was an excess of deaths in the treatment limb due to bleeding and the trial was stopped prematurely. This post hoc analysis should be treated with caution but no neuro-protective benefit of nimodipine has been reported from this trial (22).

Glutamate excitotoxicity and NMDA antagonists

Part of the sequence of events in ischaemic brain damage is that an excess of excitatory neurotransmitters, particularly glutamate accumulates and prolonged excitation of the post synaptic cells via N-methyl-D-aspartate (NMDA) "excites cells to death". An authoritative and accessible account of this subject in the context of cardiac surgery is available (4).

Pretreatment of the brain with the experimental NMDA antagonist MK-801 (or dizocilpine) has been undertaken at Johns Hopkins with striking beneficial results (13). Dogs were exposed to a 2-h period of circulatory arrest at 18 °C in a situation that closely mimicked clinical practice except that the time was deliberately chosen to be well into the damaging range, in fact near lethal. Of the 18 dogs, nine were given a prearrest intravenous bolus of 0.75 mg/kg of dizocilpine. The dogs were recovered and assessed neurologically for 3 days and then the brains of six in each group were perfusion fixed. The unprotected dogs had a sustained severe neurological injury. They were alive and conscious but could not walk or feed. Four had choreoathetosis and two had recurrent seizures. In contrast treated dogs were near normal with two having mild abnormality of gait (Fig. 7, Table 4).

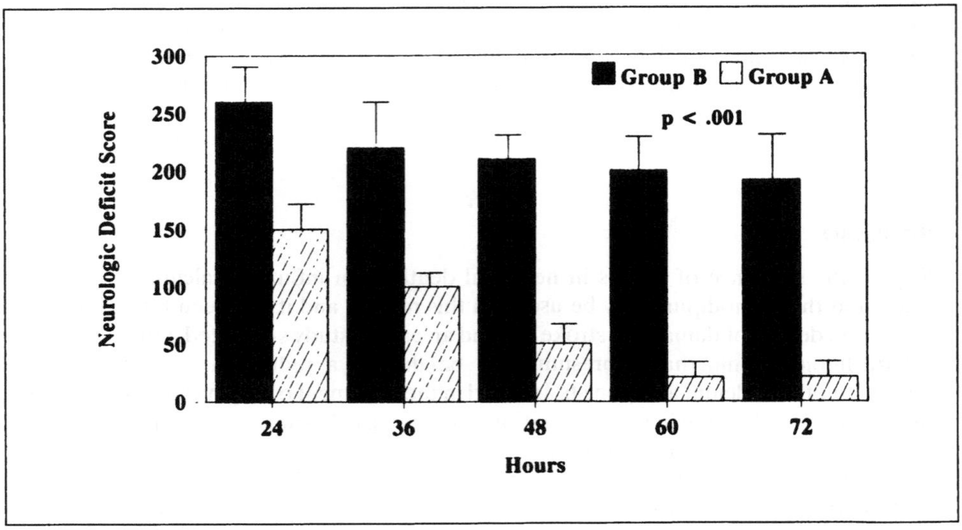

Fig. 7. Neurological deficit scores in experimental animals (see text for details) (Redmond et al. 1994).

Table 4. Circulatory arrest for 120 min in dogs at 18 °C (13)

	MK-801	Control
CNS deficit at 72 h (Brain dead = 500)	21 (SD:15)	192 (SD:40)
Histopathology (Total injury = 100)	7.3 (SD:3)	48.3 (SD:9)

The pathological injury scores were also very different with the most extensive damage appearing in the neocortex, the cerebellum and the basal ganglia.

Unfortunately the benefits of NMDA antagonists have not been confirmed in another study (3) in which MK-801 was added to cerebroplegia and gave no evident advantage.

Cerebroplegia

The development and refinement of reliable techniques to protect the myocardium seemed to bring about a sea change in the results of cardiac surgery. Although modifications, revisions and reversions continue there is little doubt that if we need to make the myocardium ischaemic for a sustained period we now know how to do it with reliable recovery by appropriate use of a number of cardioplegic techniques. Similarly, if we have to halt the circulation to the brain, it would be useful to have a reliable means of protecting it.

Jonas' group in Boston have reported on an experiment in 1-week-old pigs subjected to circulatory arrest for 2 h at 15 °C (3). They looked at a variety of vascular and biochemical indices after 3 h of normothermic reperfusion. Cerebral perfusion of cold saline at 30-min intervals was better than simply arresting the circulation as judged by recovery towards baseline of ATP and phosphocreatine and the rate of consuming oxygen but not glucose (Table 5). University of Wisconsin solution improved all of these indices further. The addition of the NMDA antagonist, MK-801 (see above) gave no further advantage.

It is hard to know how to interpret these results for practical application. Is it that cold saline has an effect because it provides better cooling or is there some advantage to washing out blood? They reperfused with saline or cerebroplegia (University of Wisconsin solution) at 30-min intervals. Resumption of antegrade flow may be an option in congenital

Table 5. Cerebroplegia for TCA at 15 °C for 120 min. Early indices of brain recovery (% baseline) in pigs (3)

	ATP	PhCr	O_2 consumption	Glucose
Control	29 %	32 %	45 %	40 %
Saline 4 °C	54 %	67 %	60 %	40 %
Wisconsin	72 %	80 %	80 %	60 %
UW+MK-801	73 %	79 %	70 %	50 %

heart surgery but is less practical if planned arrest is being used for a major construction on the aortic arch. Did MK-801 fail to show an advantage because it had no benefit or because no further benefit was discernible over UW solution?

Conclusions

1) One has to conclude that it is better to maintain as near physiological perfusion to the brain as one can. Flow is better than no flow, with the probable exception of extremely low (or trickle) flow. Low flow (50 mls/kg/min) is better for the brain than arrest in babies.
2) Some surgery, such as that involved in reconstructing the aortic arch requires interruption to normal cerebral perfusion if only for long enough to establish some alternative. Hypothermia is the best mode of protection and temperatures below 18 °C may add further protection. Retrograde perfusion is a valuable adjunct in aortic arch surgery.
3) At 18 °C 20 min seems to be the point at which metabolism becomes anaerobic. At 30 min some permanent damage may occur in some patients. By 40 min neurones are being sacrificed.
4) Barbiturate appears to have a protective effect and a protocol of 50 mg/kg/min has support.
   NMDA antagonists look promising but are yet to be proven.
   Nimodipine seems to cause serious bleeding problems
   Other pharmacological strategies are unproven.

References

1. ABPI Data Sheet Compendium P171. Datapham Publications Limited, London 1994
2. Allen GS, Ahn HS, Preziosi TJ, Battye R, Boone SC, Chou SN et al. (1983) Cerebral arterial spasm – a controlled trial of nimodipine in patients with subarachnoid haemorrhage. New England Journal of Medicine 308: 619–624
3. Aoki M, Jonas RA, Nomura F, Stromski ME, Tsuji MK, Hickey PR, Hotzman D (1994) Effects of cerebroplegic solutions during hypothermic circulatory arrest and short-term recovery. Journal of Thoracic and Cardiovascular Surgery 108: 291–301
4. Corbett D, Evans S (1993) The use of glutamate receptor antagonists P234-244. In: "Cardiac Surgery and the Brain" (eds.) Taylor KM, Smith P. Hodder and Stoughton
5. Fessatidis I Th, Thomas VL, Shore DF, Sedgwick ME, Hunt RH, Weller RO (1993) Brain damage after profoundly hypothermic circulatory arrest: correlation between neurophysiological and neuropathological findings – an experimental study in vertebrates. Journal of Thoracic and Cardiovascular Surgery 106: 32–41
6. Gelmers HJ, Gorter K, de Weerdt CJ, Wiezer HJA (1988) A controlled trial of nimodipine in acute ischaemic stroke. New England Journal of Medicine 318: 203–7
7. Jonas RA (1994) Cerebral protection in infants: state of the art In: "Annual of cardiac surgery" 7th Edition p 153–160. Edited by Yacoub M, Pepper J. Published by Current Science
8. Kimura T, Muraoka R, Chiba Y, Ihaya A, Morioka K (1994) Effect of deep hypothermic circulatory arrest on brain metabolism. Journal of Thoracic and Cardiovascular Surgery 108: 658–63
9. Mezrow CK, Midulla PS, Sadeghi AM, Gandsas A, Wang W, Dapunt OE, Zappulla R, Griepp (1994) Evaluation of cerebral metabolism and quantitative electroencephalography after hypothermic circulatory arrest and low-flow cardiopulmonary bypass at different temperatures. Journal of Thoracic and Cardiovascular Surgery 107: 1006–19

10. Michenfelder JD, Milde JH (1992) The effect of profound levels of hypothermia (below 14 °C) on canine cerebral metabolism. Journal of Cerebral Blood Flow and Metabolism 12: 877–880
11. Newburger JW, Jonas RA, Wernovsky G, Wypij D, Hickey PR, Kuban KCK et al. (1993) A comparison of the perioperative neurological effects of hypothermic circulatory arrest versus low-flow cardiopulmonary bypass in infant heart surgery. New England Journal of Medicine 329: 1057–64
12. Oates RK, Simpson JM, Turnbull JAB, Cartmill TB (1995) The relationship between intelligence and the duration of circulatory arrest with deep hypothermia. Journal of Thoracic and Cardiovascular Surgery 110: 786–92
13. Redmond JM, Gillinov AM, Zehr KJ, Blue ME, Troncoso JC, Reitz BA, Cameron DE, Johnston MV, Baumgartner WA (1994) Glutamate excitotoxicity: a mechanism of neurological injury associated with hypothermic circulatory arrest. Journal of Thoracic and Cardiovascular Surgery 107: 776–87
14. Scheller MS, Branson PJ, Cornacchia LG, Alksne JF (1992) A comparison of the effects on neuronal Golgi morphology, assessed with electron microscopy, of cardiopulmonary bypass, and circulatory arrest during profound hypothermia. Journal of Thoracic and Cardiovascular Surgery 104: 1396–1404
15. Souttar HS (1925) The surgical treatment of mitral stenosis. Brit Med J ii: 603–7
16. Svensson LG, Crawford ES, Hess KR, Coselli JS, Raskin S, Shenaq SA, Safi HJ (1993) Deep hypothermia with circulatory arrest. Determinants of stroke and early mortality in 656 patients. Journal of Thoracic and Cardiovascular Surgery 106: 19–31
17. Tan PSK, Aveling W, Pugsley WB, Newman SP, Treasure T (1989) Experience with circulatory arrest and hypothermia to facilitate thoracic aortic surgery. Ann R Coll Surg Engl 71: 81–86
18. Treasure T (1982) The safe duration of total circulatory arrest with profound hypothermia: an experimental study in the Mongolian gerbil. M.D. Thesis. University of London
19. Treasure T (1984) The safe duration of total circulatory arrest with profound hypothermia. Ann R Coll Surg Engl 66: 235–240
20. Treasure T, Naftel DC, Conger KA, Garcia JH, Kirklin JW, Blackstone EH (1983) The effect of hypothermic circulatory arrest time on cerebral function, morphology, and biochemistry: An experimental study. J Thorac Cardiovasc Surg 86: 761–770
21. Usui A, Oohara K, Liu T-l, Murase M, Tanaka M, Takeuchi E, Abe T (1994) Comparative experimental study between retrograde cerebral perfusion and circulatory arrest. Journal of Thoracic and Cardiovascular Surgery 107: 1228–36
22. Wagenknecht LE, Furberg CD, Hammon JW, Legault C, Troost BT (1995) Surgical bleeding: unexpected finding of a calcium antagonist. Brit Med J 310: 776–7
23. Weir DL (1993) The use of thiopentone and propofol P245-251 in "Cardiac Surgery and the Brain" (eds.) Taylor K, Smith P. Hodder and Stoughton

Authors' address:
T. Treasure, M.D., MS, FRCS
St. George's Hospital
Dept. of Cardiothoracic Surgery
Blackshaw Road
London, SW17 0QT, England

Cerebral oxygenation during cardiac surgery

G. Nollert, P. Möhnle, P. Tassani-Prell*, M. Schmoeckel, A. Welz, B. Reichart

Clinic of Cardiac Surgery and *Institute for Anesthesiology, University of Munich, Munich

Introduction

Despite approximately 40 years of experience, there are many unresolved questions concerning the "ideal" cardio-pulmonary bypass (CPB) method. Neurological and neuropsychological deficits are not uncommon after cardiac surgery and have been attributed to the adverse effects of CPB on cerebral perfusion and oxygenation (22).

Cerebral perfusion and oxygenation are regulated under physiological conditions, but it is well known that profound hypocarbia and hypotension (8) may impair oxygen delivery to the brain. Other factors such as temperature, acid-base status, arterial PO_2 and hemodilution as well as flow-pattern, duration and flow rate of the extracorporeal circulation may influence cerebral perfusion; the degree of the influences and the interactions of all these parameters are, however, unsatisfactorily understood (21, 24).

During hypothermia oxygen metabolism of the brain is reduced and oxygen transport to the tissue is affected by the leftshift of the hemoglobin binding curve. In order to obtain information on cerebral oxygenation we therefore monitored three different parameters representing oxygen delivery to the brain, cellular oxygenation and brain venous oxygen saturation. In recent years, near infrared spectrophotometry (NIRS) has been shown to be useful in measuring cerebral oxygenation in children and adults. NIRS obtains information on oxygen delivery (oxygenated and deoxygenated hemoglobin) and cellular oxygenation (oxidized cytochrome a,a3, the terminal enzyme of the respiratory chain) (7). Cerebral venous oxygen saturation can be estimated by oxygen saturation measurement in the jugular bulb ($S_{BJ}O_2$). Information on cerebral oxygen uptake may be obtained by taking arterial oxygen saturation, flow and hemoglobin into consideration.

In this study parameters of operative management were analyzed in order to quantify their influence on cerebral oxygenation with and without CPB.

Patients and methods

Forty-one consecutive patients undergoing cardiac operations with CPB were investigated. The study was approved by the ethics committee of the Ludwig-Maximilians-University in Munich and informed consent of these patients was obtained. The group comprised 9 female and 32 male patients with an age range at operation from 32 to 76 years, the mean age being 61.2 years. Twenty-five patients underwent coronary artery bypass grafting, 14 patients had valve replacements (aortic valve n = 10, mitral valve n = 4); two patients had a combination of coronary artery bypass grafting and valve replacements. The cardiological diagnosis was confirmed by a preoperative cardiac catheterization in all patients. In addition, all patients underwent Doppler sonography of the carotid arteries and, in the event of pathological findings, brain CT scan and single photon emission computerized tomography after inhalation of xenon-133 (SPECT) were carried out. All patients were free of cerebral infarction preoperatively; however, in nine cases significant stenoses of one or both internal carotid arteries were detected. Two of the nine patients had a severe and five a moderate stenosis on the left side, where the NIRS-measurements were obtained. Before operation and on the first, second and third post-operative days, thorough neurological examinations and neuropsychological testings (Mini-Mental-State Test (MMS) (4)) were performed. The MMS has a maximum score of 30 points; a score equal or less than 23 points or a decline of more than five points in consecutive measurements indicate neuropsychological deficits. No neurological or neuropsychological deficits were detected preoperatively.

General anesthesia and operative management

Anesthesia was induced with etomidate 0.3 mg/kg and 3 μg/kg fentanyl. Each patient received 0.1 mg/kg pancuronium for muscle relaxation. After induction of anesthesia, controlled ventilation with an FiO_2 of 0.5 was instituted. Anesthesia was maintained with isoflurane 0.6 – 1.0 % and fentanyl in increments of 0.5 mg as required. A Sarns 9000 heart-lung machine with non-pulsatile flow mode and membrane oxygenators (Maxima, Medtronic Inc.) was used for extracorporeal circulation. The priming volume of the heart-lung machine was 1800 ml and consisted of a balanced electrolyte solution and 20 % mannitol (3 ml/kg body weight). The average cardiopulmonary bypass time was 96.1 $\pm$ 26.8 min. During CPB a cardiac index of 2.4 l/min/m^2, alpha-stat blood gas values and systemic hypothermia to an esophageal temperature of 25.5 $\pm$ 3.8 °C were utilized. Alpha-stat blood gas values were later corrected for esophageal temperature (13) in order to correlate the PCO_2 and pH to CtO_2 shifts.

Near-infrared spectrophotometry

Using an NIRS-monitor (NIRO 500, Hamamatsu Corp., Osaka, Japan), the cerebral oxygenation was measured photometrically intraoperatively in all 41 patients. Two optodes were placed in a paramedian and frontotemporal position on the left forehead 5 cm apart. The emitted laser light (wavelength 770 – 910 nm) is able to penetrate the skull and is dispersed in brain tissue, where light of specific wavelengths is absorbed by oxygenated and deoxygenated hemoglobin (HbO_2, Hb) and oxidized cytochrome a,a3 (CtO_2). The optical pathlength in brain tissue can be estimated within 29.7 cm. The amount of reflected light of the specific wavelengths, the optical pathlength and the brain specific gravity (1.05) allow the measurement of chromophores in brain tissue in concentration (μMol). The NIRS system also provides the parameter of total hemoglobin (tHb) (using the formula $tHb = Hb + HbO_2$). The measurements were displayed and recorded every 2 s.

Oxymetry in the internal jugular vein

Only 11 of the 41 patients consented to the intraoperative measurement of jugular venous oxygen saturation. In three cases monitoring of oxygen saturation showed major artefacts; therefore measurements in eight patients were analyzed. Correlation coefficients of $S_{BJ}O_2$

to other data were calculated only for these cases. Four of these patients underwent coronary artery bypass grafting and four heart valve replacement. For the measurements a fiberoptic catheter (Abbott Lab.) was introduced into the left internal jugular vein and advanced into the jugular bulb under x-ray control. Oxygen saturation in the jugular bulb was measured and displayed continuously on an oxygen saturation monitor; this measurement reflects the venous oxygen saturation of the brain.

Standard intraoperative data

Mean arterial pressure, heart rate and temperature (rectal and esophageal) were displayed and recorded continuously. For each measuring time (see Fig. 1) arterial blood-gas samples were analyzed (hemoglobin concentration, PO_2, PCO_2, oxygen saturation, pH and base excess). The data of the heart-lung machine (flow rate, gas flow and FiO_2) were recorded simultaneously.

Statistical evaluation

All parameters are expressed as mean values ± standard error of the mean. For statistical analysis the data was obtained from thirteen standardized points of measurement in each operation. The values of point 1, obtained 10 min before thoracotomy were used as baseline values. The points of measurements were as follows: Before CPB: 1) 10 min before thoracotomy, 2) thoracotomy, 3) 10 min after thoracotomy, 4) aortic cannulation. During CPB: 5) onset of CPB, 6) aortic clamping on, 7) 15 min after onset of CPB, 8) beginning of rewarming, 9) 15 min after beginning of rewarming, 10) aortic clamping off, 11) end of CPB. After CPB: 12) 15 min after end of CPB, 13) closure of thorax.

A p value of 0.05 was taken as the level of significance. The Wilcoxon rank sum test served for statistical analysis. Spearman correlation coefficients were used for statistical correlation. Parameters of operative management were first tested in a univariate regression model. Every univariate significant parameter was tested in a multi-regression model and removed stepwise if no significant influence was proved. Statistical analyses were facilitated with the help of SPSS (SPSS Inc., Chicago, IL) statistical software.

Results

One patient died on the second postoperative day because of myocardial infarction due to early graft closure. No patient suffered from central neurological deficits postoperatively; one patient had a transient peripheral paresis of the left arm due to operative placement. Four patients showed transient neuropsychological deficits postoperatively diagnosed by a score of 23 or less in the Mini-Mental-State-test obtained on the first to the third postoperative day. These patients had a lower CtO_2 minimum compared to those without these deficits (-4.5 μMol v. -0.7 μMol; $p < 0.05$). All other measured parameters showed no significant differences between the groups.

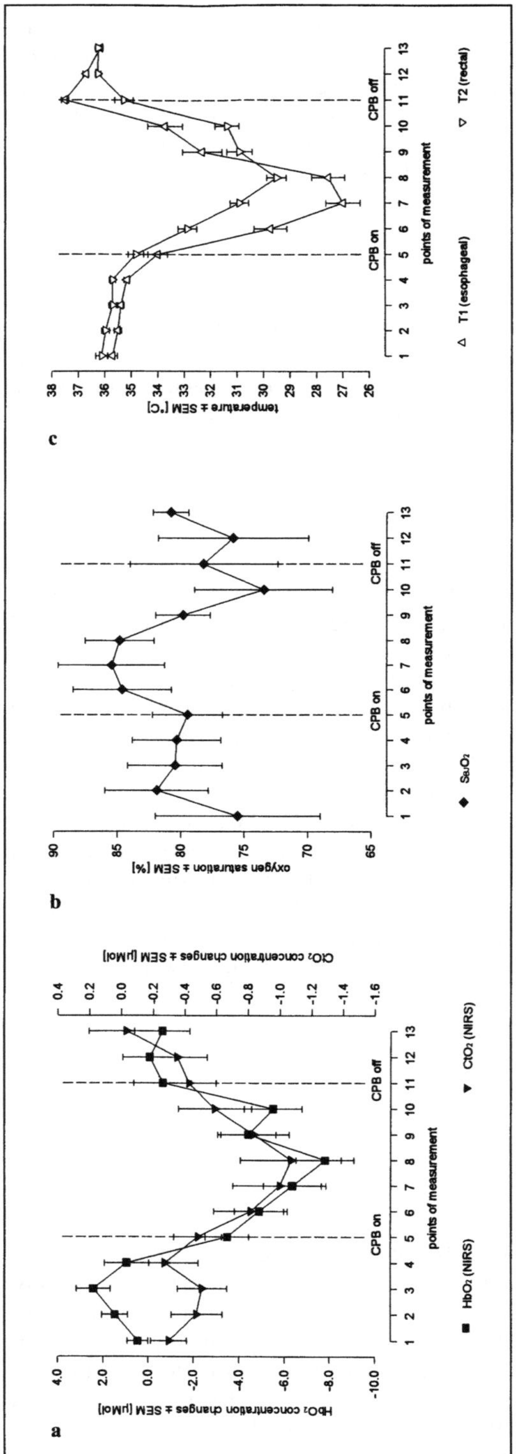

Fig. 1. Near-infrared-spectrophotometry (NIRS) and jugular bulb oxymetry ($S_{BJ}O_2$) in operations with cardiopulmonary bypass (CPB). The x-axis is split up in standardized manner in 13 points of time during the operations (see methods section). **Fig. 1a** provides the mean values of the NIRS measurements in 41 patients. The changes of the parameters oxygenated hemoglobin (HbO_2) and oxidized cytochrome a,a3 (CtO_2) are plotted. Asteriks (* for HbO_2 + for CtO_2) indicate significant changes compared to point 1 (10 min before thoracotomy). **Fig. 1b** gives changes in jugular bulb oxygen saturation ($S_{BJ}O_2$) in eight patients. **Fig. 1c** provides the course of esophageal and rectal temperature in all 41 operations. For all points of measurement except for point 12 and 13 (15 min after end of CPB and closure of thorax) the values obtained for rectal and esophageal temperature significantly differ from values on point 1 (10 min before thoracotomy).

NIRS-Monitoring and oxygen saturation measurements in the jugular bulb

The parameters HbO_2 and CtO_2 obtained by NIRS and oxygen saturation in the jugular bulb showed characteristic changes during cardiac operations (Fig. 1): At the onset of CPB the parameters CtO_2 and HbO_2 decreased continuously (CtO_2: $p = 0.104$; HbO_2: $p = 0.001$) reaching the minimum (CtO_2: -1.07 ± 0.32 μMol; HbO_2: -7.81 ± 1.29 μMol) at the beginning of the rewarming phase. During rewarming the parameters rose constantly, reaching initial levels again at the end of the operation. Oxygen saturation values in the jugular bulb increased at the onset of CPB and remained elevated (85 ± 4 %) during hypothermia. At the beginning of the rewarming phase, a decrease to minimum values of 73 ± 5 % (end of aortic clamping) was seen; at thorax closure the parameters had regained initial levels (80 ± 3 %).

Correlations to parameters of intraoperative management

The correlations of NIRS and $S_{BJ}O_2$ values to standard intraoperative data during CPB were dependent on whether CPB was on or off.

Influences on cerebral oxygenation during the period before and after CPB

During the period without CPB, temperature (ranging from 35.5 °C to 36.7 °C), mean arterial pressure (75 mmHg – 87 mmHg), heart frequency (82 l/min – 101 l/min), arterial oxygen pressure (310 mmHg – 390 mmHg) and carbon dioxide pressure (33 mmHg – 40 mmHg), pH (7.39 – 7.44) as well as arterial hemoglobin (96 g/l – 128 g/l) showed no significant influence on cerebral oxygenation in univariate analysis. Thus multiregression models were not calculated.

Influences on cerebral oxygenation during the CPB period

In order to calculate the influences of blood gases on brain oxygenation, pH, PO_2 and PCO_2 were corrected for temperature (13). A survey of the univariate correlation coefficients between the parameters of operative management and cerebral oxygenation is given in Table 1. Mean arterial pressure, arterial PO_2 and blood flow did not affect oxygenation.

By means of multiregression analysis of all probable influencing factors (with a univariate $p < 0.05$), equations were calculated in order to explain changes in cerebral oxygenation from changes in operative management. HbO_2 (measured by NIRS) depends significantly only on PCO_2 (see Fig. 2). The following equation is estimated to explain 75 % of all changes in HbO_2: $HbO_2\,(NIRS) = 0.518 \times PCO_2 - 19.9$ ($r = 0.88$; $p = 0.075$).

CtO_2 the measure for cellular oxygenation, was influenced by temperature (T), arterial Hb, PCO_2 and pH (see Fig. 3). These parameters are estimated to determine 99 % of the fluctuations of CtO_2:

$CtO_2\,(NIRS) = 0.0018 \times Hb - 6.697 \times pH - 0.025 \times PCO_2 + 0.024 \times T$
($r = 1.0$; $p < 0.001$).

The oxygen saturation in the jugular bulb was affected by PCO_2 and pH (see Fig. 4). Ninety-three percent of the $S_{BJ}O_2$ variations are explained by these parameters.

$S_{BJ}O_2 = 288.815 * pH + 2.322 * PCO_2 - 2143.35$ ($r = 0.98$; $p < 0.01$).

In Fig. 5 the measured values are plotted against values derived from the multiregression analysis in order to visualize the fit of the multiregression models.

Influences on cerebral oxygenation by open heart surgery and stenosis of the left carotid artery

The duration of CPB as well as the time of aortic clamping lasted longer in valve surgery than in coronary surgery (103.2 ± 3.2 min vs. 91.1 ± 5.0 min and 55.7 ± 3.4 min vs. 70.3 ±

Table 1. Survey of univariate correlation coefficients (Spearman) between the parameters of cerebral oxygenation and operative management for the time CPB; significant values ($p < 0.05$) are in bold type.

		CtO_2 (NIRS) [μMol]	HbO_2 (NIRS) [μMol]	$S_{BJ}O_2$ [%]
CtO_2 (NIRS) [μMol]	range −1.1 to −0.4		r = 0.857 p = 0.014	r = −0.821 p = 0.023
HbO_2 (NIRS) [μMol]	range −7.8 to −0.6	r = 0.857 p = 0.014		r = −0.607 p = 0.148
$S_{BJ}O_2$ [%]	range 73.4 to 85.4	r = 0.821 p = 0.023	r = −0.607 p = 0.148	
T (esophageal) [°C]	range 27.0 to 37.5	r = 0.929 p = 0.003	r = 0.857 p = 0.014	r = −0.893 p = 0.007
PCO_2 [mmHg]	range 24.8–35.8	r = 1.000 p = 0.001	r = 0.857 p = 0.014	r = −0.821 p = 0.023
pH	range 7.405–7.519	r = 0.964 p = 0.001	r = 0.750 p = 0.052	r = 0.893 p = 0.007
hemoglobin [g/dl]	range 8.4–12.7	r = 0.786 p = 0.036	r = 0.714 p = 0.071	r = −0.571 p = 0.180

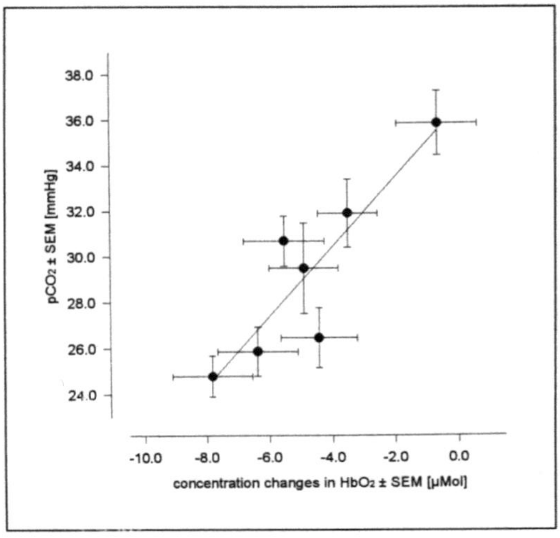

Fig. 2. During CPB HbO_2 as measured by NIRS correlates significantly univariate to esophageal temperature, arterial carbon dioxide pressure (PCO_2) values and inversely to arterial pH values. In multiregression analysis the parameter HbO_2 depends only on arterial carbon dioxide pressure. Mean values of HbO_2 ± SEM are plotted against mean values of PCO_2 ± SEM for the time of CPB.

3.0 min). In valve surgery minimal esophageal temperatures were also lower (26.5 ± 0.5 °C) than in coronary surgery (27.8 ± 0.6 °C and 24.8 ± 1.2 °C). No significant differences were found between the groups with respect to brain tissue oxygenation.

In seven patients a significant carotid artery stenosis of the left side was detected preoperatively; five of these patients underwent coronary revascularisation, two valve replacement. Patients with carotid artery stenosis differed only with respect to age from those without (70.9 ± 1.7 years vs. 58.8 ± 1.9; $p < 0.05$). The stenosis of the carotid artery showed no influence on the NIRS-measurements.

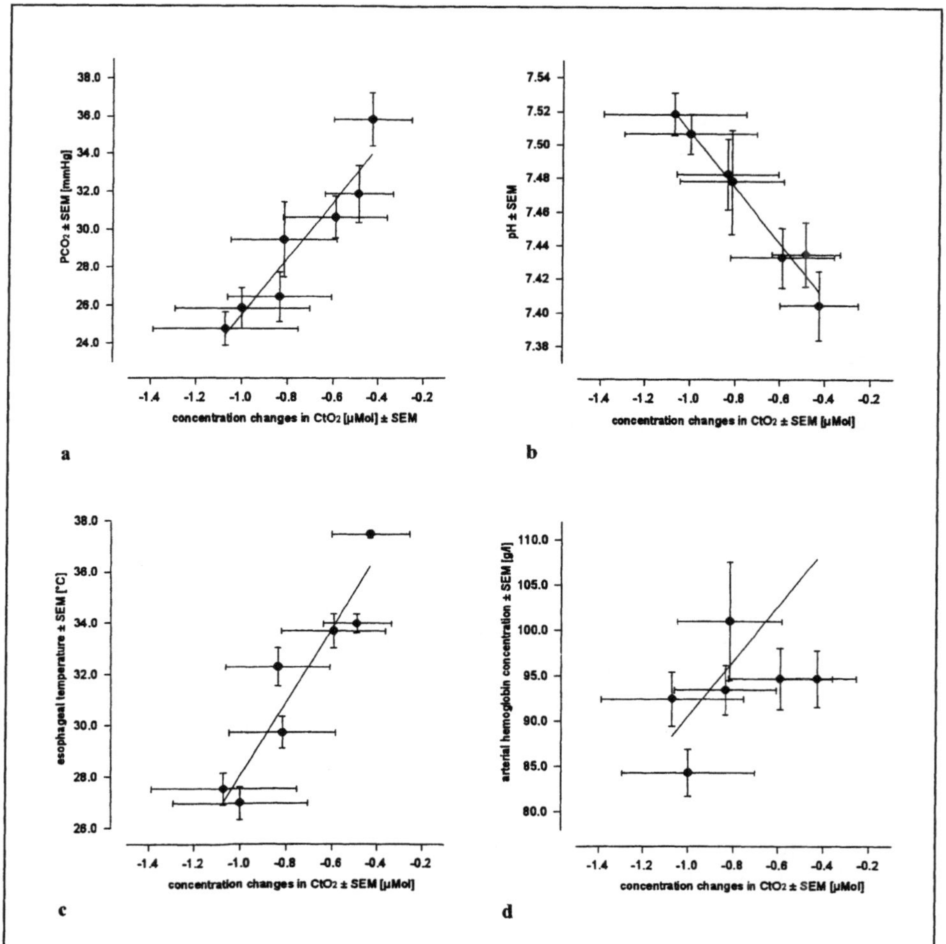

Fig. 3. Changes in CtO_2 as measured by NIRS correlate significantly to esophageal temperature, arterial carbon dioxide pressure and hemoglobin concentration in arterial blood for the time of CPB. The arterial pH values show an inverse correlation to CtO_2. Figures 3 a–d illustrate the correlations between these parameters and CtO_2 during CPB.

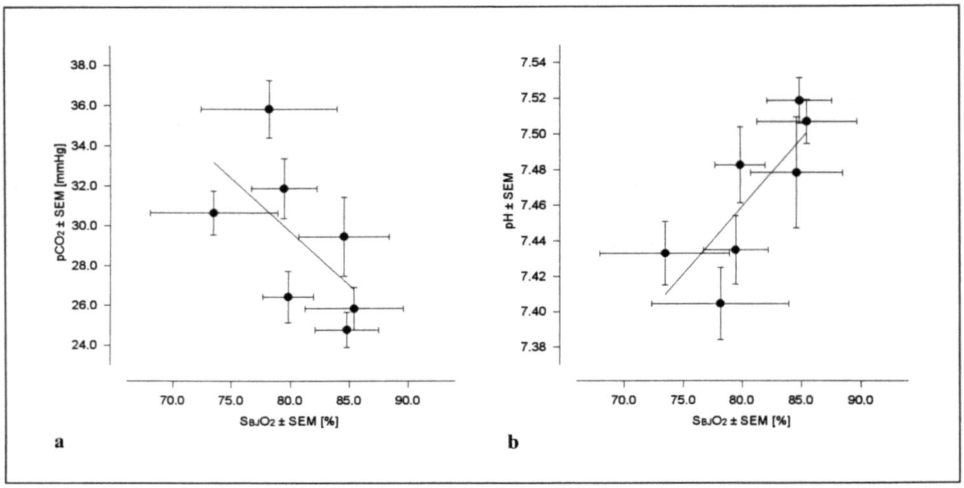

Fig. 4. The time of CPB oxygen saturation in the jugular bulb ($S_{BJ}O_2$) depends univariately on arterial pH and PCO_2 values and temperature. Since in multiregression analysis $S_{BJ}O_2$ only depends on PCO_2 and pH, the scatterplots 4a and b illustrate the relationships.

Discussion

Measurements of cerebral oxygenation – limitations

In this presented study cerebral oxygenation was assessed by three different parameters. NIRS measurements revealed information on oxygen delivery to brain (HbO_2) and cellular oxygenation (CtO_2). Information on venous oxygen saturation of the brain were provided by monitoring of $S_{BJ}O_2$. Obviously, it is difficult to compare NIRS and $S_{BJ}O_2$ recordings since NIRS measurements give only local information on brain oxygenation whereas $S_{BJ}O_2$ indicates the saturation of venous blood of one half of the brain. The optodes for the NIRS measurements were placed on the left forehead. Since brain tissue scatters light to a large extent, the average pathlength of the infrared light in brain tissue is long and might be estimated at 29.7 cm (3), if the distance between the optodes is 5 cm. One may thus assume that our NIRS measurements provide information about the left frontal brain. However, we found a correlation between the CtO_2 values obtained by NIRS with the gross neuropsychological outcome of these patients.Therefore the local measurements might be representative for the whole brain.

In this study cerebral blood flow was not measured limiting the interpretation of the results, since it is not possible to differentiate between changes of flow and oxygen consumption. Cerebral blood flow is discussed to decrease during cardio-pulmonary bypass as a function of time (11). The influences of these time-dependent changes on our multivariate models cannot be ruled out, since our data is derived from a clinical study and other parameters as for example temperature also change in time. Therefore some interrelations might be falsified or concealed by this effect.

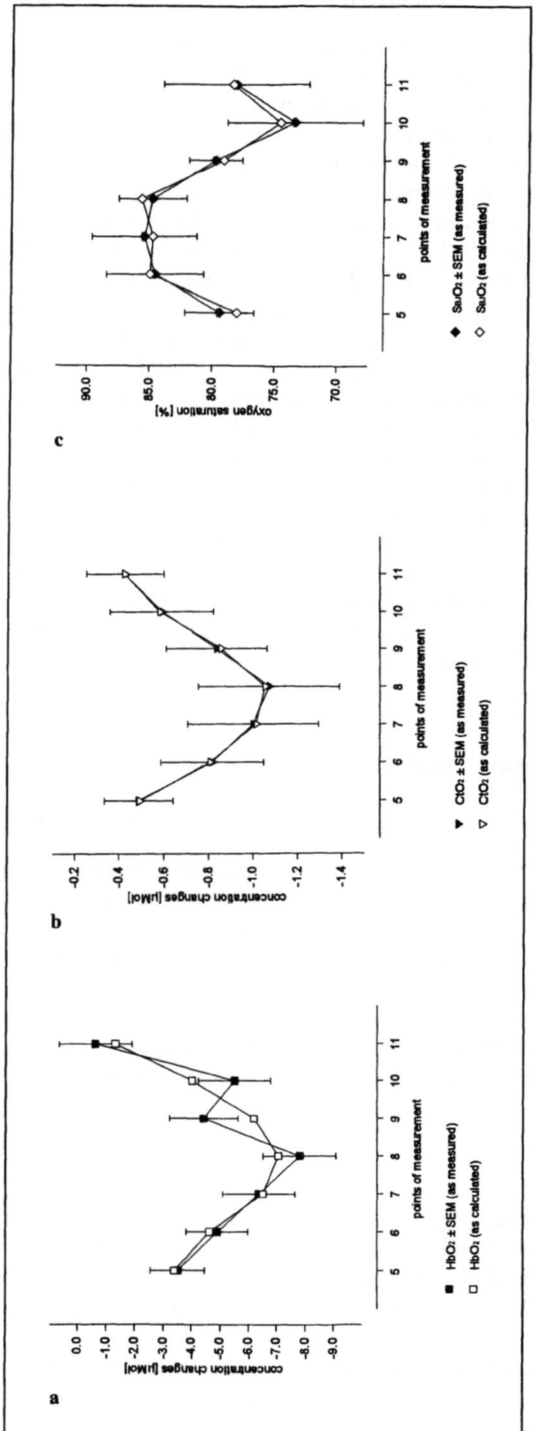

Fig. 5. In the Figs. 5a, 5b and 5c the measured values of the parameters HbO_2, CtO_2 and $S_{BJ}O_2$ for the time of CPB are compared to the values calculated with the equations derived from multiregression analysis. The equations are described in detail in the text.

Cerebral oxygenation before and after cardiopulmonary bypass

For the periods of the operation before and after extracorporeal circulation, no significant influence on any parameter of cerebral oxygenation was found. These findings underline the fact that cerebral blood flow and oxygenation are autoregulated not only within a wide variety of mean arterial pressure, but also with respect to changes in temperature, pH, PCO_2 and hemoglobin. It is important to mention that this autoregulation could be proved only for certain ranges of these parameters. We measured the autoregulation for a mean arterial pressure between 75 and 86 mmHg which is a small section of the pressure range of 60 to 125 mmHg reported in the literature (18). Esophageal temperature during this time ranged from normal values to mild hypothermia of 35.2 °C, which is reported not to affect the autoregulation (6).

Temperature corrected pH was always within the scope of normal values. Mild hypocarbia with temperature corrected PCO_2 values ranging between 30 mmHg and normal values did not significantly affect cerebral oxygenation in our study. Data from the literature suggest that the metabolic needs of the brain are met with a PCO_2 value of as low as 33 mmHg (12). The hemoglobin values of 100 g/l to 120 g/l resemble the hematocrit level of 33 % which is optimal for oxygen delivery to the brain (16). Cerebral oxygenation seems to be autoregulated during the operation periods before and after extracorporeal circulation. The cause for this finding might be that the determinants of cerebral oxygenation are close enough to normal values, unless they are not physiological. With CPB established, the oxygenation of the brain depends on parameters of the operative management, but it remains uncertain whether CPB itself is the cause for this dependency or the – under these circumstances – unphysiological determinants of cerebral oxygenation.

Cerebral oxygenation during cardiopulmonary bypass

Oxygen delivery

During extracorporeal circulation, HbO_2, the parameter for oxygen delivery to the brain, was only significantly influenced by arterial PCO_2. Using alpha-stat management, PCO_2 values corrected for temperature ranged from 25 to 36 mmHg and were thus much lower than those obtained without CPB. This moderate hypocarbia causes vasoconstriction in the brain and decreases cerebral blood flow (21). Arterial pressure had no influence on oxygen delivery in our patients; mean arterial pressure was on average always above 55 mmHg. Autoregulation of cerebral blood flow during alpha-stat management and mild hypothermia is described for a perfusion pressure range as great as 20 – 100 mmHg (5).

Cellular oxygenation

Cerebral CtO_2 representing cellular oxygenation, was influenced by esophageal temperature, arterial pH, PCO_2 and hemoglobin values. Hypothermia as well as alkalotic pH causes a displacement of the oxygen blood dissociation curve to the left leading to possible impaired tissue oxygenation. Similar observations were made by measuring PO_2 in the brain (1).

Vasoconstriction of brain vessels and consequently reduced cerebral blood flow as seen during hypocapnia is assumed to be mainly mediated by increasing the pH of the perivascular space (14). Surprisingly, in our multiregression model, CtO_2 was correlated inversely to PCO_2 indicating slightly better cellular oxygenation during mild hypocarbia provided that still stable pH, temperature and hemoglobin levels existed. In the literature only few attempts were made to differentiate between the effects of alkalosis and hypocarbia on cerebral oxygenation; inverse effects of these parameters, to our knowledge, have not been published. It therefore remains unclear whether the differentiation between the closely related parameters PCO_2 and pH in their effects on cerebral oxygenation has a physiological significance or is simply an error of our mathematical multiregression model.

The hemoglobin values during extracorporeal circulation decreased below 90 g/l. Oxygen transport to tissue is impaired when hemoglobin values fall below 100 g/l because decreasing oxygen transport capacity cannot be balanced by further improved rheological attributes (16).

Oxygen saturation in the jugular bulb

An increase in $S_{BJ}O_2$ is – according to the multiregression model – associated with alkalosis and increasing PCO_2. As discussed above the calculated inverse effects of hypocarbia and alkalosis remain unclear especially because univariate regression showed an opposite result with respect to PCO_2 (see Fig. 3); increased cerebral blood flow and impaired oxygen uptake might be the causes. CtO_2 and $S_{BJ}O_2$ showed an inverse correlation during CPB (see Table 1).

Therefore, increasing $S_{BJ}O_2$ during hypothermia must not be interpreted as an improved tissue oxygenation (7), since oxygen delivery to the brain at lower temperatures depends on dissolved oxygen and is a function of PO_2 and flow, not of saturation (17). On the contrary, during CPB a high $S_{BJ}O_2$ may give a hint of impaired oxygen uptake. For these reasons the postulated luxury perfusion of the brain during pH-stat management (9) diagnosed by a high jugular bulb venous saturation (25) is questionable.

Four patients showed transient neuropsychological deficits after the operation. Three of these patients underwent coronary artery bypass grafting and one, mitral valve replacement. The only parameter differing significantly between these patients and patients without severe neuropsychologic deficits was CtO_2, which decreased on average $-4.5\ \mu$Mol from the beginning of the operation to the beginning of rewarming (compared to $-0.7\ \mu$Mol in patients without severe neuropsychological deficits; $p < 0.05$). These data support the hypothesis that neuropsychological deficits are a direct consequence of intraoperative cerebral hypoxia. The decrease of CtO_2 was continuous during hypothermia, no sudden step in CtO_2 values could be detected. This indicates that macroembolism is not likely to be the cause of hypoxia, since in that case a sudden onset of hypoxia after embolism would be expected. Recent echo-Doppler studies revealed that microembolism does not occur continuously during heart surgery but a distinct points of time: at cannulation, declamping of the aorta and decannulation (26). CtO_2 increased in all patients during rewarming, declamping and decannulation manoeuvres. This implies that there is no correlation between microembolism and CtO_2 values. If the CtO_2 values reflect the oxygenation status of the brain, then one may conclude that microembolism during heart operations does not cause general brain hypoxia.

In summary, the described multiregression models are plausible and explain at least 85 % of all measured changes in cerebral oxygenation. They may give the surgical team practical hints to improve oxygen availability to the brain, when no direct monitoring of cerebral oxygenation is available. The invasive measurements of venous saturation are only reliable in about 80 % of the time during nonpulstile bypass (2) and difficult to interpret, because in hypothermia and alkalosis a high jugular venous saturation does not imply a sufficient oxygenation of the brain. However, in a recent study (2) the correlation between desaturation in the jugular bulb and impaired postoperative neuropsychological outcome was demonstrated stressing the importance of cerebral oxygenation monitoring. NIRS measurements – to the contrary – are noninvasive, do not delay the operation and provide detailed information on cerebral oxygenation; artefacts are rare. Our neuropsychological examinations also revealed a correlation between neuropsychological outcome and intraoperative brain hypoxia measured as a reduction in CtO_2 (19). This illustrates that this new method might have an important diagnostic value for postoperative neuropsychologic dysfunction; further investigations have to prove this promising possibility (20).

References

1. Bloor BM, Neville WE, Hellinger FR, Clowes GHR (1963) Oxygen tension of the brain and its modifications with hypothermia. Arch Psychiat Nervenkr 204: 310–316
2. Croughwell ND, Newman MF, Blumenthal JA, White WD, Lewis WD, Lewis JB, Frasco PE, Smith LR, Thyrum EA, Hurwitz BJ, Leone BJ, Schell RM, Reves JG (1994) Jugular bulb saturation and cognitive dysfunction after cardiopulmonary bypass. Ann Thorac Surg 58: 1702–1708
3. Delpy DT, Cope M, van der Zee P, Arridge S, Wray S, Wyatt J (1988) Estimation of optical pathlength through tissue from direct flight time measurement. Phys Med Biol 33: 1433–1442
4. Folstein MF, Folstein SE, McHugh PR (1975) "Mini-Mental State", A practical guide for grading the cognitive state of patients for the clinician. J psychiatr Res 12: 189–98
5. Govier AV, Reves JG, McKay RD, Karp RB, Zorn GL, Morawetz RB, Smith LR, Adams M, Freman AR (1984) Factors and their influence on regional cerebral blood flow during nonpulsatile cardiopulmonary bypass. Ann Thorac Surg 38: 592–600
6. Greeley WJ, Ungerleider RM, Smith R, Reves JG (1989) The effects of deep hypothermic cardiopulmonary bypass and total circulatory arrest on cerebral blood flow in infants and children. J Thorac Cardiovasc Surg 97: 737–745
7. Griepp RB, Ergin MA, Lansman SL, Galla JD, Pogo G (1991) The Physiology of hypothermic circulatory arrest. Seminars in Thoracic and Cardiovascular Surgery 3: 188–193
8. Henriksen L (1984) Evidence suggestive of diffuse brain damage following cardiac operations. Lancet 8381: 816–820
9. Henriksen L (1986) Brain luxury perfusion during cardiopulmonary bypass in humans: effect of carbon dioxide tension. J Cereb Blood flow Metab 6: 366–378
10. Jöbsis FF (1977) Noninvasive infrared monitoring of cerebral and myocardial oxygen sufficiency and circulatory parameters. Science 198: 1264–1267
11. Johnston WE, Vinten-Johansen J, DeWitt DS, O'Steen WK, Stump DA, Prough DS (1991) Cerebral perfusion during canine hypothermic cardiopulmonary bypass: effect of arterial carbon dioxide tension. Ann Thorac Surg 52: 479–89
12. Kern FH, Greely WJ, Ungerleider RM, Quill TJ, Baldwin B, White WD, Reves JG (1991) Cerebral blood flow response to changes in PaCO2 during hypothermic cardiopulmonary bypass in children. J Thorac Cardiovasc Surg 101: 618–622
13. Kern FH, Schell RM, Greeley WJ (1993) Cerebral monitoring during cardiopulmonary bypass. J Neurosurg Anesthesiol 213: 213–217
14. Kuschinsky W, Wahl M (1978) Local chemical and neurogenic regulation of cerebral vascular resistance. Physiol Rev 58: 656–689
15. McCormick PW, Stewart M, Goetting MG, Dujovny M, Lewis G, Ausman JI (1991) Noninvasive cerebral optical spectroscopy for monitoring cerebral oxygen delivery and hemodynamics. Crit Care Med 19: 89–97
16. Messmer K, Gornandt L, Jesch F, Sinagowitz E, Sunder-Plassmann L, Kessler M (1973) Oxygen transport and tissue oxygenation during hemodilution with dextran. Adv Exp Med Biol 33: 669–680
17. Mohri H, Martin WE, Sato S, Sands MP, Dillard DH, Merendino KA (1974) Oxygen utilization during surface induced deep hypothermia. Ann Thorac Surg 18: 494–503

18. Mutch WAC, Sutton IR, Teskey JM, Cheang MS, Thomson IR (1994) Cerebral pressure-flow relationship during cardiopulmonary bypass in the dog at normothermia and moderate hypothermia. J Cereb Blood Flow Metab 14: 510–518
19. Nollert G, Möhnle P, Tassani-Prell P, Borasio GD, Uttner I, Schmoeckel M, Reichart B (1995) Postoperative neuropsychological dysfunction and cerebral oxygenation during cardiac surgery. Thorac Cardiovasc Surg 43: 260–264
20. Nollert G, Möhnle P, Tassani-Prell P, Reichart B (1995) Determinants of cerebral oxygenation during cardiac surgery. Circulation; 92: I-327–II-333
21. Schell RM, Kern FH, Greeley WJ, Schulman SR, Frasco PE, Croughwell ND, Newman M, Reves JG (1993) Cerebral blood flow and metabolism during cardiopulmonary bypass. Anesth Analg 76: 849–65
22. Shaw PJ, Bates D, Cartlidge NEF, French JF, Heaviside D, Julian DG, Shaw DA (1987) Neurologic and neuropsychological morbidity following major surgery, comparison of coronary artery bypass surgery and peripheral vascular surgery. Stroke 18: 700–707
23. Siggaard-Andersen O, Siggaard-Andersen M (1990) The oxygen status algorithm: a computer program for calculating and displaying ph and blood gas data. Scand J Lab Invest 50: Suppl 203: 29–45
24. Swain JA (1993) Cardiac surgery and the brain. N Engl J Med 329: 1119–1120
25. Van der Linden J, Priddy R, Ekroth R, Lincoln C, Pugsley W, Scallan M, Tyden H (1991) Cerebral perfusion and metabolism during profound hypothermia in children. J Thorac Cardiovasc Surg 114: 102–103
26. Van der Linden J, Casismir-Ahn H (1991) When do Cerebral emboli appear during open heart operation? a transcranial doppler study. Ann Thorac Surg 51: 237–241

Authors' address:
G. Nollert, M.D.
Klinikum Großhadern
University of Munich
Marchioninistr. 15
81366 Munich
Germany

Cerebral ischemia and brain related complications after cardiac surgery

F. Isgro, Ch. Schmidt, G. Grimm, W. Saggau

Herzzentrum Ludwigshafen, "Clinic for Cardiac surgery", Klinikum Ludwigshafen
(Director: Prof. Dr. med. W. Saggau)

Introduction

The prognostic estimation of cerebral complications after cardiac surgery is a major problem in the early postoperative period. Neuropsychologic testing and neurologic examination have been common methods of assessing cerebral injury (2, 6). Recent investigations have found clinically significant neurologic or neuropsychologic residuals in 5 % to 15 % of the patients (5, 10, 14, 17, 19 – 23). But we have been interested in finding biochemical markers capable of detecting and quantifying the extent of cerebral injury. Neuron specific enolase (NSE) is an enzyme involved in glycolysis which is localized in neurons and axonal processes, S-100 is an astroglial specific protein with calcium-binding capacity and a molecular weight of 21 000. Both peptides escape into the blood and cerebrospinal fluid at the time of neural injury (3, 8, 9, 11, 17, 21). Very recently, increased NSE serum levels in human cerebral infarction, subarachnoid hemorrhage and head injury have been reported and also preliminary findings of NSE and Protein S-100 in blood after open-heart surgery (1, 3, 4, 7, 12 – 14). Primary goal of the study was to assess the value of NSE and S-100 as markers for brain ischemia after cardiac surgery.

Materials and methods

The experimental group consisted of 250 patients undergoing cardiac surgery with extracorporeal circulation during the last 22 months. 81 % of the patients were treated with CABG, 11 % with aortic valve replacement, 5 % with mitral valve replacement and 3 % with a combined aortic and mitral valve replacement. Average time of the operation was 153 min (range from 92 min to 300 min). Average cross-clamping time was 46 min (range from 19 min to 121 min). The mean lowest central body temperature was 32 °C. The surgical control group consisted of 50 patients having operations in general and vascular surgery. Thirteen patients received cholecystectomy, 14 patients a Y-prosthesis, 8 patients a strumectomy, and 15 patients other surgical interventions. The average time for operations was 190 min (range from 90 min to 250 min). Seventy percent of experimental group and 50 % of control group were men.

For psychometric measurements we performed the Mini Mental Status Test (MMST), which is an easy, practicable instrument to explore cognitive dysfunctions disregarding the emotional aspects of the patient. The test has a very high interrater-reliability (Pearson-correlation coefficient r = 0.887) with a sensitivity of 87 % and a specificity of 82 %. The neuropsychologic testing was typically completed within 1 day before operation for each patient. Postoperative testing was done 48 h and 72 h after operation. NSE serum levels were examined with Cobas Core NSE EIA Kit (Roche). This EIA is a solid phase enzyme immunoassay based on the sandwich technique. S-100 determinations were performed with Sangtec S-100 IRMA (Byk Sangtec) a monoclonal two-sites immunoradiometric assay. Periphery venous blood samples were taken preoperatively, direct after disconnection of ECC, right postoperatively, 8 h and 24 h postoperatively.

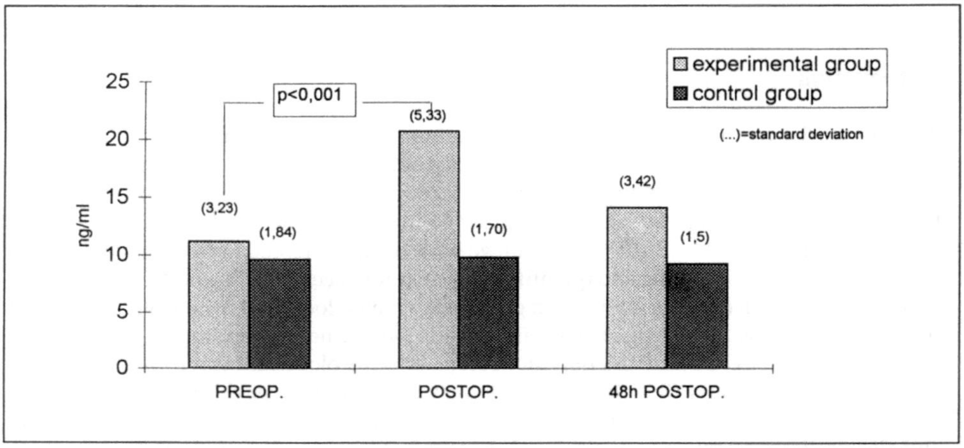

Fig. 1. Mean values and standard deviation of NSE serum levels in experimental and control group. Statistical analysis with *t*-test, significant p-value < 0.05

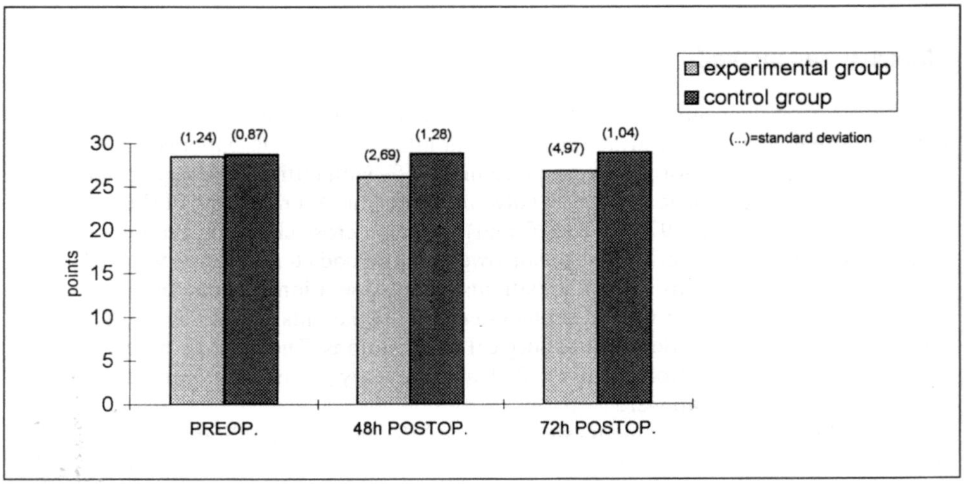

Fig. 2. Mean values and standard deviation of psychometric testing with MMST in experimental versus control group

Results

As shown in Fig. 1 NSE mean level in experimental group increases significantly ($p < 0.005$) in 191 patients from 11.2 ng/ml preoperatively to 20.7 ng/ml right postoperatively and declines to a nearly normalized mean value of 14.1 ng/ml, 48 h postoperatively. In the control group we detected no significant changes of NSE serum levels. Overall differences between experimental and control group were significant ($p = 0.002$). A shown in Fig. 2,

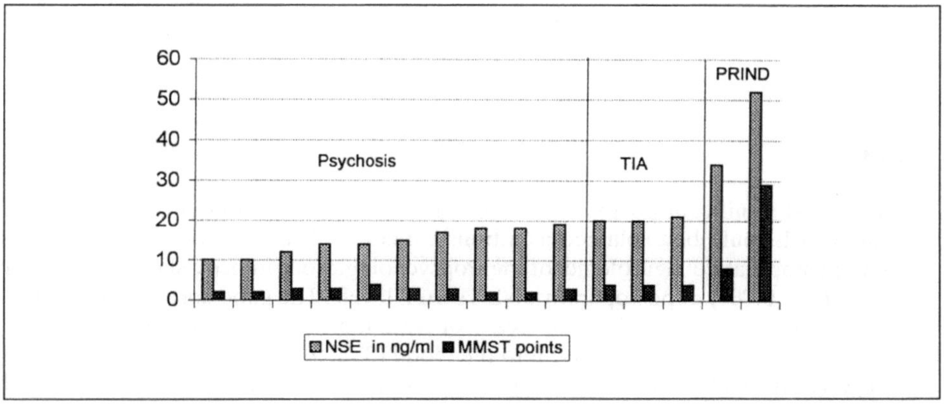

Fig. 3. Differences between preoperative and postoperative NSE serum levels and loss of points in MMST. Superscripts show the corresponding neurologic disorders

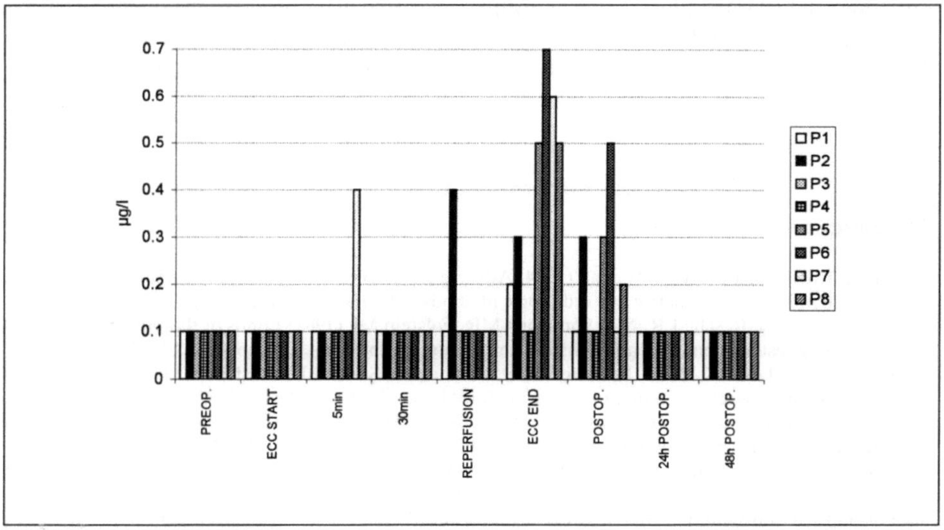

Fig. 4. Protein S-100 serum levels of 8 patients without neurologic and/or neuropsychologic disorders. Demonstrated values < 0.2 µg/l are below the detection limit of the RIA.

postoperative mean scores in MMST of experimental group differed from preoperative examination by about a 2.38 points loss. Points losses were examined in 173 patients of group I. Preoperative and postoperative mean scores of control has nearly similar point levels. Figure 3 demonstrates the changes of preoperatively to right postoperatively NSE values and points loss of 15 patients in experimental group. In these patients we measured the highest postoperative NSE serum levels. In 10 of these patients we found signs of an exogene psychosis, 3 patients had transient ischemic attack, 2 patients suffered from incomplete hemiparesis which was fully reversible in the following 14 days. There is a high correlation of $r = 0.91$ between the postoperative loss of points in MMST and the increase of the postoperative NSE serum levels. We determined in 6 of the 8 patients demonstrated in Fig. 4 elevated protein S-100 serum levels up to 0.7 μg/l.

Discussion

We measured significant postoperative NSE increases ($p < 0.001$) in over 80 % of the patients which could be explained as a transient cerebral stress response. Patients with evident postoperative neurologic or neuropsychologic occurences showed maximum increases ($p < 0.001$) of postoperative NSE serum levels. The good correlation ($r = 0.96$) between point loss in MMST and increase of NSE indicates that the extent of cerebral injury correlates to the NSE release into the blood (3, 8, 9). The mechanism of how NSE is transferred through the hemato-encephalic barrier is still not clear, but there seems to be a relationship between the elevated NSE levels in cerebrospinal fluid and blood serum. Therefore, NSE can probably size up the dimension of cerebral injury after cardiac surgery. The first analysis with S-100 indicates a speedy response to cardiopulmonary bypass and may give implications for an early therapeutical intervention. NSE values exceeding 35 μg/l point to an unfavorable postoperative neurologic and neuropsychologic outcome. In order to validate this hypothesis we are still working on the development of a new concept of cerebral monitoring which includes: 1) Near-infrared Spectroscopy, 2) Bubble Detection, 3) Protein S-100 and NSE, and 4) Neuropsychologic Testing.

References

1. Aberg T, Ronquist G, Tyden H et al. (1984) Adverse effects on the brain in cardiac operations as assessed by biochemical, psychometric and radiologic methods. J Thorac Cardiovasc Surg 87: 99–105
2. Anthony JC, Le Resche LR, Niaz von Korff MR, Folstein MF (1982) Limits of the Mini Mental State as a screening test for dementia and delirium among hospital patients. Psychol Med 12: 397–408
3. Barone FC, Clark RK, Price JP, White RF, Feuerstein GZ, Storer BL, Ohlstein EH (1993) NSE increases in cerebral and systemic circulation following focal ischemia. Brain Research 623: 77–82
4. Cunningham RT, Morrow JI, Johnston CF, Buchanan KD (1994) Serum neurone-specific enolase concentrations in patients with neurological disorders. Clin Chim Acta 230/2: 117–124
5. Folks DG, Franceschini J, Sokol RS, Freeman AM, Folks DM (1986) Coronary artery bypass surgery in older patients: psychiatric morbidity. South Med J 79: 303–306
6. Folstein MF, Folstein SE, McHugh PR (1975) Mini Mental State: A practical method for grading the cognitive state of patients for the clinician. J Psychiat Res 12: 189–198
7. Gruener N, Gross B, Gozlan O, Barak M (1994) Increase in superoxide dismutase after cerebral vascular accident. Life Science 54: 711–713

8. Hardemark HG, Ericsson N, Kotwica Z, Rundstrom G, Mendel-Hartwig I, Olsson Y, Pahlmann S, Persson L (1989) S-100 Protein and NSE in CSF after experimental traumatic or focal ischemic brain damage. J Neurosurg 71: 727–731
9. Hardemark HG, Persson L, Bolander HG, Hillered L, Olsson Y, Pahlmann S (1988) NSE is a marker of cerebral ischemia and infarct size in rat cerebrospinal fluid. Stroke 19: 1140–1144
10. Harrison DC (1981) Coronary bypass: the first 10 years. Hosp Pract 16: 49–56
11. Hay E, Royds JA, Davies Jones GAB, Timperley W, Lewtos N, Taylor C (1984) Cerebrospinal fluid enolase in stroke. J Neurol Neurosurg Psychiatry 47: 724–729
12. Kuroiwa T, Tanabe H, Takatsuka H, Arai M, Negasawa S, Ohta T (1993) Significance of serum NSE levels after head injury. No-Shinkei-Geka 21: 1021–1024
13. Mokuno K, Kato K, Kawai K, Matsuoko Y, Yanagi T, Sabue I (1983) NSE and S-100 protein levels in CSF in patients with various neurological diseases. J Neurol Sci 60: 443–451
14. Nussmeier N (1994) Neuropsychiatric complications after cardiac surgery. J Cardiothoracic vasc Anesth 8: 13–18
15. O'Connor DW, Pollitt PS, Hyde JB, Fellows JL, Miller ND, Brook CPB, Reiss BB (1989) The reliability and validity of Mini Mental State in a British community survey. J Psychiat Res 23: 87–96
16. Prange HW (1994) Pathophysiology, treatment and prognosis of cerebral hypoxic-ischemic brain damage. Z Kardiol 83/Suppl 6: 127–
17. Savageau JA, Stanton B, Jenkins CD, Klein MD (1982) Neuropsychologic dysfunction following elective cardiac operation. I Early assessment. J Thorac Cardiovasc Surg 84: 585–594
18. Schaarschmidt H, Prange HW, Reiber H (1994) NSE concentrations in blood as a prognostic parameter in cerebrovascular disease. Stroke 25: 558–565
19. Shaw PJ, Bates D, Cartlidge NE, Heaviside D, Julian DG, Shaw DA (1985) Early neurological complications of coronary artery bypass surgery. Br Med J 291: 1384–87
20. Shaw PJ, Bates D, Cartlidge NE et al. (1986) Neurological complications of coronary artery bypass graft surgery: six months follow up study. Br Med J 293: 165–167
21. Sotaniemi KA (1983) Cerebral outcome after extracorporeal circulation. Arch Neurol 40: 75–77
22. Sotaniemi KA, Juolasmaa A, Hokkanen ET (1981) Neuropsychologic outcome after open-heart surgery. Arch Neurol 38: 2–8
23. Taylor KM (1986) Pathophysiology of brain damage during open heart surgery. Texas Heart Inst J 13: 91–95
24. Hammeke TA, Hastings JE (1988) Neuropsychologic alterations after cardiac operation. J Thorac Cardiovasc Surg 96: 326–331

Author's address:
OA Dr. med. Frank Isgro
Klinikum Ludwigshafen
Klinik für Herzchirurgie
Bremserstr. 79
67063 Ludwigshafen, Germany

The role of cardiopulmonary bypass technique in cerebral protection

C. Blauth

Department of Cardiothoracic Surgery, Guy's and St. Thomas' Hospitals, London, England

Introduction

Cardiopulmonary bypass is neccessary for most operations on the thoracic aorta, and optional for some cerebrovascular operations. In this context it is probable that the contribution of the bypass circuit itself to cerebral injury is small compared to the intrinsic risks imposed by the arterial pathology being treated. Particular patient related hazards for the brain include aortic atherosclerosis, flow limiting stenoses in extracranial and intracranial cerebral arteries, and previous cerebral infarcts.

Nevertheless, the surgeon needs a perfusion strategy which recognises cerebral protection, particularly in operations when the pump time may be prolonged, and where cerebral injury is either already known to exist or is anticipated from planned hypothermic circulatory arrest. The special circumstances arising from circulatory arrest and cardiopulmonary bypass in small children are described elsewhere in this volume.

Bypass related hazards for the brain which need to be taken into account include atheroembolism from the aorta, unphysiological cerebral blood flow, pump generated embolism, and haemorrhage. Intracerebral haemorrhage is a rare postoperative complication but is a recognised risk for patients with recent cerebral infarction or victims of multiple trauma requiring emergency aortic surgery in the presence of head injury.

Perfusion strategy

The selection of bypass circuit components, their connection to the patient, and the conduct of the perfusion present a number of options and variables which require the surgeon to make strategic decisions (Fig. 1).

Component selection

Oxygenators are of two main types: bubble and membrane. Usage of bubble oxygenators is now diminishing as costs are reduced, but most membrane oxygenators are in fact microporous bubblers with no barrier separation between the blood and gaseous compartments. The exception is the silicon membrane oxygenator which is selected for ECMO and prolonged perfusions expected to last for several days. Arterial line filters have two main functions: firstly to reduce microembolism, and secondly to act as a barrier against major gas embolism. The efficacy of a filter depends on the magnitude of the microembolic load

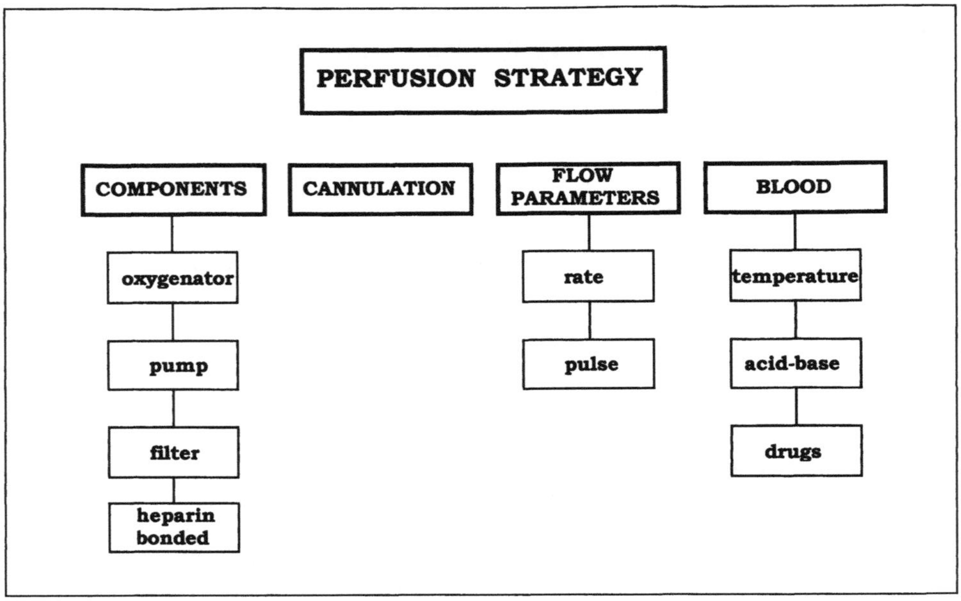

Fig. 1. Options and variables for cardiopulmonary bypass.

generated by the pump-oxygenator, and its pore size. Since all contact with foreign surfaces activates platelets, arterial line filters may in fact generate platelet aggregates. Recent developments starting to feature in clinical practice but still under evaluation include centrifugal pumps which cause less damage to blood cells than the traditional roller pump, and heparin bonded circuits.

Cannulation

Both arterial and venous cannulation may effect cerebral perfusion and embolism. The site of arterial cannulation is usually determined by the operative procedure, therefore the main considerations are selecting a cannula of sufficient size and avoidance of atheroembolism. Venous cannulation must allow complete venous drainage, especially from the superior vena cava, otherwise cerebral perfusion pressure and blood flow are reduced irrespective of the total pump blood flow.

Flow parameters

The pump flow rate and pressure are under the direct control of the perfusionist and anaesthetist unless obstruction to venous return forces reduced flow. The optimum flow rate on CPB at various temperatures has been described elegantly by Kirklin and Barratt-Boyes (1). Various modifications have been suggested, and in most patients lower flows and perfusion pressures appear to be safe, but the relationship between pump flow rate and pressure and optimum cerebral perfusion in the presence of cerebrovascular disease remains complex. Much research has also been done on the potential benefits of pulsatile perfusion, but this issue is also complex (2). Interpretation of studies in this field requires appraisal of the quality of the pulse produced (pulse pressure and waveform), the magnitude of any benefit proposed (significant improvement of clinical outcome as opposed to statistical significance of the measurements made), and appreciation that pulsatile flow may only be applied for that fraction of the total perfusion time when the heart is arrested or the aorta is clamped. Certain pump-oxygenator configurations with membrane oxygenators may substantially dampen the pulse, and pulsatile mode is not achievable with the centrifugal pump.

Blood control

Adjustment of the blood perfusate is inevitable during CPB as the circulating volume is increased up to 150 % by the pump prime, its temperature falls, and the blood gases are controlled by gas flows through the oxygenator. Optimum haematocrit for maximum oxygen delivery is determined by a combination of rheological and oxygen carrying considerations both of which are temperature dependent. Apart from surgery requiring profoundly hypothermic circulatory arrest, normothermic bypass is becoming fashionable in some centres, but even a mild degree of hypothermia increases the tolerance of the brain to ischaemia thereby improving the safety margin in the event of unexpected perfusion problems, and increased neurological morbidity has been reported after normothermic bypass (3).

Acid-base management during CPB is simple until hypothermic conditions blur the definition of acid-base neutrality by shifting the ionic dissociation of water. At hypothermia blood gases may be measured either with or without temperature correction, leading to two different strategies of acid-base management: pH-stat and alpha-stat (Table 1). Improved understanding of the intracellular mechanisms following neuronal ischaemia and their inhibition by drugs including calcium channel blockers are described elsewhere in this symposium.

Table 1. Comparison of the different characteristics of pH-stat and alpha-stat acid-base management during hypothermic cardiopulmonary bypass.

pH-stat	alpha-stat
temperature corrected blood gas mesasurements	no temperature correction
added CO_2	no added CO_2
hibernating mammal	poikilotherm

Atheroembolism

Embolisation of atheromatous debris from the wall of the atherosclerotic aorta or extracranial cerebral vessels may be produced either by trauma of cannulation or the "sand blasting" effect of the high velocity jet of blood leaving the arterial cannula. Selection of an appropriate cannula with side holes which is fixed in the centre of the aortic lumen may minimise this effect. Femoral artery cannulation may not reduce the risk as the retrograde flow of blood to the brain passes over a larger area of aortic atheroma which is usually most frequent and most severe in the abdominal region. The propensity of atheroma to embolise may be related to its morphology, particularly the texture and surface contour. Clinical experience suggests that soft atheroma which is not palpable externally is more prone to embolise than a hard palpable plaque. For this reason epiaortic echo has been advocated for the intraoperative detection of ascending aortic disease, and specific interventions to prevent atheroembolism when detected in this way have been encouraging (4). An autopsy study from the Cleveland Clinic demonstrated the wide dispersal of atheroembolism and the distinctive histological appearance. The incidence of atheroembolism after cardiac surgery correlated with the presence of severe atherosclerosis of the ascending aorta, which was predicted by a clinical history of hypertension and peripheral vascular disease. The most interesting observation was the highly significant increased incidence of clinically evident stroke before death in those patients with histological evidence of brain atheroembolism (Fig. 2) (5).

Perioperative stroke is the most feared complication of cardiovascular surgery. Generally recognised patient related risk factors include advancing age and a previous history of stroke. The relationship between stenotic disease of the carotid arteries and perioperative stroke following coronary surgery has been surprisingly difficult to establish despite numerous comprehensive studies, and any association appears rather weak. In this context the strong correlation between brain atheroembolism, aortic atherosclerosis, and stroke seems to have important implications for clinical practice.

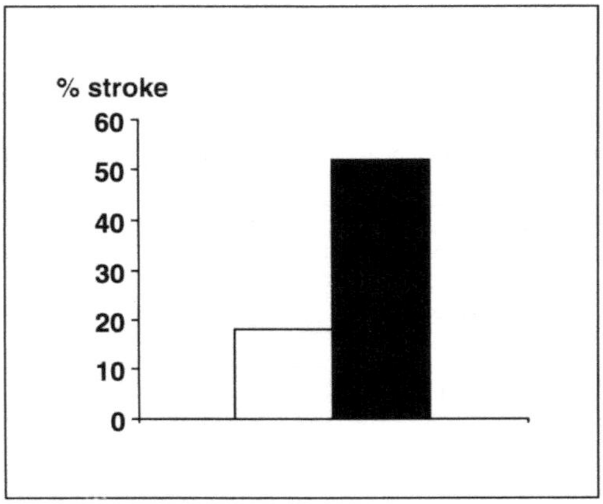

Fig. 2. Incidence of stroke before death in 129 consecutive patients. At postmortem examination, brain studies showed a significantly higher incidence of stroke in patients with brain atheroemboli (52 %; n = 21; black bar) than in those without brain atheroemboli (18 %; n = 108; white bar) (p = 0.001). (Reproduced by permission of the Annals of Thoracic Surgery (6).)

Pump generated embolism

The extracorporeal circuit may generate macroemboli and microemboli of gas, platelet-fibrin microaggregates, and inorganic debris, primarily from the oxygenator (6). Major emboli are usually the result of perfusion accidents, either overtly pumping air, or inadvertently pumping thrombus, and are fortunately very rare. Microemboli are probably universal but their effect on global and regional blood flow and pathological significance remains unclear (7).

Numerous methods have been used to detect and quantify microembolism. Histopathological changes were frequent in the early days of clinical perfusion when rotating disc oxygenators and large volume stored blood primes were used, but more sophisticated techniques indicate that histopathological changes are still in evidence in the current era (8). The disadvantage of histopathological techniques in the study of cerebral injury is that comparative studies of perfusion techniques are not readily available. *In vivo* methods include ultrasound Doppler or observation and imaging of the microcirculation. Ultrasound Doppler has the advantage of on-line analysis, but quantification may be misleading due to calibration difficulties, and distinction between gas bubbles and particulate emboli is unreliable. Comparative studies using signals from the middle cerebral artery in clinical practice have indicated the superiority of membrane over bubble oxygenators in terms of the generation of microemboli (9), and have also suggested a beneficial effect from arterial line filtration (10).

The retina provides an accessible microvascular bed within the central nervous system in which imaging by fluorescein angiography has revealed arteriolar and capillary occlusions during clinical cardiopulmonary bypass. The number and extent of the resulting areas of focal ischaemia was substantially reduced with a membrane oxygenator compared to a bubbler, but arterial line filtration with a 40 μm pore size had no discernible effect (11).

Cerebral blood flow

The aims of cerebral perfusion during bypass are primarily to avoid watershed ischaemia and to match flow to metabolic demand. Cerebral autoregulation may be altered not only by the artifical perfusion conditions associated with bypass, but also by patient related factors such as hypertension and diabetes (12). Ensuring adequate regional blood flow to all territories of the brain is not feasible by currently available clinical monitoring, and the perfusionist must rely on adjusting total flows and mean arterial pressure in the absence of generally recognised safe upper and lower limits for either of these parameters. There is some evidence in primates without atherosclerosis that perfusion pressure is a more important determinant of global cerebral blood flow than pump flow rates (13). When stenotic cerebrovascular disease is present, standard practice remains to increase mean arterial pressure to 70 – 90 mm Hg with vasoconstrictors, and addition of pulsatile flow may further improve distal perfusion.

Measurement of global cerebral blood flow by radioisotope clearance techniques is cumbersome and presents methodological difficulties, but middle cerebral blood flow velocity measurements can show good correlation and have the added advantage of rapid instantaneous measurement which enables real-time monitoring of acute changes (14).

Metabolic demand of the brain is assessed by measurement of oxygen uptake and extraction using jugular bulb venous saturation analysis combined with flow measurements. This remains a research tool, but has provided useful information on the effects of pH-stat and alpha-stat blood gas management. Alpha-stat management results in better matching of cerebral blood flow to demand, and pH-stat provides increased cerebral blood flow, which has been termed "luxury perfusion" although this concept has been questioned (15). Excessive perfusion may theoretically lead to an additional unnecessary microembolic burden, and there is some evidence that early postoperative cognitive function may be better preserved by alpha-stat management (14).

Measuring cerebral injury

Numerous methods have been used to quantify cerebral injury related to cardiopulmonary bypass, but the relationships between the different modalities and their impact on clinical outcome and quality of life have not been adequately evaluated. Interpretation of reported studies must consider pre-existing injury and dysfunction, which makes prospective preoperative and multiple repeated postoperative assessments essential for reliable data.

Manifestations of cerebral injury may be categorised as those which are clinically definite, those which present mild dysfunction of unknown significance, and those which consist of abnormalities detected by special investigations. The clinically definite category comprises all unequivocal neurological deficits: stroke, transient ischaemic attack, and new visual field defect. Detailed clinical examination by neurologists and neuropsychologists can reveal soft neurological signs, behavioural disorders and impaired performance on neuropsychological tests. In a minority of cases there may be a parallel deterioration in quality of life measures, but in the majority these mild detected impairments appear in patients who have returned to a normal lifestyle, and most of the impairments resolve after a few weeks or months. Neuropsychological data is often presented as unequivocal evidence of cerebral injury, but there is no evidence to support this conclusion. The long-term consequences of short-term impaired performance on neuropsychological tests have not yet been established, and such data would be valuable (16).

Special investigations which have been used to demonstrate cerebral injury include histopathological techniques; brain imaging by computerised tomography (CT), magnetic resonance imaging (MRI), and positron emission tomography (PET); retinal angiography; and neuronal enzyme measurements in blood and cerebrospinal fluid (creatine kinase brain isoenzyme (CKBB), adenylate kinase (AK) and S-100b). Brain imaging by MRI has revealed a high incidence of preoperative abnormalities in patients undergoing coronary surgery, and very impressive immediate postoperative changes which resolve within days (17). In this regard the findings are similar to the microvascular occlusions seen in the retina, and in the absence of clinically identifiable problems, the implications remain speculative. Regional metabolic activity of the brain during CPB can be studied by PET, which has the potential to define safety limits for cerebral perfusion under various conditions by assessing watershed zone changes.

Current recommendations and future possibilities

Safe cannulation, optimum blood flow, and minimal embolism are the key issues for the protection of the brain on bypass. The current recommendations for achieving these aims are generally accepted. These include assessment of ascending aortic atherosclerosis, and careful handling of the aorta. The arterial cannula should be selected and positioned to minimise the "sandblasting" effect of the blood jet, and the end of the cannula should lie in the centre of the aortic lumen. Venous drainage should be complete so that the cerebral venous pressure is zero or slightly subatmospheric. A membrane oxygenator should be used, and alpha-stat blood gas management appears preferable. An arterial line filter is an optional extra but probably unnecessary with a membrane oxygenator. At normothermia the conventional flow rate of 2.4 litres/m^2 with a mean arterial pressure of 50 – 60 mm Hg has stood the test of time. Moderate hypothermia (28 – 32 °C) has no appreciable disadvantage and increases the margin of safety in the event of perfusion difficulties.

Future improvements in cerebral protection during bypass will depend primarily on better definition of cerebral injury, its causes and consequences for the patient. Better understanding of the intracellular events leading to irreversible structural changes in the ischaemic neurone may soon produce effective cerebroprotective drugs for clinical use. While control of the coagulation system using heparin appears satisfactory, we still have very little reversible control over platelet function during bypass. The ability to do so may reduce microembolism and improve postoperative haemostasis. Imaging of regional cerebral blood flow and metabolism during bypass with PET may answer questions about optimum pump flow rates, arterial pressures, and the effects of pulsation in patients with cerebrovascular disease.

Acknowledgements

I am indebted to numerous colleagues for assistance with this presentation, notably Drs Saundrie Padayachee and Graham Venn of Guy's and St Thomas' Hospitals, and Drs Peter Smith, Mark Ali, and David Harris of the Royal Postgraduate Medical School, Hammersmith Hospital.

References

1. Kirklin JW, Barratt-Boyes BG (1993) Cardiac Surgery, 2nd Edition, Churchill Livingstone, New York, pp 89–91
2. Edmunds LH (1982) Pulseless cardiopulmonary bypass. J Thorac Cardiovasc Surg 84: 800–804
3. Craver JM, Bufkin BL, Weintraub WS, Guyton RA (1995) Neurologic events after coronary bypass grafting: further observations with warm cardioplegia. Ann Thorac Surg 59: 1429–1434
4. Wareing TH, Davila-Roman VG, Barzilai B, Murphy SF, Kouchoukos NT (1992) Management of the severely atherosclerotic ascending aorta during cardiac operations: a strategy for detection and treatment. J Thorac Cardiovasc Surg 103: 453–462
5. Blauth CI, Cosgrove DM, Webb BW, Ratliff NB, Boylan M, Piedmonte MR, Lytle BW, Loop FD (1992) Atheroembolism from the ascending aorta. J Thorac Cardiovasc Surg 103: 1104–1112
6. Blauth CI (1995) Macroemboli and microemboli during cardiopulmonary bypass. Ann Thorac Surg 59: 1300–1303

7. Johnston WE, Stump DA, DeWitt DS, Vinten-Johansen J, O'Steen WK, James RL, Prough DS (1993) Significance of gaseous microemboli in the cerebral circulation during cardiopulmonary bypass in dogs. Circulation 88: II 319–329
8. Moody DM, Bell MA, Challa VR, Johnston WE, Prough DS (1990) Brain microemboli during cardiac surgery or aortography. Ann Neurol 28: 477–486
9. Padayachee TS, Parsons S, Theobold R, Linley J, Gosling RG, Deverall PB (1987) The detection of microemboli in the middle cerebral artery during cardiopulmonary bypass: a transcranial Doppler ultrasound investigation using membrane and bubble oxygenators. Ann Thorac Surg 44: 298–302
10. Pugsley W, Klinger L, Paschalis C, Treasure T, Harrison M, Newman S (1994) The impact of microemboli during cardiopulmonary bypass on neuropsychological functioning. Stroke 25: 1393–1399
11. Blauth C, Smith PL, Arnold JV, Jagoe JR, Wootton R, Taylor KM (1990) Influence of oxygenator type on the incidence and extent of microembolic retinal ischaemia during cardiopulmonary bypass. Assessment by digital image analysis. J Thorac Cardiovasc Surg 99: 61–69
12. Schell RM, Kern FH, Greeley WJ, Schulman SR, Frasco PE, Croughwell ND, Newman M, Reves JG (1993) Cerebral blood flow and metabolism during cardiopulmonary bypass. Anesthesia and Analgesia 76: 849–865
13. Schwartz AE, Sandhu AA, Kaplon RJ, Ypung WL, Jonassen AE, Adams DC, Edwards NM, Sistino JJ, Kwiatkowski P, Michler RE (1995) Cerebral blood flow is determined by arterial line pressure and not cardiopulmonary bypass flow rate. Ann Thorac Surg 60: 165–170
14. Venn GE, Patel RL, Chambers DJ (1995) Cardiopulmonary bypass: perioperative cerebral blood flow and postoperative cognitive deficit. Ann Thorac Surg 59: 1331–1335
15. Dexter F, Hindman BJ (1995) Theoretical analysis of cerebral venous blood hemoglobin oxygen saturation as an index of cerebral oxygenation during hypothermic cardiopulmonary bypass. A counterproposal to the "luxury perfusion" hypothesis. Anesthesiology 83: 405–412
16. Newman S (1995) Analysis and interpretation of neuropsychologic tests in cardiac surgery. Ann Thor Surg 59: 1351–1355
17. Toner I, Peden CJ, Hamid SK, Newman S, Taylor KM, Smith PL (1994) Magnetic resonance imaging and neuropsychological changes after coronary artery bypass graft surgery: preliminary findings. J Neurosurg Anesthesiol 6: 163–169

Author's address:
Christopher Blauth
Consultant Cardiac Surgeon
Cardiothoracic Unit
Guy's and St Thomas' Hospitals
London SE1 7EH
England

Cerebral protection in aortic arch surgery

Antegrade versus Retrograde Cerebral Perfusion – A review of the recent literature

J. Ennker, A. St. Bauer

Heart Institute Lahr/Baden, Germany

In October 1995, a symposium on "Cerebral Protection in Cerebrovascular and Aortic Surgery" was held at the Schloßhotel Bühlerhöhe in Baden-Baden. At this international symposium prominent authorities concentrated on cerebral physiology, monitoring and protection in association with operations of the supra-aortic vessels and the aortic arch. Many controversial issues such as modes of cerebral monitoring in cerebrovascular surgery or antegrade versus retrograde perfusion in aortic arch surgery have been disscussed.

One of the most discussed points during the symposium was the question: antegrade or retrograde perfusion during repair of aortic arch aneurysms? Is there a superior method? In this article we want to give a review of the literature between 1995 and the publication of this book dealing with this still controversial theme.

The protection of the brain from hypoxic or ischemic injury is among the greatest perioperative challenges for repair of aortic arch aneursyms. Repair poses one of the most complicated technical challenges in surgery today. First reported by DeBakey et al. in 1957 (8), the procedure has carried a high morbidity and mortality rate until the 1980s. Griepp et al. reported in 1975 (11) the use of deep hypothermic circulatory arrest (DHCA) for the replacement of the aortic arch pathology.

With popularization of the profound hypothermic circulatory arrest the results of aortic arch surgery improved. This method provides a dry and motionless surgical field in which the difficult surgical procedure can be performed, thus eliminating the majority of uncontrollable perioperative bleedings. However the cerebral protection produced by hypothermia alone has its limits. The analysis of large series of adult patients undergoing aortic arch operations demonstrated an increased risk of cerebral complications with more than 40 min of DHCA; Griepp and colleagues (11) noted that evidence of diffuse cerebral injury increased in frequency and a marked increase in mortality appeared as the time of circulatory arrest approached 60 min. The results were also supported by investigations of Svensson et al. in 1993 (25). These findings demonstrated that the ability to protect the heart during surgical procedures on the aortic arch using DHCA has not kept pace with our ability to protect the brain.

Out of this dilemma arose the need for new cerebroprotective strategies which allowed a prolonged safe cerebral preservation time. One strategy involves selective cerebral antegrade perfusion using the brachiocephalic or the right axillary artery and the left common carotid or left subclavian artery (7, 17). In this technique arterial blood is perfused in an antegrade way with a pressure around 50 mmHg through the arterial site and drained through the right atrium. An advantage of this method is that perfusion-time can be extended to hypothermic cerebral perfusion-times of 120 min with a low risk for brain damage, especially when a complicated aortic arch repair has to be performed (13, 21). The disadvantages of this method are that a complicated manipulation process is required to establish cannulation for SCP and that arch vessels which may be involved in a dissection must be cannulated. This could result in fragmentation of the fragile vessel wall. For that reason some easier cannulation techniques have been proposed (2). Furthermore, it is difficult to decide in cases of dissection of the aortic arch which lumen has to be cannulated (13). Another point that has drawn attention is that especially in atherosclerotic, diseased aortas the dislodgement of debris by the perfusion cannulae from the vessels or air bubbles can embolize to the brain causing a high incidence of stroke (26).

The second strategy is that of retrograde cerebral perfusion via the superior vena cava. Arterial blood is perfused in the superior vena cava with a pressure of not more than 25 mmHg. The blood is returning through the arterial arch vessels and is then recirculated in the extracorporeal circuit. This method of retrograde cerebral perfusion (RCP) was initially described by Mills and Ochsner (20) as a treatment for air embolization during cardiopulmonary bypass. Intermittent RCP was used by Lemole and associates (16). Ueda and colleagues used continuous RCP during aortic arch operations in 1987 (27), a strategy that is now evaluated by many surgical groups. The advantage of this method is that it can be performed without additional clamping or cannulation of the cervical arteries, which reduces the incidence of cerebral embolism (26, 18). The disadvantage of the RCP is the limitation of time. The “safe“-perfusion time for RCP is believed to be around 60–80 min (18, 28) and that the operative view field might be slightly poorer because of the reflux of blood from the arch vessels.

In the following, we want to have a closer look at the most recent literature concerning antegrade and retrograde cerebral perfusion.

There are still concerns about the real distribution of blood injected in the superior vena cava to the brain, especially when the internal jugular vein is valvulated. In an cadaver study, de Brux and coworkers (6) could demonstrate by injection of opacified latex that the brain was perfused even if competent valves in the internal jugular vein system were present. In this study jugular valves were found in 100 % of the cadavers. The brain was perfused in a retrograde manner through the azygos venous connections. As stated by Ergin (9) in an invited commentary, the greatest portion of blood infused through the superior vena cava does perfuse the systemic venous bed and only a very small fraction comes back through the carotid arteries, so that he proposes a total body retrograde perfusion in order to perfuse the whole body and then the brain. The fact that retrograde perfusion of the brain only results in an apparently small backflow fraction has often been a point of discussion. Some authors did state that a perfusion of the brain is not possible (5). In a investigation of Pagano et al. (23), it could be demonstrated that a technetium (TC-99m)-labeled brain perfusion agent, which is able to diffuse freely through the blood-brain barrier, perfused the brain of human beings under the condition of RCP and deep hypothermic circulatory arrest during aortic arch replacement. In this experiment the authors demonstrated that retrograde cerebral perfusion for a mean perfusion time of 32 ± 7 min perfuses the brain. In that article no neurologic complication was detected. But the question that remains to be answered is whether the metabolic demand of the brain may be met with the technique of retrograde perfusion.

In animal experiments research groups tried to answer this question. In a pig experiment a workgroup (29) exposed the animals to 120 min of hypothermic circulatory arrest (HCA), 120 min of retrograde cerebral perfusion (RCP) and 120 min of antegrade cerebral (ACP) perfusion. After perfusion was finished all animals were reperfused and rewarmed with the aid of cardiopulmonary bypass. The brains of the animals were perfusion fixed at the end of the experiment and examined by light microscopy. The control group consisted of animals that were only anesthetized without any surgical intervention. The result of the study was that no changes were found in the normothermic anesthesia group and only very little changes in the hypothermic antegrade perfusion group. Varying severity of neuronal damage was found in the brains of the HCA- and RCP-group. The damage in the RCP-group was less severe relative to the HCA group. The conclusion the authors draw is that antegrade perfusion prevented ischemic damage to the brain and retrograde cerebral perfusion provided some protection but moderately to severe damage occurred.

In a study of Safi et al. (24) carried out with pigs the authors evaluated the use of RCP under profound hypothermia. The animals were under normothermic circulatory arrest for 60 min (NCA), profound hypothermia and circulatory arrest (PHA) and profound hypothermia circulatory arrest and RCP. The results were that none of the animals in the normothermic group with CA awoke. In the PHA-group only 2 of the 5 animals awoke and in the group with retrograde perfusion all animals awoke, but some had slight neurological deficits that were significantly lower than those compared to the PHA-group. The brain tissue oxygen level, jugular venous blood oxygen-saturation and the cerebral blood-flow was significantly better in the retrograde cerebral perfusion group. The conclusion of this article is that in pigs RCP in combination with profound hypothermia during circulatory arrest significantly reduces neurologic dysfunction, providing superior brain protection. The study also shows that profound hypothermia reduces the brain metabolism (19) and preserves stores of high-energy phosphates, but there is still an obligatory energy requirement even during hypothermic circulatory arrest. The brain will continously consume oxygen until it depletes the energy storages (ATP) and with this depletion brain damage ensues. This leads to postischemic impaired cerebral microcirculation known as non reflow phenomenon (1) or the development of "misery perfusion" characterized by uncoupled changes of flow and metabolism (3).

Exactly regarding this point Filgueiras and coworkers (10) contributed an animal study that investigated the metabolism during antegrade and retrograde cerebral perfusion using 31P-magnetic resonance spectroscopy. Pigs were perfused using an antegrade or retrograde technique for 120 min under profound hypothermic circulatory arrest. In the group receiving antegrade perfusion cerebral metabolites and intracellular pH were unchanged throughout the experiment. During circulatory arrest in the retrograde perfusion group the intracellular pH decreased to 6.4 ± 0.1 and recovered fully during reperfusion. High energy phosphates also returned to their initial levels during reperfusion. These studies showed that deep hypothermic circulatory arrest with antegrade brain perfusion provides best brain protection under the investigated conditions.

Yerlioglu and coworkers (30) showed that pigs in an embolization experiment recovered better by using deep hypothermia and retrograde cerebral perfusion then they did with antegrade cerebral perfusion. The primary aim of the research was to evaluate the efficacy of retrograde cerebral perfusion in migitating the effects of particulate cerebral embolism occuring during aortic surgery. After embolization, unequivocal neurologic injury occurred in both groups (antegrade and retrograde perfusion). Although it was noted that neurologic outcome was not significantly better in the retrograde perfusion group, it became apparent that some of the animals in the retrograde perfusion group recovered almost completely after retrograde cerebral perfusion. These animals were found to have been perfused with much lower perfusion pressures then the rest of the animals in the retrograde perfusion group. Perfusion pressures of less than 40 mmHg did beneficially influence the neurological outcome. The animals with high perfusion pressures after embolization had behavioral scores comparable to those of the antegrade perfusion group and showed a high incidence of histopathological lesions, significantly higher than the retrograde perfusion group with low venous pressure. This result suggests that retrograde cerebral perfusion provides some degree of cerebral protection after embolization in the ascending aorta.

Yet unclear is the question of how long the safe time for retrograde cerebral perfusion can be.

A survey of 49 institutions in Japan was performed by Usui et al. (28) concerning the "early clinical results of retrograde cerebral perfusion for aortic arch surgery in Japan". The background of the investigation was to find out which perfusion technique and which optimal perfusion conditions have the best results for cerebral retrograde perfusion (15, 21). Two hundred twenty-eight patients were collected of whom 46 patients sustained brain complications. Twenty-seven patients had permanent and 19 temporary neurological dysfunctions; 45 patients died. The results of the study were that the duration of RCP was the single RCP-related factor predictive for brain complications. The incidence of permanent neurologic dysfunction was less than 10 % when the RCP time was shorter than 60 min but increased abruptly when the RCP time exceeded 100 min and it remained approximately 15 % between 60 and 99 min. In this survey, superior vena cava (SVC) pressure was not a significant predictor of brain complication, but SVC pressure between 15 and 24 mmHg showed the least risk for neurologic dysfunction. When SVC pressure exceeded 35 mmHg, the risk of brain complications increased significantly. The author draws the conclusion that retrograde perfusion is not the complete answer to brain protection but, with guidelines, may help to prolong the safe time for circulatory arrest.

In this content Bavaria et al. (4) demonstrated that the addition of retrograde cerebral perfusion to deep hypothermic circulatory arrest reduced the stroke rate from 12 % to 0 %. The perfusion pressures were the same as mentioned above.

In a publication of Kazui et al. (14) a modified method of selective cerebral perfusion was used for the operation of 30 patients with aortic aneurysms. After institution of SCP into both innominate and left common carotid arteries the distal graft anastomosis and left subclavian reconstruction was performed while the descending aorta was left open. The antegrade perfusion with rewarming was started via a fourth limb attached to the main graft instead of the femoral artery. Out of these patients no neurologic complication was found.

In a publication of Niinami et al. (22) both SCP and RCP were used to treat 20 patients undergoing aortic arch surgery. Eleven patients were perfused with the SCP-technique the others were treated with the RCP. The result was that in three patients cerebral complications occured postoperatively and all patients were supported with selective cerebral perfusion. The author also found that the retrograde perfusion technique shortened the cardiopulmonary bypass time, heart ischemic time and brain ischemic time. In another article, Higami et al. (12) reported a comparative study of RCP versus SCP in 14 patients which they screened with infrared spectroscopy for changes in rSO_2. They found that RCP time was almost half as short as the SCP time, but they found a significant decrease in the rSO_2 in the RCP-group, whereas the rSO_2 in the SCP-group. No data was given about the neurological outcome.

When comparing the results of antegrade cerebral perfusion and retrograde cerebral perfusion there is no great difference between these results, but there seems to be a tendency that retrograde cerebral perfusion has certain advantages. Coselli demonstrated that by the routine use of retrograde cerebral perfusion a mortality of 0 % can be achieved, a result that mirrors the unique experience reached in this institution as well.

Cardiovascular centers that do not operate routinely on the ascending aorta or the aortic arch are often reluctant in using antegrade perfusion, because it seems to be more difficult to establish and it definitely require experience. The excellent results of Kazui and Bachet are in particular due to a very extensive experience with the method of antegrade cerebral perfusion. In centers where antegrade perfusion is seldom used results may not be that satisfactory. In this context retrograde cerebral perfusion gives also "inexperienced" centers the possibility to provide an effective, safe and simple method of brain protection during operations of the ascending aorta or the aortic arch.

There are still some points of interest that have to be investigated by further studies. One of these points is the question of how long cerebral perfusion can be done without any damage to the neurons. What is definitely the best retrograde perfusion pressure for the brain? And, is the addition of antiischemic drugs of any advantage?

Summing up all the recent studies no absolute recommendation can be given about which of the two methods, RCP or SCP, guarantees the best result. However, we can draw conclusions concerning venous perfusion pressures and time limits of RCP. New studies should be planned to demystify the work mode of RCP. In particular it is important to find out if the perfusion time can be prolonged by infusion of cerebroplegic solutions or improved cerebroprotective substances.

References

1. Ames A, Wright RL, Kowada M, Thurston JM, Manjo G (1968) Cerebral ischemia II. The non-reflow phenomenon. Am J Pathol 52: 437–448
2. Aoyagi S, Akashi H, Kubota Y, Momosaki M, Tayama K, Hanamoto Y, Oryoji A, Kosuga K, Oishi K (1994) Surgical treatment of aneurysms of the aortic arch using a simplified selective cerebral perfusion technique. Thorac Cardiovasc Surg 42: 279–284
3. Baron JC, Bousser MG, Rey A, Guillard A, Comar D, Castaigne P (1981) Reversal of focal "misery perfusion syndrome", by extracranial arterial bypass in hemodynamic cerebral ischemia. Stroke 12: 454–459
4. Bavaria JE, Woo YJ, Hall RA, Carpenter JP, Gardner TJ (1995) Retrograde cerebral and distal aortic perfusion during ascending and thoracoabdominal aortic operations. Ann Thorac Surg 60: 345–353
5. Boeckxstaens CHJ, Flameng WJ (1995) Retrograde cerebral perfusion does not perfuse the brain in nonhuman primates. Ann Thorac Surg 60: 319–328
6. Brux de JL, Subayi JB, Pegis JD, Pillet J (1995) Retrograde cerebral perfusion: anatomic study of the distribution of blood to the brain. Ann Thorac Surg 1294–1298
7. Cooley DA, Ott DA, Frazier OH, Walker WE (1981) Surgical treatment of the transverse aortic arch: experience with 25 patients using hypothermic techniques. Ann Thorac Surg 32: 260–272
8. DeBakey ME, Cooley DA, Crawford ES, Morris GC (1957) Successful resection of fusiform aneurysm of the aortic arch with replacement by homograft. Surg Gynecol Obst 105: 656–664
9. Ergin MA (1995) Invited commentary. Ann Thorac Surg 60: 1294–1298
10. Filgueiras CL, Winsborrow B, Ye J, Scott J, Aronov A, Kozlowski P, Shabnavard L, Summer R, Saunders JK, Desaulier R, et al. (1995) A 31p-magnetic resonance study of antegrade and retrograde cerebral perfusion during aortic arch surgery in pigs. J Thorac Cardiovasc Surg 110: 1, 55–62
11. Griepp RB, Stinson EB, Hollinsworth JF, Buehler D (1975) Prosthetic replacement of the aortic arch. J Thorac Cardiovasc Surg 70: 1051–1063
12. Higami T, Kozawa S, Asada T, Mukohara N, Obo H, Gan K, Iwahashi K, Ogawa K (1995) A comparison of changes of cerebrovascular oxygen saturation in retrograde and selective cerebral perfusion during aortic arch surgery. Nippon Kyobu 43: 1919–1923
13. Kazui T, Kimura N, Yamada O, Komatsu S (1994) Surgical outcome of aortic arch aneurysms using selective cerebral perfusion. Ann Thorac Surg 57: 904–911
14. Kazui T, Kurimoto Y, Umami T, Tanaka T, Morishita K, Komatsu S, Yanaginya A, Tanaka H, Yamada O, Yamaguchi T, et al. (1995) Aortic arch aneurysm: new modifications of aortic arch reconstruction and selective cerebral perfusion. Koybu Geka 48: 519–525
15. Kitamura M, Hashimoto A, Akimoto T, Tagusari O, Aomi S, Koyanagi H (1995) Operation for type A aortic dissection: introduction of retrograde cerebral perfusion. Ann Thorac Surg 59: 1195–1199
16. Lemole GM, Strong MD, Spagna PM, Karmilowicz NP (1982) Improved results for dissecting aneurysms. Intraluminal sutureless prosthesis. J Thorac Cardiovasc Surg 83: 249–255
17. Livesay JJ, Coooley DA, Duncan JM, Ott DA, Walker WE, Reul GJ (1982) Open aortic anastomosis: improved results in the treatment of aneurysms of the aortic arch. Circulation 66 (Suppl 1): 122–127
18. Lytle BW, McCarthy PM, Meaney KM, Steward RW, Cosgrove DM (1995) Cardiopulmonary bypass, myocardial management and support techniques. J Thorac Cardiovasc Surg 109: 738–743

19. Mault JR, Ohtake S, Klingensmith ME, Heinle JS, Greeley WJ, Ungerleider RM (1993) Cerebral metabolism and circulatory arrest: effects of duration and strategies for protection. Ann Thorac Surg 55: 57–64
20. Mills NL, Ochsner JL (1980) Massive air embolism during CPB: causes, prevention and management. J Thorac Cardiovasc Surg 80: 708–717
21. Mohri H, Sadahiro M, Akimoto H, Haneda K, Tabayashi K, Ohimi M (1993) Protection of the brain during hypothermic perfusion. Ann Thorac Surg 56: 1493–1496
22. Niinami H, Hashimoto A, Aomi S, Takazawa A, Imamiki M, Noji S, Koyanagi H (1995) Selection of the surgical methods and surgical outcome of the distal arch aneurysm. Nippon Kyobu 43: 1963–1941
23. Pagano D, Boivin CM, Faroqui MH, Bonser RS (1996) Retrograde perfusion through the superior vena cava perfuses the brain in human beings. Thorac Cardiovasc Surg 111: 270–272
24. Safi HJ, Iliopoulos DC, Gopinath SP, Hess KR, Asimacopoulos PJ, Bartoli S, Rashkind SA, Shaibani AT, Leveque CM, Yawn DH (1995) Retrograde cerebral perfusion during profound hypothermia and circulatory arrest in pigs. Ann Thorac Surg 1107–1112
25. Svensson LG, Crawford ES, Rashkind SA, et al. (1993) Deep hypothermia with circulatory arrest: determinants of stroke and early mortality in 656 patients. J Thorac Cardiovasc Surg 106: 19–31
26. Rashkind SA, Coselli JS (1995) Retrograde cerebral perfusion: overview, techniques and results. Perfusion 10: 51–57
27. Ueda Y, Miki S, Kusuhara K, Okita Y, Tahara T, Yamanaka K (1990) Surgical treatment of aneurysm of dissection involving the ascending aorta and aortic arch, utilizing circulatory arrest and retrograde cerebral perfusion. J Cardiovasc Surg (Torino) 31: 553–558
28. Usui A, Toshio A, Murase M (1996) Early clinical results of retrograde cerebral perfusion for aortic arch operations in Japan. Ann Thorac Surg 62: 94–104
29. Ye J, Yang L, Bigio MR, Filgueiras CL, Ede M, Summers R, Salerno T, Desauliers R (1996) Neuronal damage after hypothermic circulatory arrest and retrograde cerebral perfusion in the pig. Ann Thorac Surg 61: 1316–1322
30. Yerlioglu ME, Wolfe D, Mezrow CK, Weisz DJ, Midulla PS, Zhang N, Shiang HH, Bodian C, Griepp RB (1995) The effect of retrograde cerebral perfusion after particulate embolization to the brain. J Thorac Cardiovasc Surg 110: 1470–1485

Author's address:
J. Ennker M.D.
Cardiothoracic Surgeon in Chief
Heart Institute Lahr/Baden
P.O.B. 1340
D-77933 Lahr
Germany

Surgery of aortic arch aneurysm – A ten-year experience with cold cerebroplegia

J. Bachet, D. Guilmet, G. Dreyfus, B. Goudot, A. Piquois

Service Chirurgie Cardio-Vasculaire Hôpital Foch – Université René Descartes, Suresnes, France

Despite the considerable progress made in the past decades with the operative management of aneurysms involving the transverse aortic arch (2, 14, 17), replacement of this portion of the vessel remains a surgical challenge and is still associated with a high rate of mortality and morbidity. This is not due to the technical difficulties of the procedure but, mainly, to the necessity of protecting the integrity of the central nervous system during the period of arch exclusion. Since our first resection of the aortic arch in 1966 (13), we have performed 190 replacements of the transverse aortic arch using three different methods of cerebral protection:

1) From 1966 to 1977, antegrade carotid perfusion at moderate hypothermia through an arterial line derived from the main arterial circuit: 27 cases.

2) From 1977 to April 1984 deep hypothermia associated with circulatory arrest: 34 cases.

3) Since then, an original technique of antegrade carotid perfusion with cold blood (10 °C) derived from the oxygenator through a separate heat exchanger: 129 cases.

For obvious reasons (number of patients at risk, period of surgery, evolution in the medical and surgical management of the patients, etc.), those three techniques cannot be compared.

The present study reports on our experience with "cold cerebroplegia" which in our opinion has proved to the more efficacious than the other methods hiterto employed.

Methods

Principle

The technique of "cold cerebroplegia" is aimed at cooling the brain independently of the rest of the body, through a selective perfusion of the brachiocephalic arteries with cold blood (6° to 12 °C) on the analogy of cold blood cardioplegia (2). Meanwhile the patient is maintained at moderate core hypothermia (25° to 28 °C). CPB is discontinued and the cerebral perfusion is maintained during the aortic repair.

Perfusion equipment

A regular CPB is modified by addition, beyond the oxygenator, of a heat exchanger usually dedicated to cold blood cardioplegia and a roller pump (Fig. 1).

By means of the heat exchanger, blood derived from the oxygenator can be cooled to 6° to 12 °C. A perfusion line distributes the cold blood to the brachiocephalic arteries and the

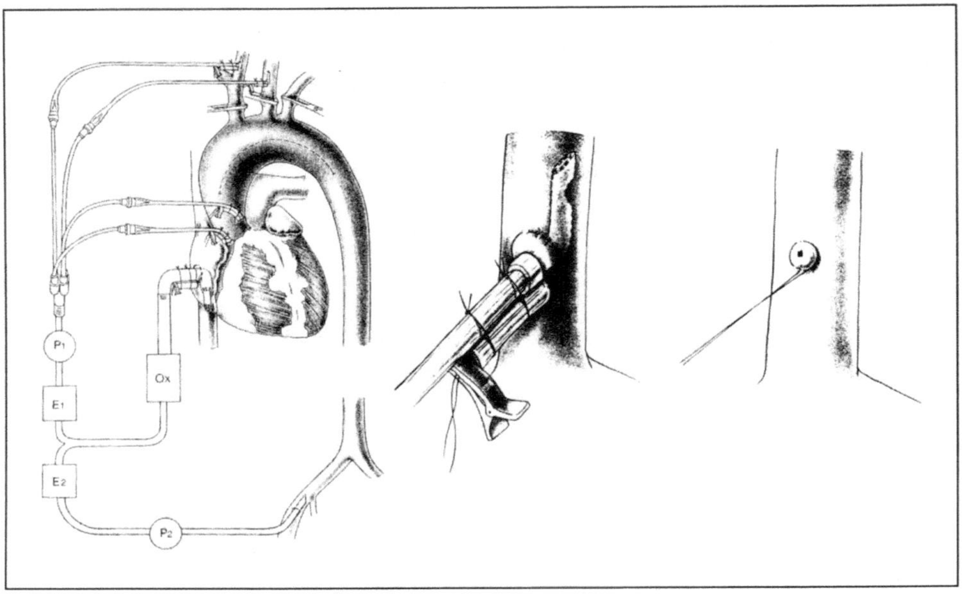

Fig. 1

coronary arteries through a quadrifurcated connector. Specially designed cannulas are available in several diameters to perfuse the carotid arteries. The blunt tip of the cannulas avoids traumatism of the cannulated vessel, whereas a lateral orifice located near the tip prevents the flow from being interrupted in case of occlusion of the main orifice. The cannulas are bent at a square angle to allow their proper placement and position during operation.

Surgical technique

The patient is prepared and anesthetized as usual. The electroencephalogram is recorded permanently throughout the procedure, as are the rectal and esophageal temperatures.

The transverse aortic arch is approached through a median sternotomy. In case of large aneurysm extending distally, a left thoracotomy (fifth or seventh intercostal space) may be associated with the sternotomy. CPB is established between the right atrium (two-stage single cannula) and one femoral artery. To avoid platelet destruction during bypass, we prefer to use a membrane oxygenator. Patient cooling is initiated. During cooling, the brachiocephalic arteries are dissected free and encircled with snares.

When the rectal temperature is lowered to 27 °C, cannulas are inserted in the innominate and left carotid arteries, or in both carotid arteries, and held by means of adventitial 5–0 polypropylene purse-string sutures. The brachiocephalic arteries are then cross-clamped, and the selective cold perfusion is initiated. When the electroencephalogram demonstrates total disappearance of activity, the main CPB is discontinued and the aortic arch is opened. Myocardial protection is achieved by perfusing cold blood through selective cannulation of the coronary ostia or the ascending aorta, if this segment is not replaced. In addition, iced sludge is placed into the pericardium.

During circulatory arrest the selective perfusion of the cerebral and coronary arteries is maintained at a flow rate of about 400 to 500 ml/min. Because of the shape and size of the coronary line and cannulas, a maximum of 150 ml/min. is perfused into the coronary arteries. The perfusion flow of the brain is, therefore, about 250 to 350 ml/min. The pressure in the perfusion line is maintained between 200 and 250 mmHg, which corresponds to a pressure of approximately 60 to 70 mmHg into the carotid arteries. During cerebral perfusion and circulatory arrest, no adjuncts, such as barbiturates or steroids, are used to enhance the cerebral protection.

When the distal anastomosis is completed, the prosthesis is crossclamped, CPB is resumed, and the patient's rewarming is started. The brachiocephalic vessels are then reimplanted into the prosthesis either in a single cuff or separately. Cerebral perfusion is discontinued, and the arteries are unclamped after careful removal of any air bubbles. The prosthesis is then secured to the ascending aorta. If the aortic valve is to be replaced, or a Bentall procedure is to be performed, those procedures are generally performed before replacement of the aortic arch.

Withdrawal of the carotid cannulas is easy, hemostasis being achieved by simply tightening the adventitial purse-string suture. The procedure is completed as usual.

Patients

Between April 1984 and June 1995, 129 patients (88 men and 41 women) underwent replacement of the transverse aortic arch with the aid of cold cerebroplegia. Ages ranged from 25 to 81 years (mean 57).

Operation was indicated for various anatomic situations; 1) 97 patients whose chronic lesions were operated on electively; 2) 32 patients were operated on urgently for acute aortic dissection necessitating replacement of the transverse arch. The causes and circumstances of operations are summarized in Table 1.

The extension of the aortic replacement varied on the basis of the anatomic lesions:

1) Forty-seven patients underwent an isolated replacement of the transverse arch. In all but five the cephalic arteries were reimplanted through a single cuff. The left subclavian artery was ligated in three patients.

2) Forty-eight patients underwent a replacement of the transverse arch associated either with a Bentall procedure (25 patients), or an ascending aorta substitution (17 patients), or an aortic valve replacement (six patients).

Table 1. Cause and circumstances of transverse aortic arch remplacement

Cause	No.	Circumstance	Repeat operation
Atheromatous aneurysm	27	Elective	2
Dystrophic aneurysm	21	Elective	5
Calcified endoaortitis	1	Elective	
Chronic aortic dissection	48	Elective	28
Acute aortic dissection	32	Urgent	1

3) Thirty-four patients underwent a replacement of the transverse arch associated with a more or less extended replacement of the descending aorta. In nine patients of this group a lateral thoracotomy was associated with the median sternotomy.

Results

CPB

Duration of CPB, circulatory arrest, perfusion of the brachiocephalic and coronary arteries, and level of rectal and esophageal temperatures are indicated on Table 2. There is a significant difference in duration of CPB and coronary perfusion according to the lesion treated and, subsequently, the procedure performed. Conversely, the extension of the aortic replacement had no influence on the duration of the cephalic perfusion, the time of circulatory arrest, and the level of rectal and esophageal temperatures.

Electroencephalogram

An intraoperative electroencephalogram has been recorded in all patients. During cooling, cerebral activity disappears completely in a mean time of 9 min (3 to 16 min) after initiation of the cold blood perfusion. During rewarming, the first electrical wave appears in a mean time of 12 min (1 to 35 min), and the cerebral activity is restored to normal in a mean time of 66 min (Fig. 2).

Neurologic complications

All patients but one showed signs of awakening within 8 h postoperatively and were fully conscious after 24 h.

Five patients had fatal neurologic complications: in three pts. the cause was unknown, and in two it was an air embolism (Table 3). We have observed 11 cases of non fatal complications: three cases of paraplegia related to cord ischemia after replacement of the descending aorta and ligation of the left subclavian artery (in one patient); in three patients the occurrence of a Brown-Séquard syndrome was related to the extension of an acute dissecting process. Two patients had transient hemianopsia 9 and 11 days postopera-

Table 2. Perfusion data

	Mean	SD	Range
Duration (min)			
CPB	131	33	65–248
Circulatory arrest	29	12	10– 51
Cerebral perfusion	60	20	16– 94
Coronary perfusion	74	25	20–158
Temperature (°C)			
Esophageal	19	3.5	11– 27
Rectal	26	3	20– 30

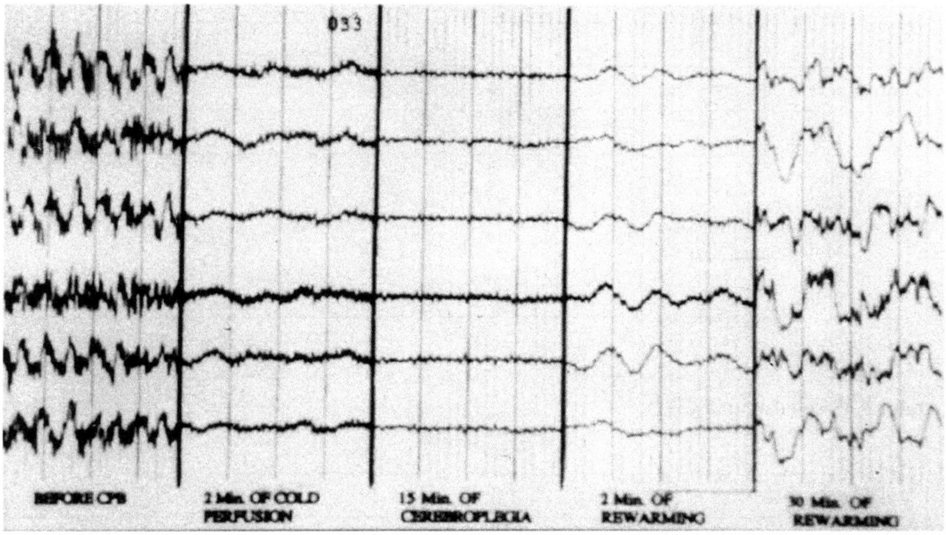

Fig. 2

tively, in probable relation to emboli; finally three patients with preoperative hemiplegia were permanently disabled.

Other complications

Five patients had major respiratory failure, necessitating prolonged ventilation. One patient had a postoperative myocardial infarction. One patient underwent a left hemicolectomy for colic ischemia. Recurrent nerve palsy was observed in seven patients, and three patients had a phrenic nerve palsy. Five patients had acute renal failure, three suffered from mediastinitis and one from peptic ulcer.

Mortality

Twenty-three patients (18 %) died during the post-operative course. Cause of death is indicated in Table 4 and 5.

Table 3. Neurological complications

Fatal		Cause	
Stroke	5	Unknown	3
		Air embolism	2
Non fatal	11		
Paraplegia	3	Resection desc. aorta?	
Brown-Sequard S.	3	Acute dissection?	
Hemiplegia	3	Preoperative	
Transient hemianopsy	2	Emboli?	

Table 4. Hospital mortality I

	No.	%
Intra operative deaths	2	1.7
Hospital deaths	21	16.4
Overall mortality	23	18.1
– Infection	4	
– Myocardial infarction	3	
– Multi organ failure	10	
– Stroke	5	
– Other	1	

Table 5. Hospital mortality II

	No.	%
Emergency	10/35	28.5
Elective surgery	13/94	12.2 $p = 0.05$

Death is directly related to a neurologic complication in five patients. The mean durations of CPB, circulatory arrest, and cerebral perfusion were 105 min, 23 min and 48 min, respectively.

Risk factors

Lesion, age, and sex had no significant influence on the outcome of the patients, nor had the duration of CPB, circulatory arrest, and cerebral perfusion. In particular, no correlation could be established between the duration of cerebral perfusion and the occurrence of neurologic complications. Conversely, the type of the performed replacement was a prominent risk factor(x^2, $p < 0.02$).

Comments

Profound hypothermia and circulatory arrest is presently the most frequently used method of cerebral protection. It has obvious advantages. It necessitates no brachiocephalic cannulation, and it can be used in almost any circumstance with a regular CPB circuit. Its main advantage, however, is to allow a total circulatory arrest and, thus, the possibility of performing an "open" bloodless replacement of the aortic arch without crossclamping the vessel.

Conversely, this method has some cumbersome drawbacks. Mostly efficient when temperature gradients between organs are absent or reduced, it requires a long time to lower the patient's temperature to a proper level and a longer time to raise it back to its physiologic value. This prolonged time of CPB has been held responsible for various disorders, especially hemorrhage and infections. It has been proposed that circulatory arrest be performed at moderate hypothermia to reduce the rate of those complications (4). The time allowed then to perform the distal aortic repair is severly limited, however, and calls the surgeon's skill into play. Besides even for deep hypothermia, uncertainty continues regarding the possible duration of the circulatory arrest and, consequently, the time of cerebral ischemia.

For all these reasons the results associated with circulatory arrest at profound hypothermia vary widely in the literature (4, 6, 7, 8, 9, 12, 20). In our experience the method has often been held responsible for delayed postoperative awakening, and transient or permanent neurologic disturbances, especially in aged patients (14).

Selective perfusion of the brachiocephalic arteries has been used to protect the central nervous system since 1957 (8) and is still advocated by some authors (11, 18). Its main advantage is to provide an unlimited time to perform the distal aortic repair. However this method is associated with several drawbacks. It may appear to be a complicated technique; it requires that the cephalic arteries be dissected free and cannulated; it necessitates specific equipment and the presence of several perfusion lines in an already encumbered surgical field. Its main disadvantages however, are linked with its very principle:

1) There is a continuing uncertainty concerning the proper perfusion flow to achieve a satisfactory cerebral protection (15, 20).

2) When the perfusion line is derived from the main arterial line, the CPB cannot be discontinued. The possibility of total circulatory arrest is suppressed, and, consequently, the distal aorta must be crossclamped to perform the repair. In many situations (large aneurysm, acute dissection, reoperations) crossclamping of the distal aorta may be a dangerous maneuver, clamp injury of the vessel resulting in an untractable hemorrhage.

Our experience with deeply hypothermic circulatory arrest has been somehow disappointing. Many patients, especially the elderly, had postoperative awakening times exceeding the usual few hours. Transient or permanent neurologic complications were not rare and were responsible for death in several instances. Our experience is in accordance with some reports in the literature (4, 14) but it contrasts sharply with the results obtained by other groups (12, 17). This disparity might be explained by the fact that in our patients deep hypothermia has always been induced through CPB and was never initiated by surface cooling. Therefore, despite the permanent monitoring of esophageal and rectal temperatures, temperature gradients between organs might have been generated by rapid cooling and the brain might not have been as cold and protected as we wanted it to be.

The most important unresolved question is the limit of time allowed for circulatory arrest. This limit of time has not be clearly defined to date. Several experimental studies have been undertaken to estimate the maximum duration of circulatory arrest that could safely be applied to animals. Despite the various methods and techniques of analysis used, they generally agree that the limit is about 60 min when temperature is below 18 °C. It seems that in man the safe limit of time is shorter and that the risk of neurologic disturbance becomes important if the period of circulatory arrest exceeds 45 min (4, 14, 19). Although most distal aortic repairs can be performed within this period of time, it is never assured that a longer time would not be required, either in case of extended and complex anatomic lesions or in case of unforeseeable difficulties.

Besides, the time required on the CPB to avoid excessive thermal gradients during rewarming of the patient (about 3 min per degree centigrade) has been held responsible for generating important coagulation disorders and, consequently, for a high rate of morbidity and mortality.

Is, then, the use of standard carotid perfusion simpler and safer? It may seem more complex. The presence of extra perfusion lines and cannulas in an already encumbered surgical area can be cumbersome. Any obstruction (kinking, malposition) of the supplying line or cannula may result in cerebral ischemia. With properly designed and placed cannulas this difficulty can be easily managed. A simplified method of cerebral perfusion through a single brachiocephalic artery has been proposed by the Stanford group (11, 18). Although it is elegant, the cannulation of only one artery may be dangerous in patients with an unfunctional circle of Willis.

Some authors have suggested that the carotid cannulation may be the cause of atheromatous or gas emboli (5, 8). We have never observed such a complication, and we believe that it can be easily avoided by choosing a proper site of cannulation and taking great care in air removal.

The procedure is not totally safe. The use of a Y-shaped junction to provide a cerebral circuit derived from the main arterial line is simple, but it does not allow independent control of cerebral flow. The proper cerebral flow at moderate hypothermia is not clearly defined. As emphasized by Crawford and colleagues (5), high flow rate administered at high pressure can be responsible for neurologic damage.

As already pointed out, however, the main drawback of this method of cerebral protection is that it precludes the possibility of circulatory arrest. The superiority of "open" bloodless repair of the transverse arch has been widely demonstrated (1, 6, 9, 17). It seems, therefore, difficult to use and commend a technique with which this advantage is suppressed.

Autoregulation of the cerebral blood flow is an important factor of maintenance of a stable environment in the brain. Recent reports (10, 22) have suggested that in deep hypothermic situations (20 °C) autoregulation on the cerebral blood flow is maintained and prevents cerebral ischemia or hypoperfusion for perfusion pressure ranging from 30 to 100 mmHg. If perfusion flow rate is reduced, the total flow brain decreases, but even at lowest perfusion flow rates, all areas of the brain appear to remain perfused (10). Normally, individual cerebral structures are perfused in proportion to the metabolic demands. At 20 °C, oxygen consumption of the brain is reduced to one-fifth of that at normothermia, as a result of the effect of hypothermia on the metabolic processes (22). It is probably suppressed at low temperatures (< 15 °C).

At this level of hypothermia, the dissociation curve of hemoglobin is displaced toward the left. The oxygen delivered to the tissues is, therefore, mainly transported in the dissolved form. The main advantage of using oxygenated blood consists, thus in the buffer capacity of the imidazole nucleus of the hemoglobin molecule. Those factors constitute the basic reasons for the beneficial effect of permanently perfusing the brain at a very low temperature. As a cerebral flow rate and pressure are maintained in a range allowing autoregulation, a safe protection against ischemia or hyperperfusion is provided, as assessed by the good results obtained in our experience, even for long perfusion times.

Our technique of "cold blood selective cerebral perfusion" has found an important experimental support in the article published by Swain and coworkers (21). In this article there is a striking difference in favor of the method of deep hypothermic perfusion at moderate flow, which shows no alteration of any of the energic components of the cerebral tissues.

Because circulatory arrest is used only to perform the distal aortic anastomosis, its duration is reduced to a minimum of time. It can therefore, be conducted at moderate hypothermia without endangering the spinal cord or the abdominal organs, as already demonstrated (1, 17).

The present study is not comparative. Absolute statistical proof would require a prospective randomized study.

However the safety of the cerebral protection provided during a nonlimited time of arch exclusion makes this technique the method of choice in frail or aged patients or in patients requiring a long or difficult operation.

References

1. Bachet J, Teodori G, Goudot B et al. (1988) Replacement of the transverse aortic arch during emergency operations for type A acute aortic disection: report of 26 cases. J Thorac Cardiovasc Surg 96: 912–24
2. Bachet J, Guilmet D, Goudot B, Termignon JL, Teodori G, Dreyfus G, Brodaty D, Dubois Cl, de Lentdecker Ph (1991) Cold cerebroplegia: a new technique of cerebral protection during operations on the transverse aortic arch. J Thorac Cardiovasc Surg 102: 85–94
3. Cooley DA, DeBakey ME (1956) Resection of entire ascending aorta in fusiform aneurysm using cardiac bypass. JAMA 162: 1158
4. Cooley DA, Ott DA, Frazier OH, Walker WE (1981) Surgical treatment of aneurysms of the transverse aortic arch: experience with 25 patients using hypotermic techniques. Ann Thorac Surg 32: 260–72
5. Crawford ES, Saleh SA, Schuessler JS (1979) Treatment of aneurysm of transverse aortic arch. J Thorac Cardiovasc Surg 78: 383–93
6. Crawford ES, Saleh EB (1981) Transverse aortic arch aneurysm: improved results of treatment employing new modifications of aorta reconstitution and hypothermic cerebral circulatory arrest. Ann Surg 194: 180–8
7. Culliford AT, Ayvaliotis B, Shemin R, Colvin B, Isom W, Spencer FC (1982) Aneurysms of the ascending aorta and transverse arch. J Thorac Cardiovasc Surg 83: 701–10
8. DeBakey ME, Henly WS, Cooley DA, Crawford ES, Morris GC, Beall AC (1962) Aneurysms of the aortic arch: factors influencing operative risk. Surg Clin North 42: 1543–54
9. Ergin MA, O'Connor J, Guinto R, Griepp RB (1982) Experience with profound hypothermia and circulatory arrest in the treatment of aneurysm of the aortic arch. J Thorac Cardiovasc Surg 84: 649–55
10. Fox LS, Blackstone EH, Kirklin JW, Bishop SP, Bergdahl LAL, Bradley EL (1984) Relationship of brain blood flow and oxygen consumption to perfusion flow rates during profoundly hypothermic cardiopulmonary bypass. J Thorac Cardiovasc Surg 87: 658–64
11. Frist WH, Baldwin JC, Starness VA et al. (1986) A reconsideration of cerebral perfusion in aortic arch replacement. Ann Thorac Surg 42: 273–81
12. Griepp RB, Stinson EB, Hollingsworth JF, Buehler D (1975) Prosthetic replacement of the aortic arch. J Thorac Cardiovasc Surg 70: 1051–63
13. Guilmet D, Scetbon V, Ricordeau G, Besse Ph, Weiss J, Devilleger H, Baumann D, Arfel G, Vigano M, Danan M, Dubost C (1966) Un cas d'anévrysme de la totalité de la crosse aortique traité avec succès par résection greffe. Mémoires de l'Académie de Chirurgie. Tome 92, 18–19, pp 479–487
14. Guilmet D, Diaz F, Roux PM et al. (1986) Anévrysmes de la crosse aortique: traitement chirurgical: 60 observations. Presse Med 15: 2191–5
15. Guilmet D, Roux PM, Bachet J, Goudot B, Tawil N, Diaz F (1986) Nouvelle technique de protection cérébrale: Chirurgie de la crosse aortique. Presse Med 15: 1096–8
16. Hou YL, Shang TY, Wu YK (1964) Surgical treatment of aneurysm of thoracic aorta. Chinese Medical Journal 83: 740–749
17. Livesay JJ, Cooley DA, Reul GJ et al. (1983) Resection of aortic arch aneurysms: a comparison of hypothermic techniques in 60 patients. Ann Thorac Surg 36: 19–28
18. Miller DC (1982) Discussion of culliford et al.[7] J Thorac Cardiovasc Surg 83: 711
19. O'Connor JV, Wilding T, Farmer P, Sher J, Ergin MA, Griepp RB (1986) The Protective effect of profound hypothermia on the canine centrale nervous system in surgery of the ascending aorta and the aortic arch. Ann Thorac Surg 41: 255–9
20. Soma Y, Kawada K, Kono N et al. (1986) Clinical results of cardiopulmonary bypass with selective cerebrale perfusion for aneurysm of the ascending aorta and the aortic arch. Ann Thorac Surg 42: 273–81
21. Swain JA, McDonald TJ, Griffith PK et al. (1991) Low-flow hypothermic cardiopulmonary bypass protects the brain. J Thorac Cardiovasc Surg 102: 76–84
22. Tanaka J, Shiki J, Asai T, Yasui H, Tokunaga K (1988) Cerebral autoregulation during deep hypothermic non pulsatil cardiopulmonary bypass with selective cerebral perfusion in dogs. J Thorac Cardiovasc Surg 95: 124–32

Authors' address:
Jean Bachet M.D.
Service Chirurgie Cardio-Vasculaire
Hôpital-Foch – Université René Descartes
40 rue Worth
92151 Suresnes Cedex, France

Aortic arch surgery using antegrade selective cerebral perfusion

H. Akashi, K. Tayama, S. Fukunaga, K. Kosuga, S. Aoyagi

Second Department of Surgery, Kurume University School of Medicine, Kurume, Japan

Introduction

The surgical management of aneurysms involving the aortic arch has been fraught with technical difficulties in the past. In only a few reports (1 – 3) has the surgical outcome in a sufficiently large number of patients with an aortic arch aneurysm been described. It is no exaggeration to say that the success of an operation for the repair of an aortic arch aneurysm mainly depends on how well the brain is protected from ischemia during aortic arch repair. For reconstruction of the aortic arch or adjacent part of the aorta, the following methods have been used as supportive techniques: hypothermic cardiopulmonary bypass (CPB) with selective cerebral perfusion (SCP) (4 – 6), hypothermic CPB with circulatory arrest (7 – 10) and hypothermic CPB with retrograde cerebral perfusion (11). From April 1989, based on results from our experimental studies (12), we have employed hypothermic CPB with SCP as the supportive method for the surgical treatment of aortic arch aneurysms. This report describes the SCP technique and results in 74 patients and includes discussion about its advantages.

Patients and methods

Between April 1989 and August 1995, 74 patients underwent surgical treatment of aortic arch aneurysms using antegrade selective cerebral perfusion at our hospital. There were 42 male and 32 female patients who ranged in age from 26 to 86 years, with a mean age of 64 years. The etiology of the aortic aneurysm was type A dissection in 44 patients, type B dissection in 4, and atherosclerotic disease in 25. In the remaining one, the cause of the aneurysm was aortitis syndrome (Table 1).

From April 1989 to August 1992, we employed hypothermic CPB with partial brachiocephlic perfusion (PBP), in which the whole brain was perfused through the right axillary artery. This method was used in 21 patients.

Until October 1994, hypothermic CPB with two-vessel selective cerebral perfusion (two-vessel SCP) was used. In this method, the right axillary and left common carotid arteries were perfused. This two-vessel SCP method was employed in 36 patients.

In the recent 17 patients, three-vessel SCP method in which all three arch vessels were perfused was used (Fig. 1).

The cardiopulmonary bypass and cannulation technique in the PBP method was shown in Fig. 2.

Electroencephalogram was monitored, and the left temporal artery was cannulated for measuring the distal stump pressure in the left common carotid artery before CPB, and the

Table 1. Patients

No.	74				
Age (years)	64.2 ± 11.5 (26 ~ 86)				
Sex (M: F)	42 : 32				
Period	April 1989 ~ August 1995				
Etiology					
Type A aortic dissection		Type B aortic dissection		Atherosclerotic aneurysm	Aortitis
acute	chronic	acute	chronic		
34	10	1	3	25	1

Period	Technique	Description
April 1989 → August 1992	PBP (n = 21)	Partial brachiocephalic perfusion; only brachiocephalic a. was perfused
August 1992 → October 1994	2 vessel SCP (n = 36)	Selective cerebral perfusion; brachiocephalic a. & common carotid a. were perfused
October 1994 → August 1995	3 vessel SCP (n = 17)	Selective cerebral perfusion; brachiocephalic a., common carotid a. and lt. subclavian a. were perfused

Fig. 1. History of cerebral protection in our hospital

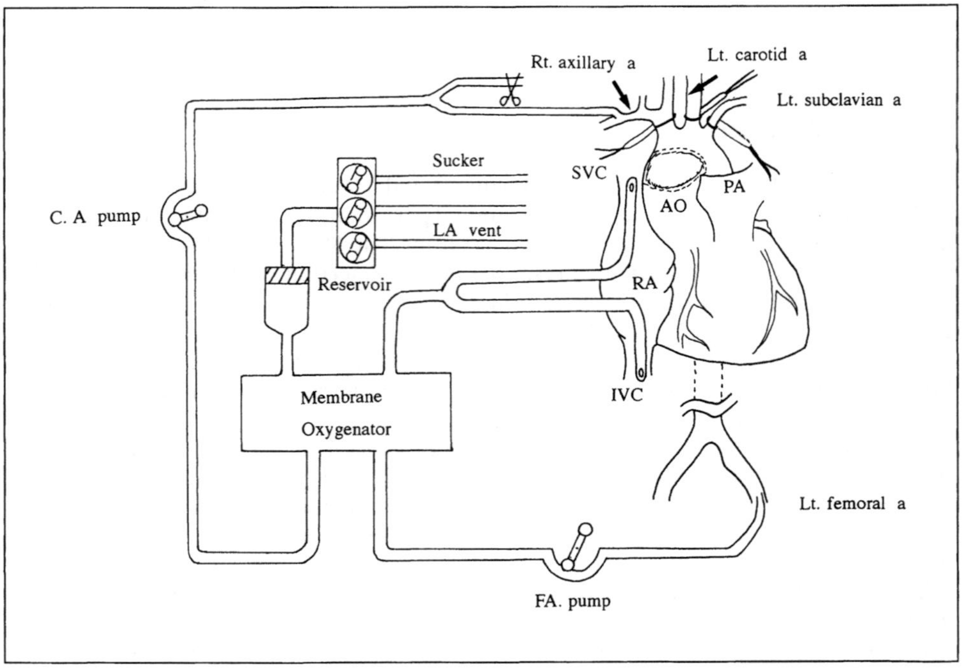

Fig. 2. Hypothermic CPB with PBP technique

cerebral perfusion pressure on SCP. If the distal stump pressure was higher than 30 mmHg or the ratio of the distal stump pressure to systemic pressure in the radial artery was greater than 0.5, the PBP through the right axillary artery was performed. An fiber-optic Oxymeter catheter was introduced to the left internal jugular vein for continuous monitoring of cerebral venous oxygen saturation. Direct cannulation to the brachiocephalic, left common carotid, and left subclavian arteries was not performed in this method. When the rectal temperature had reached between 20° and 23 °C and the electronencephalogram showed an absence of activity, the PBP was started with a perfusion flow rate of about 10 ml/kg/min.

The operative procedures in the three groups are shown in Table 2. In all patients who underwent antegrade selective cerebral perfusion, graft replacement of the partial and total aortic arch was performed on 44 and 24 patients respectively, on 4 of the other 6 patients were performed primary repairs, the remaining 2 patients underwent patch-grafting of the aortic wall.

In two-vessel SCP and three-vessel SCP group, extensive operative procedures, for example, total aortic arch replacement, were used in many patients.

Results

As the operative results (Table 3), 12 of the 74 patients, 4 in the PBP group, 6 in the two-vessel SCP group, and 2 in the three-vessel SCP group died within 30 days after surgery.

Table 2. Operative procedure

	PBP	2 vessel SCP	3 vessel SCP	total
Primary repair	4	0	0	4
Hemiarch replacement	16	20	8	44
Total aortic arch replacement	1	14	9	24
Patch glafting	0	2	0	2
total	21	36	17	74

Table 3. Operative results in all patients

Early death	12/74 (16.2 %)
Cerebral complication	2/74 (2.7 %)
Transient lethargy	3/74 (4.1 %)
Causes of early death	
LOS (low output syndrome)	2
MNMS (myonephropathic metabolic syndrome)	3
Peritonitis	2
MOF (multiple organ failure)	2
Respiratory failure	1
ARDS (adult respiratory distress syndrome)	1
Unknown	1

The early mortality rate was 16.2 %. Three patients with acute aortic dissection died of myonephropathic metabolic syndrome resulting from preoperative malperfusion of the legs, and 2 patients died of acute peritonitis due to perforation of the colon. The other 6 early deaths were related to operative procedures.

According to the cerebral perfusion data (Table 4) in our three antegrade cerebral perfusion methods, cerebral perfusion flow rate was generally regulated to about 10 ml/kg/min (range 10.4 to 12 ml/kg/min) in all three groups. The mean cerebral perfusion pressure was 39.4 mmHg in the PBP group, 45.4 mmHg in the two-vessel SCP group, and 51.6 mmHg in the three-vessel SCP group. The mean cerebral perfusion time was 68.8 min in the PBP group, 91.3 min in the two-vessel SCP group and 104.5 min in the three-vessel SCP group. The mean cerebral perfusion time in the three-vessel SCP group was significantly longer than that in the PBP group, because extensive graft replacement of aorta, for example total aortic arch replacement, was performed on many patients in the three-vessel SCP group as mentioned above.

Regarding the cerebral complications (Table 5) in the 74 patients: Stroke occurred in one each patient who underwent PBP or two-vessel SCP. No stroke was seen in the three-vessel SCP group. Three patients required more than 24 h for recovering consciousness. There were no significant differences in the incidence of cerebral complications among the three groups.

We monitored changes of oxygen saturation in the internal jugular vein (SjO2), during hypothermic CPB with selective cerebral perfusion in the PBP group and the three-vessel SCP group (Fig. 3). The mean values of SjO2 during cerebral perfusion were kept over 90 % in the three-vessel SCP group, and they were maintained between 80 and 90 % in the PBP group. The mean values of SjO2 during cerebral perfusion were kept higher in the three-vessel SCP group than those in the PBP group, however, there were no significant differences between any values of SjO2 in the two groups.

The mean cerebral perfusion pressure and cerebral perfusion time in the 74 patients are shown in Fig. 4. When the mean perfusion pressure was kept over 30 mmHg and perfusion time was within 160 min, no cerebral complications occurred.

Tabe 4. Data of cerebral perfusion

	flow	pressure		duration	rectal temperature
PBP	10.4 ± 1.9	39.4 ± 16.9	┌	68.8 ± 39.3	21.5 ± 1.2
2 vessel SCP	10.7 ± 1.2	45.4 ± 9.9	*	91.3 ± 49.5	23.3 ± 2.2
3 vessel SCP	12.0 ± 1.4	51.6 ± 13.1	└	104.5 ± 51.4	23.6 ± 2.5
	(ml/kg/min.)	(mmHg)		(min.)	(°C)

* $p < 0.05$

Table 5. Cerebral complication

	PBP (n = 21)	2 vessel SCP (n = 36)	3 vessel SCP (n = 17)	total (n = 74)
Stroke	1 (4.7 %)	1 (2.8 %)	0	2 (2.7 %)
Transient lethargy	1 (4.7 %)	1 (2.8 %)	1 (5.9 %)	3 (4.1 %)

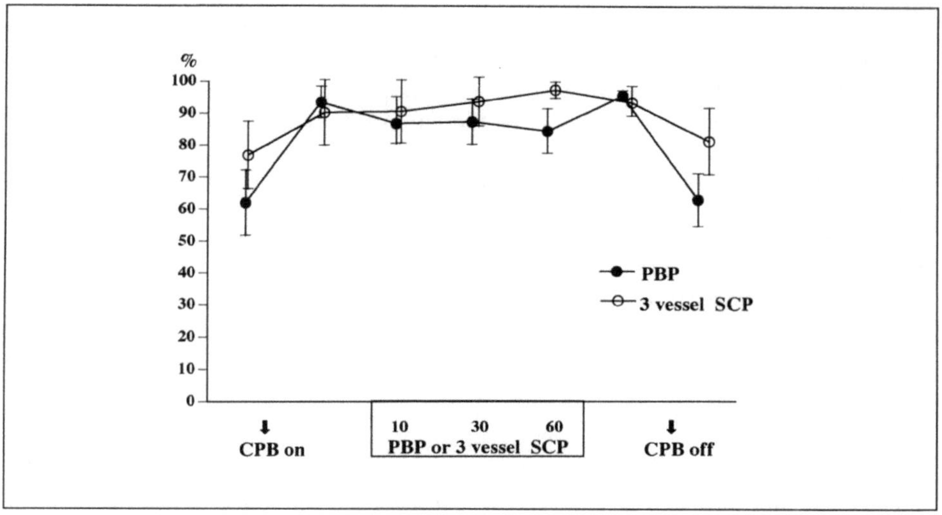

Fig. 3. SjO_2 during hypothermic CPB with cerebral perfusion

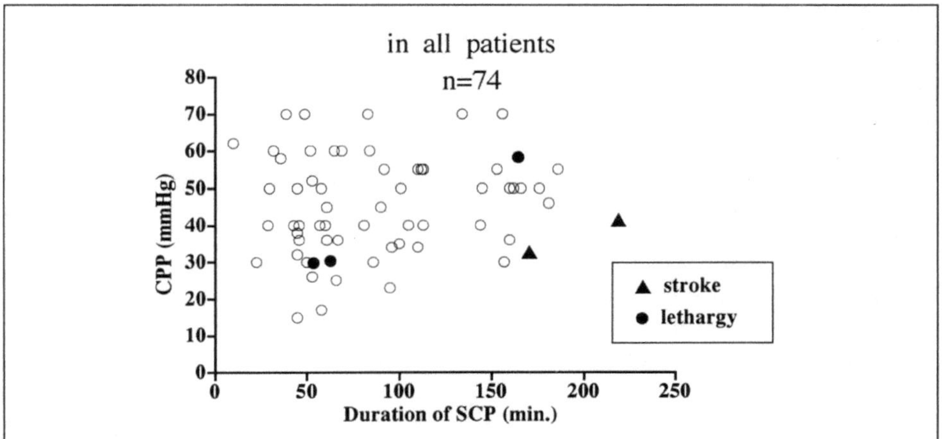

Fig. 4. Cerebral perfusion pressure and duration of SCP

Discussion

For reconstruction of the aortic arch, selective cerebral perfusion (4 – 6), retrograde cerebral perfusion (11) and hypothermic circulatory arrest (7 – 10) have recently been employed as supportive techniques. The method of profound hypothermia and circulatory arrest is easy to carry out without the need for special equipment or cannulation of the arch vessels, but the time allowed for cerebral circulatory arrest is restricted. The method of profound hypothermia and retrograde cerebral perfusion made it possible to prolong the circulatory arrest time slightly, however, safety for that method has not been established. On the other hand, SCP has the advantage of permitting less restricted cerebral protection, making it suitable for treating patients who require a complicated aortic arch repair.

In our hospital, we began to use PBP as the supportive method during circulatory arrest. However, our 21st patient suffered a cerebral infarction of left occipital lobe, therefore, we began using two-vessel and three-vessel SCP as our method of cerebral protection. But, there was one patient with a stroke in the two-vessel SCP group and no patients with stroke in the three-vessel SCP group. Although the cause of those strokes, we still believe that perfusion in the left vertebral artery is important.

According to the perfusion data in patients with SCP, when the mean perfusion pressure was kept over 30 mmHg and perfusion time was within 160 min, no cerebral complications occurred. Matsuda and assosiates (5) described the mean perfusion flow rate as 12.9 ml/kg/min when perfusion pressure has been controlled to approximately 50 mmHg. In our perfusion data, the mean perfusion pressure and flow rate in the three-vessel SCP group were 51.6 mmHg and 12.0 ml/kg/min, respectively, therefore we think that our perfusion method is appropriate and safe.

The early mortality and incidence of a postoperative stroke for the entire series of 74 patients was 16.2 % and 2.7 % respectively. Coseli and associates (13) reported results for 227 patients with aortic arch operation; in their large series they reported the inhospital mortality and incidence of a stroke as 6.17 % and 3.1 %, respectively. It was found that our unsatisfactory early mortality rate was caused by a difference of the etiology in this series. Hypothermic CPB with SCP was a satisfactory and safe method for cerebral protection.

In conclusion, we studied the selective cerebral perfusion technique and its results in 74 consecutive patients.

1) Hypothermic CPB with selective cerebral perfusion was a safe and reliable procedure as a supportive method for aortic arch surgery
2) A stroke occurred perioperatively in 2 patients who received the operation under hypothermic CPB with PBP or two-vessel SCP, however, no patient suffered a stroke in the three-vessel SCP group.
3) The overall early mortality rate was 16.2 %, however, there were no deaths related to our cerebral protective methods.
4) When the mean perfusion pressure was kept over 30 mmHg and perfusion time was within 160 min, no cerebral complications occurred.

References

1. Livesay JJ, Cooly DA, Reul GJ, Walker WE, Frazier OH, Duncan JM, Ott DA (1983) Resection of aortic arch aneurysms: a comparison of hypothermic techniques in 60 patients. Ann Thorac Surg 36: 19–28
2. Crawford ES, Svensson LG, Coselli JS, Safi HJ, Hess KR (1989) Surgical treatment of aneurysm and/or dissection of the ascending aorta, transverse aortic arch. Factors influencing survival in 717 patients. J Thorac Cardiovasc Surg 98: 659–74
3. Bachet J, Guilmet D, Goudot B, Termignon JL, Teodori G, Dreyfus G, Brodaty D, Dubois C, Delentdecker P (1991) Cold cerebroplegia. A new technique of cerebral protection during operation on the transverse aortic arch. J Thorac Cardiovasc Surg 102: 85–94
4. Aoyagi S, Akashi H, Kubota Y, Momosaki M, Suzuki S, Ohryoji A, Kosuga K, Ohishi K (1993) Partial brachiocephalic perfusion in aortic arch replacement. Jpn J Surg 23: 331–337
5. Matsuda H, Nakano S, Shirakura R, Matsuwaka R, Ohkubo N, Ohtani M, Hirose H, Kawashima Y (1989) Surgery for aortic arch aneurysm with selective cerebral perfusion and hypothermic cardiopulmonary bypass. Circulation 80 (suppl I): 243–248

6. First WH, Baldwin JC, Starnes VA, Stinson EB, Oyer PE, Miller DC, Jamieson SW, Mitchell RS, Shumway NE (1986) A reconsideration of cerebral perfusion in aortic arch replacement. Ann Thorac Surg 42: 273–81
7. Griepp RB, Stinson EB, Hollingsworth JF, Buehler D (1975) Prosthetic replacement of the aortic arch. J Thorac Cardiovasc Surg 70: 1051–63
8. Cooley DA, Ott DA, Frazier OH, Walker WE (1981) Surgical treatment of aneurysms of the transverse aortic arch: experience with 25 patients using hypothermic techniques. Ann Thorac Surg 32: 260–72
9. Crawford ES, Snyder DM (1983) Treatment of aneurysms of the aortic arch: a progress report. J Thorac Cardiovasc Surg 85: 237–46
10. Mahfood S, Qazi A, Garcia J, Mispireta L, Coaso P, Smyth N (1985) Management of aortic arch aneurysm using profound hypothermia and circulatory arrest. Ann Thorac Surg 39: 412–7
11. Ueda Y, Miki S, Kusuhara K, Okita Y, Tahara T, Yamanaka K (1990) Surgical treatment of aneurysm of dissection involving the ascending aorta and aortic arch, utilizing circulatory arrest and retrograde cerebral perfusion. J Cardiovasc Surg 31: 553–8
12. Kubota Y, Akashi H, Aoyagi S, Yamana K, Nishimi M, Uraguchi K, Fujino T, Koga M, Suzuki S, Kenmochi K, Kosuga K, Ohishi K (1990) An experimental study of hypothermic cardiopulmonary bypass with partial brachiocephalic perfusion (in Japanese). J Jpn Assoc Thorac Surg 38: 1975
13. Coselli JS, Buket S, Djukanovic B (1995) Aortic arch operation: Current treatment and results. Ann Thorac Surg 59: 19–27

Author's address:
H. Akashi, M.D.
Second Department of Surgery
Kurume University School of Medicine
67 Asahi-machi
Kurume, Japan

Selective cerebral perfusion for brain protection during surgery of the aortic arch

T. Kazui

Department of Thoracic and Cardiovascular Surgery, Sapporo Medical University School of Medicine, Japan

Introduction

The methods for protecting the brain during surgery of the aortic arch differ from institution to institution at present. We have used the antegrade selective cerebral perfusion in the treatment of aortic arch aneurysm requiring complicated arch repair because of unlimited duration of cerebral protection (4, 5).

In the present paper, we describe the operative technique of aortic arch reconstruction with an aid of selective cerebral perfusion in the operation of aortic arch aneurysm.

Material and methods

During the period between January 1986 and August 1995, 161 patients underwent operation for aortic arch aneurysms using selective cerebral perfusion as a cerebral protection method.

The patient profiles are listed in Table 1. Their mean age (± standard deviation) was 60.2 ± 12.2 years, and about two-thirds of them were male. The etiology of the aortic aneurysm was aortic dissection in 99 patients including 52 cases of acute dissection, and atherosclerotic and degenerative aneurysms in 47 patients.

Table 1. Patient profiles

no. of patients	161
Age (mean ± SD)	60.2 ± 12.2
Gender (male/female)	103/58
Etiology	
Aortic dissection	99
acute	52
chronic	47
Atherosclerotic and degenerative	62
Previous operation	30 (19%)
Emergency operation	63 (39%)

Thirty patients had undergone operations on the great vessels. Of these, 17 patients had undergone operations on the ascending aorta and/or aortic arch, 2 on the descending aorta, and 11 on the aorto-iliac artery.

Sixty-three patients (39 %) had an emergency operation within 24 h after hospitalization to treat either an acute type A dissection (52 patients) or aneurysm rupture (11 patients). The operations were performed through the median sternotomy and left supraclavicular incision in all patients except six in which an additional thoracotomy was made to expose the distal portion of the descending aorta. After systemic heparinization, extracorporeal circulation was instituted with the arterial return cannula placed in a femoral artery and a single two-stage cannula for venous drainage in the right atrium (Fig. 1). The left side of the heart was vented through the right superior pulmonary vein. Myocardial protection was provided with cold blood cardioplegia.

Selective cerebral perfusion (SCP) was used in all patients to prevent cerebral ischemia during the aortic arch repair. When the patient was cooled to 22 °C rectal temperature by extracorporeal circulation, systemic circulation from the femoral artery was arrested and the aorta was opened. SCP cannulae (Fig. 2) were then inserted into the innominate and left common carotid arteries via the aortic lumen. Blood was perfused into both arteries at the rate of 10 ml/kg/min using a single roller pump separated from the systemic circulation. The cerebral perfusion pressure was adjusted to maintain a right radial arterial pressure of 40 to 70 mmHg.

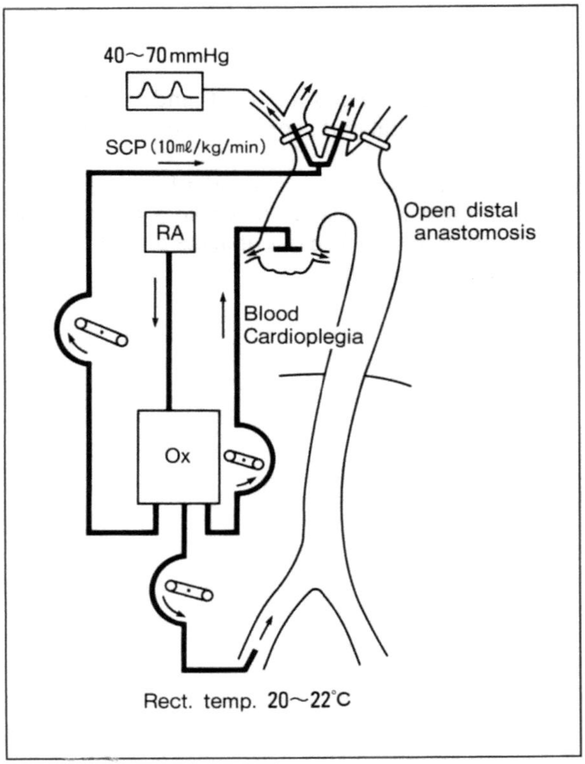

Fig. 1. Schema of extracorporeal circulation and selective cerebral perfusion (Ox: oxygenator, RA: right atrium)

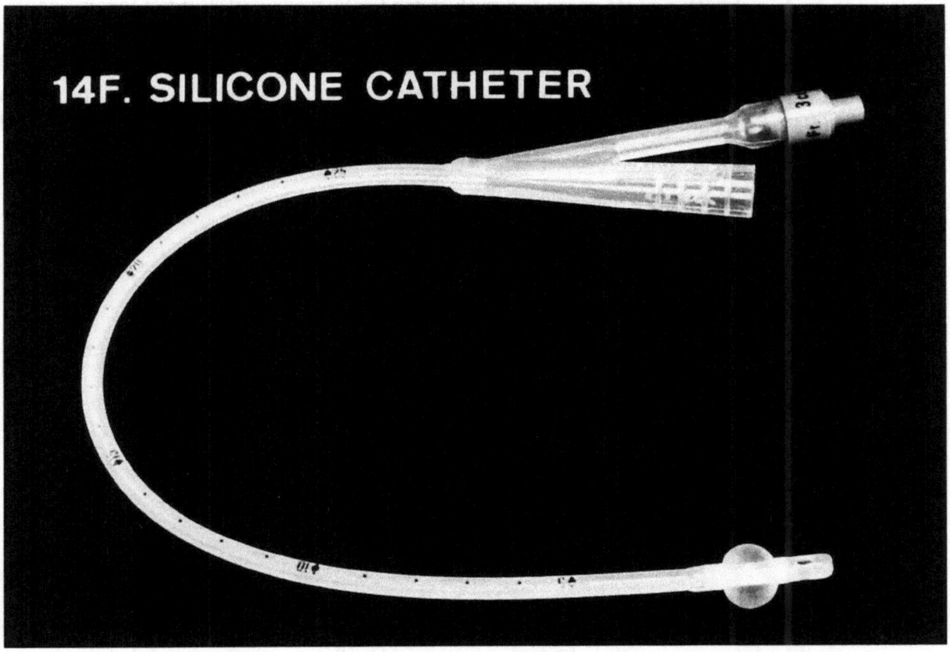

Fig. 2. Selective cerebral perfusion cannula made of flexible silicone tube with balloon at its end. Eighteen French size cannula is used for innominate artery perfusion, and 14 French size for left common carotid artery perfusion.

In the majority of the cases, open aortic anastomosis was concomitantly used for distal graft anastomosis. The operative techniques used are shown in Table 2. Patch angioplasty of the aortic arch was performed in four patients, partial arch replacement in 13, and total arch replacement in 144 (90 %). As the operative technique of total arch replacement, the "en bloc" repair technique in which the orifices of the arch vessels were anastomosed to the opening made on the graft in an end-to side fashion, was used in the first 22 patients. In the rest of 122 patients, the separated graft technique in which the aortic arch and arch ves-

Table 2. Operative technique

technique	no. of patients
Patch	4 (2%)
Partial Arch	13 (8%)
Total Arch	144 (90%)
en bloc	22
Separated graft	122
Total	161

sels were replaced with a graft provided with three limbs was used. Since December 1993, we have modified our technique of aortic arch reconstruction using the separated graft to reduce the occurrence of cerebral complication as illustrated in Fig. 3. With the aid of the antegrade selective cerebral perfusion and systemic circulatory arrest at 22 °C rectal temperature (B), the distal graft was anastomosed to the descending aorta (C) and then the

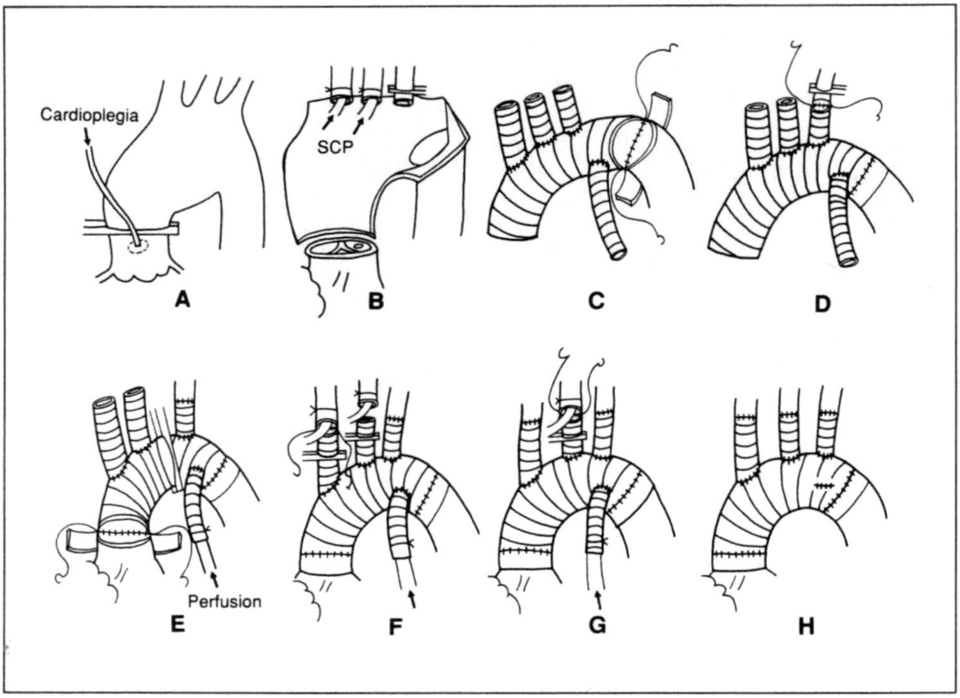

Fig. 3. Operative technique of total arch replacement using the separated graft (see the text).

Table 3. Concomitant procedures

procedures	no. of patients
Composite graft	27 (4)
A/V suspension	20
CABG	17
AVR	5
MVR/MAP	2
Extended aortoplasty	1
Total	72 (45 %)

( ): re-do case

left subclavian artery was sutured to the 3rd limb of the graft (D). After the proximal graft was cross-clamped, the antegrade systemic perfusion with rewarming through the 4th limb attached to the graft instead of femoral artery perfusion was started (E). The proximal graft was anastomosed to the ascending aorta and coronary circulation was started. The innominate and left common carotid arteries were then anastomosed to each limb in succession (F, G). Prior to completion of the anastomosis, each cerebral perfusion cannula was removed. The 4th limb used as the antegrade systemic perfusion was resected after the extracorporeal circulation was terminated (H). Concomitant procedures are listed in Table 3. They included composite graft replacement with coronary reimplantation in 27 patients including four re-do operations, aortic valve suspension in 20 with acute type A aortic dissection, CABG in 17, AVR in five, and miscellaneous in three.

Results

The surgical results of aortic aneurysm operation in 161 patients are listed in Table 4. The overall 30-day survival rate was 90.1 %, and the 30-day mortality rate 9.9 %. As post-operative complications, cerebral complication occurred in three patients. One patient who was preoperatively in profound shock secondary to rupture of aneurysm suffered from massive stroke postoperatively. This patient's stroke was apparently related to his critical condition, and not related to SCP procedure. One patient had brain stem infarction due to left vertebral-basilar artery ischemia, which recently caused us to modify the operative technique of arch reconstruction. The remaining one patient suffered from minor cerebral embolism resulting from migration of the atherosclerotic debris from the injection site of myocardial protection.

Table 5 shows the preoperative and perioperative predictors of early mortality determined by univariate and multivariate analysis. Eight variables were found to have a significant influence on early mortality through the univariate analysis. They were studied by multivariate analysis to confirm that these variables could influence early mortality. The results of this analysis showed preoperative intubation for cardiopulmonary resuscitation, preoperative stroke episode, and previous ascending aorta and/or arch operation to be significant predictors of early mortality rate.

Early mortality according to risk factors determined by multivariate analysis is shown in Table 6. None of these risk factors was present in 119 patients (74 %), and the early mortal-

Table 4. Surgical results

No. of Patients	161
30-day Survival	145 (90.1 %)
30-day Mortality	16 (9.9 %)
Postoperative Complications	
Cerebral complication	3 (1.9 %)
Hemorrhage	6 (3.7 %)
LOS	9 (5.5 %)
Respiratory failure	20 (12.4 %)
Hepatic failure	2 (1.3 %)
Infection	7 (4.3 %)

Table 5. Risk factors of early mortality

Risk factors	Univariate A. p value	Multivariate A. p value
Rupture	0.049	0.361
Renal/mesenteric ischemia	0.004	0.299
Leg ischemia	0.024	0.126
Preop. intubation	0.001	0.020
Renal failure	0.019	0.101
Preop. stroke	0.024	0.010
Pump time	0.018	0.198
Previous Asc. Ao/Arch Op.	0.034	0.007

Table 6. Early mortality according to risk factors determined by multivariate analysis

No. of risk factors	No. of patients	Early mortality	
		no.	%
0	119 (74%)	3	2.5%
1	40 (25%)	11	27.5%
2	2 (1%)	2	100.0%

Table 7. Surgical results

Period	Dec. 1993 ~ Aug. 1995
No. of Patients	58
Op. Survival	58
30-day Mortality	0
Hospital Death	2 (3.4%)
Post op. complication	
Cerebral complication	0
Respiratory failure	11
Infection	2
Renal failure	1
G1 Bleeding	1

ity rate in these patients was as low as 2.5 %. On the other hand, the early mortality in 40 patients with one risk factor and in two patients with two risk factors were 27.5 %, and 100 %, respectively.

The causes of early death included multiple organ failure in four patients, hemorrhage in three, low cardiac output in three, respiratory failure in three, and infection, G1 bleeding, and sudden death in one patient each.

The data concerning extracorporeal circulation were as follows: mean total bypass time was 202 min, aortic cross clamp time 128 min, selective cerebral perfusion time 91 min, and circulatory arrest time 44 min at the lowest rectal temperature of 22.1 °C.

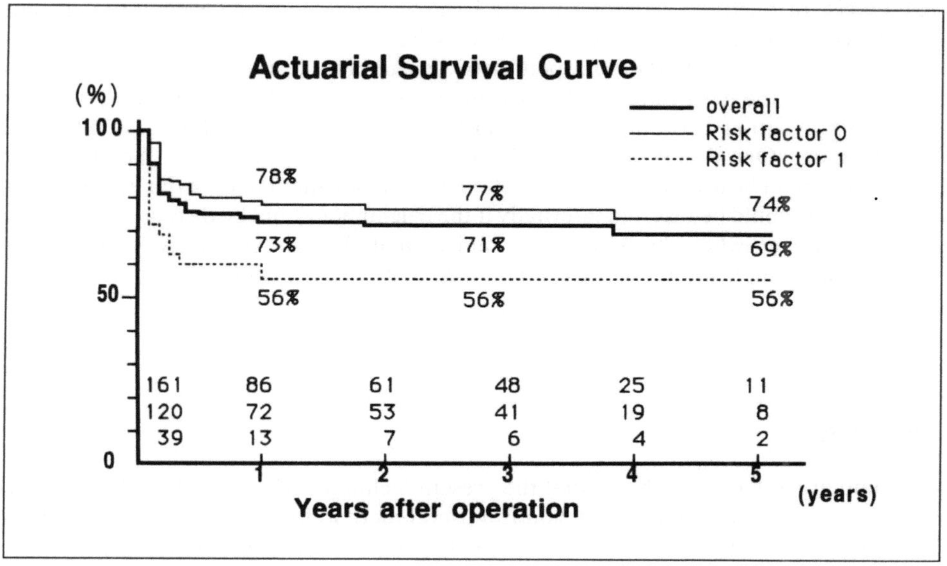

Fig. 4. Actuarial survival curve following aortic arch aneurysm operation using selective cerebral perfusion

Figure 4 shows the actuarial survival curve calculated by the Kaplan-Meier method. The 5-year survival rate, including early mortality, was 69 % for overall patients. The 5-year survival rate in 120 patients without any risk factors was 74 %. On the other hand, the 5-year survival rate in 39 patients with one risk factor was 56 %.

Discussion

As the methods for protecting the brain during the reconstruction of the aortic arch, antegrade selective cerebral perfusion (1), profound hypothermia with circulatory arrest (3, 6), or retrograde cerebral perfusion (2, 7) have been used in many institutions. During the last years, we have used selective cerebral perfusion in more than 160 patients with satisfactory results. In order to simplify the operative technique and to improve the surgical outcome, with an aid of two arch vessels perfusion of innominate and left common carotid arteries with right radial arterial pressure monitoring and systemic circulatory arrest at 22 °C rectal temperature, total aortic arch was replaced with the separated graft.

The present technique has several advantages as follows:

1) The unlimited duration of cerebral protection allows us to perform more radical and extended operation such as "total arch replacement" or "total thoracic aortic replacement".
2) This method is simpler than that in which three arch vessels are perfused or bilateral carotid arteries are perfused with two pumps and bilateral superficial temporal artery pressures are monitored.

3) Precise reconstruction of the aortic arch can be performed even in cases of acute aortic dissection with severely involved arch vessels.
4) The combined technique of open distal anastomosis has the advantage of not only extending the graft as far as the descending aorta through a median sternotomy, but also preventing crush injury to a fragile aorta in acute aortic dissection by avoiding clamping. One disadvantage of selective cerebral perfusion is that the arch vessels, which might be involved in the dissection, should be cannulated. In our experience, the cannulae could be inserted internally if the true lumen could be distinguished from the aortic lumen when the branches to be cannulated were extensively involved. There were no complications due to cannulation in any of our patients.

Summary

In summary, it has been shown that the present technique of total arch replacement with an aid of selective cerebral perfusion is a useful method for preventing the neurological complications in the treatment of aortic arch aneurysm requiring complex repair.

References

1. Bachet J, Guilmet D, Goudot B et al. (1991) Cold cerebroplegia. A new technique of cerebral protection during operations on the transverse aortic arch. J Thorac Cardiovasc Surg 102: 85–94
2. Coselli JS (1994) Retrograde cerebral perfusion via a superior vena cava cannula for aortic arch aneurysm operations. Ann Thorac Surg 53: 1668–1669
3. Griepp RB, Stinson EB, Hollingsworth JF, Buehler D (1975) Prosthetic replacement of the aortic arch. J Thorac Cardiovasc Surg 70: 1051–1063
4. Kazui T, Inoue N, Yamada O, Komatsu S (1992) Selective cerebral perfusion during operation for aneurysms of the aortic arch: A reassessment. Ann Thorac Surg 53: 109–114
5. Kazui T, Kimura N, Yamada O, Komatsu S (1994) Surgical outcome of aortic arch aneurysms using selective cerebral perfusion. Ann Thorac Surg 57: 904–911
6. Svensson LG, Crawford ES, Hess KR et al. (1993) Deep hypothermia with circulatory arrest. Determinants of stroke and early mortality in 656 patients. J Thorac Cardiovasc Surg 106: 19–31
7. Ueda Y, Miki S, Kusuhara K et al. (1990) Surgical treatment of aneurysm or dissection involving the ascending aorta and aortic arch, utilizing circulatory arrest and retrograde cerebral perfusion. J Cardiovasc Surg 31: 553–558

Author's address:
T. Kazui, M.D.
Sapporo Medical University
School of Medicine
Dept. of Thoracic and
Cardiovascular Surgery
South 1, West 16, Chuc-ku
Sapporo 060
Japan

Brain monitoring during retrograde cerebral perfusion in operations on the thoracic aorta

M. Ehrlich, M. Grabenwöger, D. Luckner, F. Cartes-Zumelzu, P. Simon, G. Grubhofer, A. Lassnig, G. Laufer, E. Wolner, M. Havel

Department Cardio-Thoracic Surgery, University of Vienna, Austria

Introduction

Surgical treatment of aneurysms of the ascending aorta and transverse arch still represent a challenging situation for cardiac surgeons. Great strides have been made since the introduction of deep hypothermia and circulatory arrest (1, 2, 5, 8) in reducing neurological complications associated with these procedure. Nevertheless, neurological injury as a result of temporary disconnection of cerebral blood flow during the period of circulatory arrest still remains an important complication in operation performed on the aortic arch.

Retrograde cerebral perfusion (RCP) via a superior vena cava (SVC) cannula is a relatively new and simply technique that can improve neurological outcome in patients requiring surgery on the aortic arch and great vessels.

Patients and methods

Patients

Between May 1993 and September 1995, a total of 22 patients with an aneurysm of the ascending aorta and arch were operated on at the Dept. of Cardio-Vascular Surgery at the University of Vienna. The average age of our patients was 60 years (range 22–78), and there were 8 female and 14 male. Nine patients had an acute, 13 a chronic dissection. One patient underwent concomitant aortic valve replacement; he received a composite aortic valve-ascending aortic conduit graft. Two patients underwent coronary artery revascularization for proximal left anterior descending coronary artery disease.

Operative technique

General endotracheal aneasthesia was used for all repairs. Spectroscopy patches placed over both cerebral hemispheres to monitor cerebral oxygen saturation throughout the whole operation (Fig. 1), as well as Doppler flow measurements in the middle cerebral artery (Fig. 2) during retrograde cerebral perfusion were performed. A median sternotomy was employed, and arterial perfusion was through the common femoral artery.

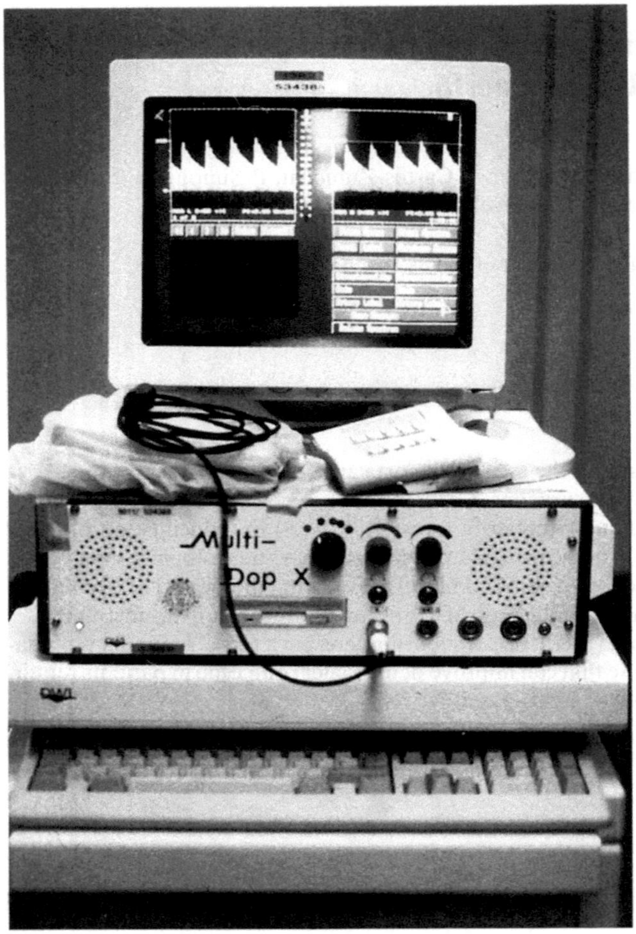

The right atrium was cannulated with a two-stage cannula for venous drainage. The left ventricle was vented through a cannula placed in the apex. All patients received, right before circulatory arrest, 1000 mg of Cortison for added cerebral protection. At a rectal temperature of 18 °C and a nasopharyngeal temperature of 12 °C, most of the intravascular blood volume was drained into the pump reservoir and circulatory arrest was induced. At this time, the cardiopulmonary bypass circuitry was converted into the retrograde cerebral perfusion system. The distal anastomosis was performed between the graft and the proximal aortic arch mostly in a hemiarch fashion. Thereafter, hypothermic body perfusion was commenced via a 8 mm Dacron graft (already anastomosed end-to-side into the prosthesis by the manufacturer). This graft was linked to a second arterial line, which was connected by a Y-adapter to the arterial line of the extracorporeal circuit. The aorta was clamped distal to the junction of the second arterial line and it was possible to start with the antegrade hypothermic perfusion (3–4 liter/min). Then, the proximal anastomosis was performed. Rewarming was started, and cardiopulmonary bypass was discontinued at 36 °C.

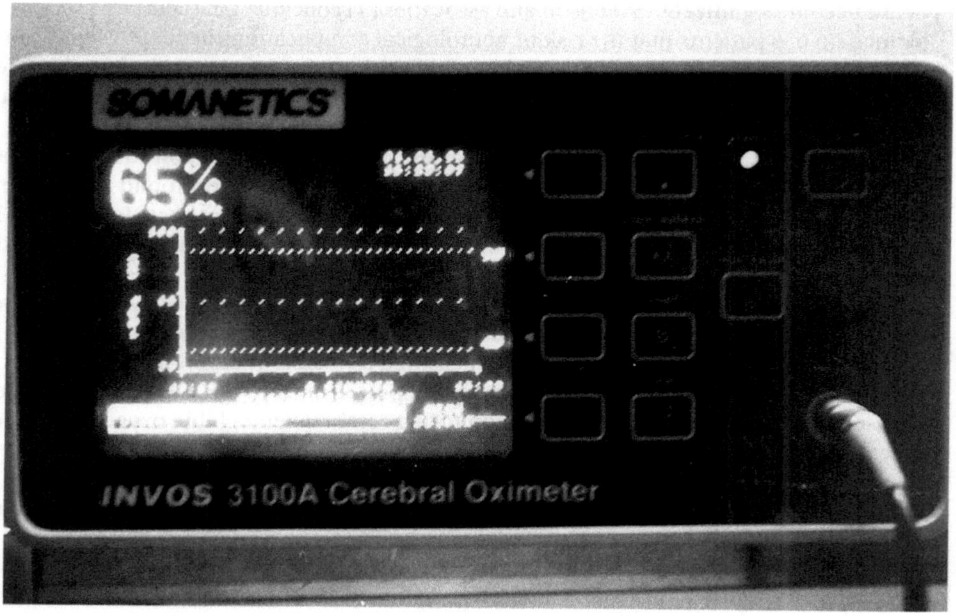

Results

All patients survived the operation. The mean duration of retrograde cerebral perfusion was 31 min (range 16 to 88 min). Two patients had RCP times greater than 45 min and one patient had RCP for a period exceeding 65 min.

Cerebral oxygen saturation was continually monitored during the time of RCP and the goal was to keep oxygen saturation within 10 % of baseline. To maintain this value, flow rates ranged from 200 to 300 ml/min with a central venous pressure between 20 and 25 mm Hg. Blood flow in the cerebral media artery showed the same reversed flow rates (mean velocity 50 cm/s) as before and after the RCP period.

All 22 patients were awake and followed simple commands within 24 h after the operation. They were all oriented to time, place and person at the time of extubation.

Postoperative cerebral complications occurred only in a single case (4.5 %) and were manifested by a transient paraparesis.

Discussion

Operations on the aorta, especially on the aortic arch still remain a formidable task for cardiac surgeons. Since the introduction of hypothermia and circulatory arrest as an valuable adjunct in aortic surgery, neurological complications have been markedly decreased in the last two decades. Nevertheless, there is a distinct time limit before neurological damage or death become significant. Svennson and assocaties (7) concluded in their large series performed on 656 patients that the risk of neurological complications increased significantly when the arrest period exceeded 40 min and the risk of death increased when the arrest period exceeded 45 min. In another series of Ergin and Griepp (4), none of their patients, whose time of cerebral ischemia was less than 40 min, had neurological complications.

Therefore the safe period of circulatory arrest is still a subject of considerable debate and has yet to be firmly established. To extend this "safe time" of profound hypothermic circulatory arrest, alternative methods have been employed in recent years to enhance the safety for this operative procedures. One of these new methods includes (RCP) via the superior vena cava.

There is evidence that RCP does deliver oxygen to the brain, and the oxygenated blood perfused into the SVC clearly desaturates before retrograde flow comes back through the cerebral vessels. Ueda and associates (9) measured a consistent difference in oxygen content between the SVC and aortic arch blood for up to 30 min of RCP. Deep and coworkers (3) used the same technique as ours in monitoring cerebral hemoglobin oxygen saturation spectroscopically.

Another important positive effect of RCP is the maintanance of hypothemia. Perfusing the brain with blood by a temperature of 15 °C will keep this region cool, and ice-bags around the head may become unnecessary.

It is likely that another aspect of the positive effect of RCP is the avoidance and treatment of embolization. Mills and Ochsner (6) first described RCP as a treatment for embolization and its benefit in preventing air embolization during operations on the aortic arch.

As a further diagnostic method, we used in this series transcranial Doppler measurement in the middle cerebral artery. This technique gives information concerning flow velocity in the cerebral vessel system. In our series, flow was measured 10 min before, during and 10 minutes after RCP. In all patients reversed flow could be observed through the whole period of RCP.

We are at an early stage in our experiences with this new technique, but we believe that RCP combined with oxygen monitoring as well as transcranial Doppler flow measurement is a very useful adjunct in the treatment of complex aortic arch procedures. It can increase the safety of circulatory arrest, especially when arrest time af greater than 45 min is expected.

References

1. Barnard CN, Schiere V (1963) The surgical treatment of acquired aneurysms of the thoracic aorta. Thorax 18: 101–5
2. DeBakey ME, Cooley DA, Crawford ES, Morris GC Jr. (1957) Succesful resection of fusiform aneurysm of aortic arch with replacement by homograft. Surg Gynec Obstet 105: 656–64
3. Deep GM, Jenkins E, Bolling SF (1995) Retrograde cerebral perfusion during hypothermic circulatory arrest reduces neurological morbidity. J Thoracic Cardiovasc Surg 109: 259–68
4. Ergin MA, Griepp RB (1980) Progress in treatment in aneurysms of the aortic arch. World J Surg 4: 535
5. Griepp RB, Stinson EB, Hollingsworth JF, Buhler D (1975) Prosthetic replacement of the aortic arch. J Thoracic Cardiovasc Surg 70: 1051–63
6. Mills NL, Ochsner JL (1980) Massive air embolism during cardiopulmonary bypass. J Thoracic Cardiovasc Surg 80: 708–17
7. Svensson LG, Crawford ES, Hess KR et al. (1993) Deep hypothermia with circulatory arrest: determinants of stroke and early mortality in 656 patients. J Thorac Cardiovasc Surg 106: 19–31

8. Ueada T, Yamamoto YL, Takara E, Diksic M (1989) Tolerance of the cerebral venous system to retrograde perfusion pressure in focal cerebral ischemia in rats. Stroke 20: 378–85
9. Ueda Y, Miki S, Kusuhara K, Okita Y, Tahata T, Yamanaka K (1992) Deep hypothermic systemic circulatory arrest and continuous retrograde cerebral perfusion for surgery of aortic arch aneurysm. Eur J Cardiothoracic Surg 6: 36–41

Authors' address:
M. Ehrlich, M.D.
Dept. of Cardio-Thoracic Surgery
University of Vienna
Währinger Gürtel 18–20
A-1090 Vienna, Austria

Impact of antegrade perfusion in aortic arch surgery

P. Kleine, C. Draeger, A. Alken, J. Laas

Department of Cardiovascular Surgery, Cardiovascular Center Bad Bevensen, Germany

Introduction

Perioperative neurological complications remain a major problem in surgery of the proximal aorta (3, 7). Deep hypothermic circulatory arrest with a nasopharyngeal temperature below 20 °C is commonly used and well accepted for brain and/or spinal protection (1, 5). In addition, various methods like continuous antegrade and/or retrograde cerebral perfusion are discussed to minimize the risk of neurological deficits (2). The following study retrospectively analyzes as to whether the site of arterial cannulation and the direction of flow during extracorporeal circulation correlate with the neurological outcome of aortic arch surgery.

Patients and methods

From June 1993 to July 1995, 41 patients (30 male, 11 female) underwent surgery of the aortic arch. Cerebral protection was performed by decreasing the nasopharyngeal temperature below 20 °C. This was achieved by extracorporeal circulation and local cooling of the head with ice. Furthermore, 4 mg/kg/h Thiopental-Na (Trapanal) (6) was given starting with induction of anesthesia. Immediately before circulatory arrest a bolus of 40 mg Dexamethason was injected, with reperfusion 3.5 mg/kg Manitol were administered.

Operative techniques included replacement of the proximal arch in 22 patients (54 %), glue repair of the arch and open anastomosis in eight patients (19 %), total arch replacement in nine patients (22 %), and finally elephant trunk technique in two patients (5 %). Accompanying aortic valve replacement had to be performed in 15 patients (37 %) and aortic valve repair in eight patients (19 %).

Continuous arterial blood pressures were recorded in both radial and the right femoral artery for immediate recognition of malperfusion (4). Cerebral monitoring was performed by continuous derivation of EEG and SEP of the median nerve.

Generally it was attempted to maintain antegrade flow throughout the procedure. Preferably the ascending aorta or arch was used as site for arterial cannulation, while after repair the vascular prosthesis was intubated. Cannulation of the femoral artery was established in acute dissections and in the chronic form of the disease with unsuitable aortic wall anatomy. Here again after repair the vascular prothesis was cannulated for the re-warming procedure. Continuous retrograde perfusion was performed as an exception.

Results

Early mortality was 7.3 %. Causes of death were multiple organ failure, pulmonary failure and right ventricular infarction in the patient after the-third re-operation of aortic dissection.

Postoperatively in six patients neurological deficits (Table 1) were observed (group II) while 35 patients were free of symptoms (group I). Statistical analyses of pre-, intra- and postoperative data were performed according to the neurological outcome of patients.

Mean age of all patients was 54.6 years. Diagnosis was aneurysmal disease in 24 (56 %), acute dissection in 14 (34 %) and chronic in six (10 %) cases. Nine patients (22 %) had had previous aortic or cardiac surgery. Neurological status of patients prior to surgery is shown in Table 2. Ten patients (24 %) had positive anamneses or findings. There were no statistically significant differences with respect to age, aortic pathology and the presence of neurological symptoms between group I and group II.

Table 3 summarizes our intraoperative data. There were no statistically significant differences with respect to nasopharyngeal temperature, duration of operation, bypass, cross clamping and circulatory arrest between the groups.

With respect to site of arterial cannulation and/or direction of blood flow during extracorporeal circulation statistically significant difference could be found (Table 4). The rate of neurological deficits was significantly higher in patients with solely retrograde and combined retrograde and antegrade perfusion. Patients with solely antegrade perfusion by cannulation of the proximal aorta and the vascular graft after repair showed the best results.

The period of intubation as well as for intensive care treatment was prolonged in case of neurological disturbances.

Table 1. Postoperative neurological deficits (n = 6 patients)

Transient paresis	2 patients
Permanent hemiparesis	1 patient
Permanent paraplegia	1 patient
Coma	1 patient
Hemianopsia	1 patient

Table 2 Preoperative neurological status

	Total	Group I	Group II
Nasopharyngeal temp. (°C)	19.4	19.6	18.6
Operation time (min)	275	250	423
Bypass time (min)	130	129	137
X-clamping time (min)	60	61	53
Circulatory arrest (min)	18.4 (8 to 46)	18.3 (8 to 44)	19.4 (9 to 46)

Table 3. Operative data

	Total	Group I	Group II
Nasopharyngeal temp. (°C)	19.4	19.6	18.6
Operation time (min)	275	250	423
Bypass time (min)	130	129	137
X-clamping time (min)	60	61	53
Circulatory arrest (min)	18.4 (8 to 46)	18.3 (8 to 44)	19.4 (9 to 46)

Table 4. Influence of cannulation technique on neurological outcome

	Total	Group I	Group II
Retrograde perfusion via Femoral artery (%)	24	14	83*
Combined perfusion (%) (intially retrograde, after repair antegrade)	30	34	0*
Antegrade perfusion (%)	46	51	17*

* = $p < 0.05$

Conclusions

With hypothermia below 20 °C nasopharyngeal temperature and periods of circulatory arrest ranging from 8 – 46 min neurological outcome could not be related to the degree of hypothermia and duration of arrest.

Retrograde perfusion during extracorporeal circulation was combined with a significantly higher rate of neurological deficits. These patients experience prolonged periods of intubation and intensive care treatment.

Our data indicate that the site of arterial cannulation significantly determines the neurological outcome of patients with reversal of flow, atheriosclerotic detritus from the whole aorta especially from the abdominal part can cause cerebral embolism. Furthermore reversed flow can provoke malperfusion syndrome (e.g., blind pocket phenomena).

Thus the preferred site of cannulation should be the ascending aorta or arch in case of acute dissections or otherwise impaired quality of the proximal aorta cannulation through the left ventriculär apex or through the right subclavian artery.

References

1. Borst HG, Laas J (1993) Surgical treatment of thoracic aortic aneurysms. Advances in Cardiac Surgery, Vol 4: pp 47 – 88, Mosby Year Book Inc.
2. Deeb GM, Jenkins E, Bolling SF, Brunsting LA, Williams DM, Quint LE, Deeb ND (1995) Retrograde cerebral perfusion during hypothermic circulatory arrest reduces neurologic morbidity. J Thorac Cardovasc Surg 109 (2): pp 259–268

3. Frist WH, Baldwin JC, Starnes VA et al. (1986) A reconsideration of cerebral perfusion in aortic arch replacement. Ann Thorac Surg 42: pp 273–281
4. Laas J, Heinemann M, Schaefers HJ, Daniel W, Borst HG (1991) Management of thoracoabdominal malperfusion in aortic dissection. Circulation 84, Suppl 3: III-20 – III-24
5. Laas J, Jurmann M, Heinemann M, Borst HG (1992) Advances in aortic arch surgery. Ann Thorac Surg 53: pp 227–232
6. Nussmeier NA, Arlund C, Slogoff S (1986) Cerebral protection by a barbiturate. Anesthesiology 64: pp 165–170
7. Okita Y, Takamoto S, Ando M, Morota T, Kawashima Y (1996) Predictive factors for postoperative cerebral complications in patients with thoracic aortic aneurysm. Europ J Cardiothor Surg (in press)

Author's address:
Dr. med. Peter Kleine
Herz-, Gefäß- und Thoraxchirurgie
Herz-Kreislauf-Klinik Bevensen
Römstedter Straße 25
29549 Bad Bevensen
Germany

Hypothermic circulatory arrest through the left chest

J. S. Coselli

The Methodist Hospital/Baylor College of Medicine, Houston, Texas, USA

Introduction

The concept of profound hypothermic circulatory arrest (HCA) through an anterior mediastinal approach has been a widely employed technique for the protection of the central nervous and other organ systems in the treatment of complex congenital and cardiac lesions, as well as aneurysms of the aortic arch. The application of this technique in the treatment of aortic disease through a posterolateral approach has received far less attention. The rationale for the use of hypothermic circulatory arrest in the treatment of patients with aortic pathology beyond the left subclavian artery includes proximal extension of the aortic pathology into the transverse aortic arch, the inability to safely place proximal aortic cross clamp for anatomical reasons (size, rupture, friability, scar tissue from prior operation), or the use of hypothermia as a modality for organ protection (most importantly, the spinal cord). A number of clinical reports have demonstrated the effective use of cardiopulmonary bypass, hypothermic circulatory arrest, and posterolateral exposure for procedures on the thoracic aorta for diverse aortic pathology (1–8). This report is a retrospective review of the author's experience using HCA for patients requiring replacement of the descending thoracic or thoracoabdominal aorta through the left chest where proximal cross clamping was not feasible or aneurysmal disease extended into the transverse aortic arch. The technique was not employed primarily for spinal cord or other organ protection in patients in whom proximal cross clamping was possible.

Operative technique

The author has previously described in detail his approach to the preoperative evaluation and surgical treatment of patients with descending and thoracoabdominal aortic aneurysmal disease (9–13). The technical aspects of aortic reconstruction with hypothermic circulatory arrest in patients with distal aortic disease through the left chest is presented in Fig. 1A–F.

Following induction of general anesthesia and placement of a right radial artery cannula, a pulmonary artery catheter and a double lumen endotracheal tube are inserted. Two 14-gauge peripheral intravenous catheters and a 12-French double lumen central venous access catheter via the right internal jugular vein are placed for intravenous access. The Rapid Infusion System (Haemonetics, Braintree, MA) is connected to these large pore catheters. During the period of time that the thoracic aorta is clamped, the pressures are controlled by the rapidly infusing volume in the form of crystalloid, packed red blood cells, fresh frozen plasma, platelets, or washed cells from the cell-saving device (or any combina-

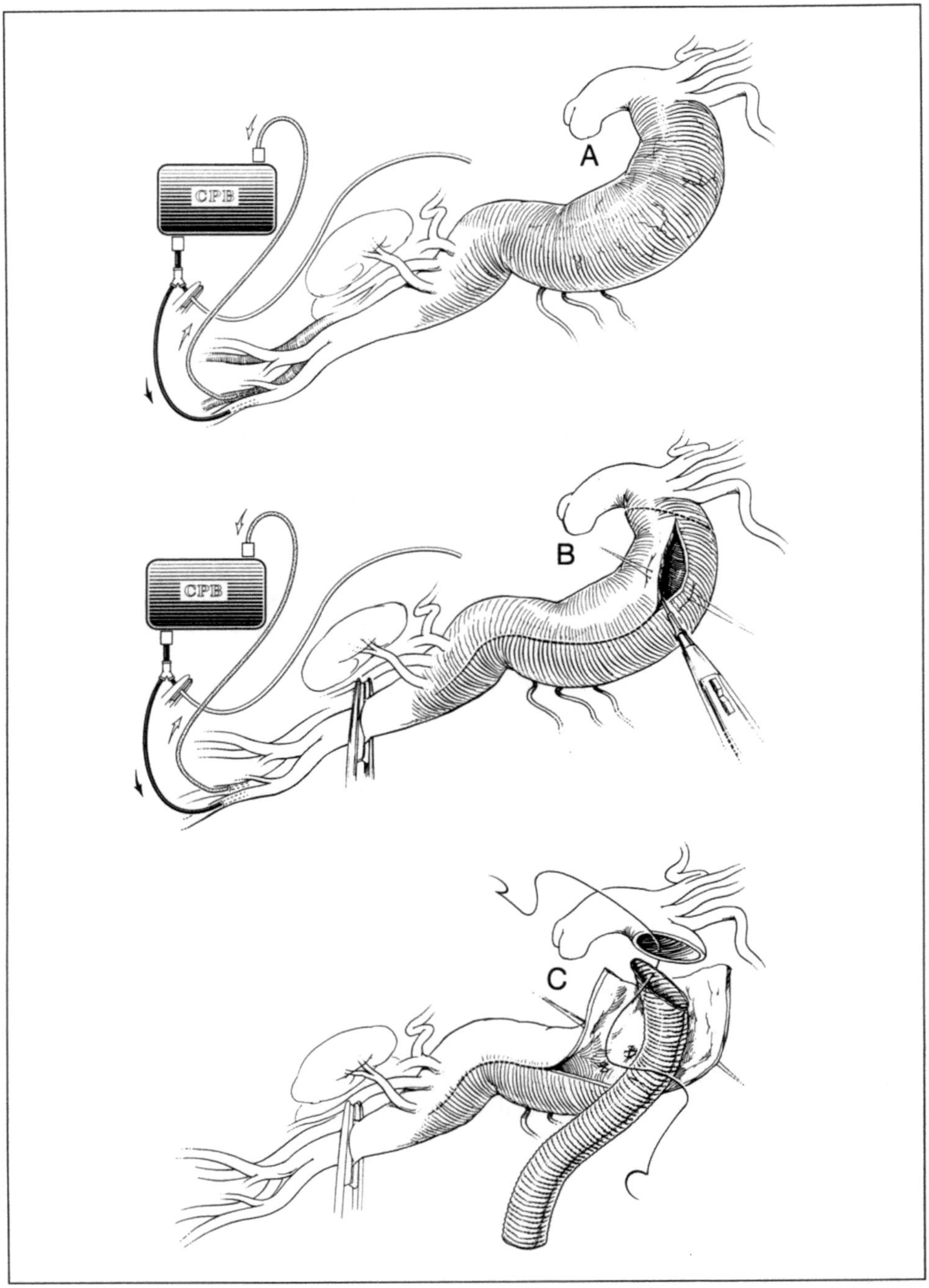

Fig. 1 A) Exposure and bypass circuit for patients undergoing aneurysm repair using hypothermic circulatory arrest via left thoracic/thoracoabdominal approach. Femoro-femoral cannulation employing partial cardiopulmonary bypass with a Y in-arterial line for secondary arterial infusion.
B) Following hypothermic circulatory arrest the distal arch and descending thoracic component of the aneurysm are opened. Distal clamping of the aorta allows low flow arterial infusion.
C) An open distal anastomosis at the arch level is carried out under circulatory arrest.

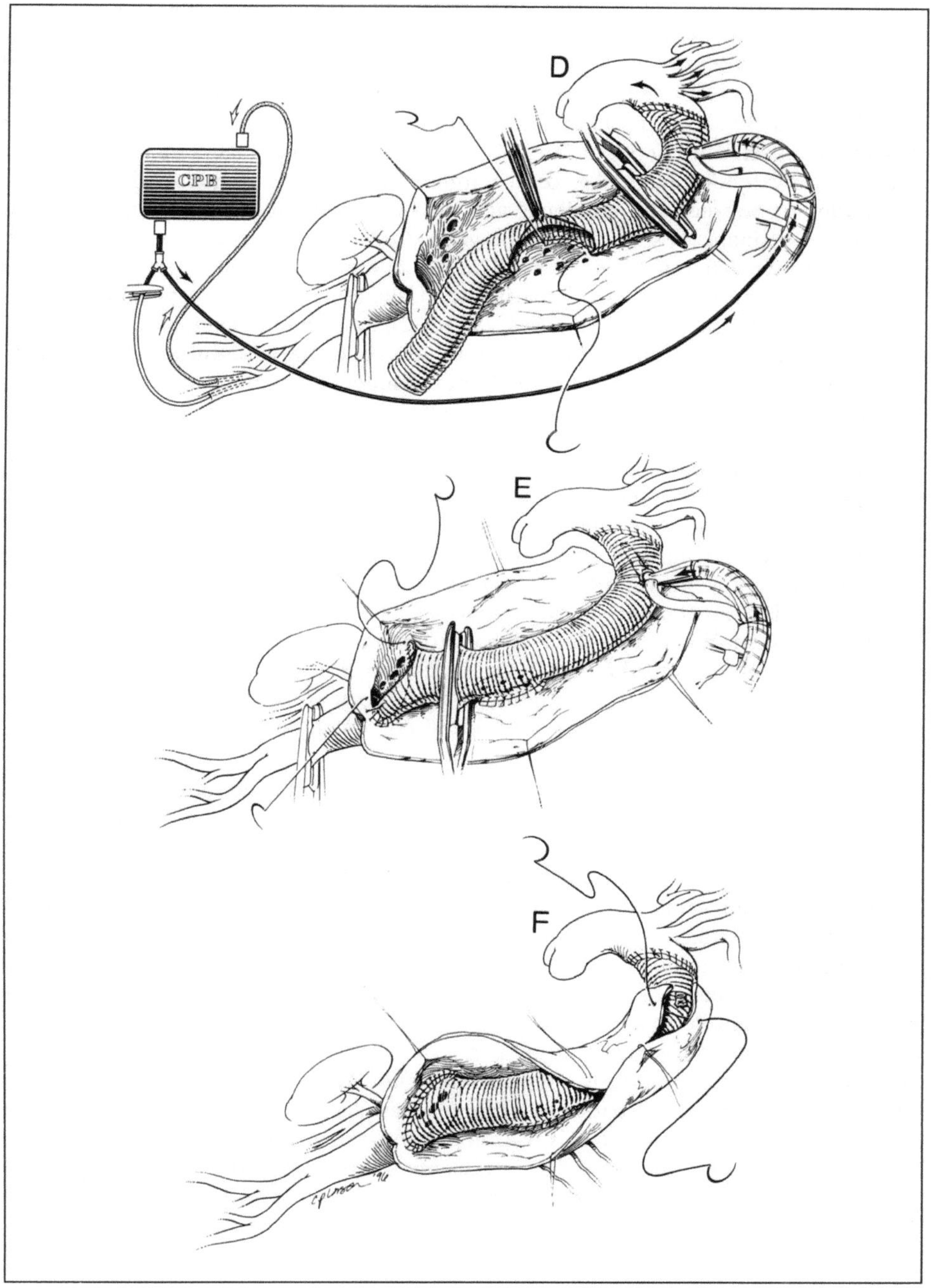

Fig. 1 D) Following completion of arch anastomosis, secondary arterial infusion catheters are placed in the aortic graft for reinstitution of cardiopulmonary bypass with perfusion of the heart and cerebral vessels. Intercostal arteries are reattached.

E) Following reattachment of intercostal arteries, the cross clamp is moved down restoring flow to the spinal cord. Distal reconstruction including reattachment of visceral vessels is carried out.

F) Following completion of aortic repair, the aneurysm wall is wrapped around the aortic graft.

tion), or by removing volume from the heart by directing blood away from the left ventricle via the left atrium into the lower extremities. The Rapid Infusion System provides warm fluid and blood products rapidly at a potential rate of 1500 mL/min.

Patients were positioned in a right lateral decubitus manner with the shoulders at 60° and the hips at 30°. A posterolateral thoracotomy incision was then carried out through the bed of the resected 5th or 6th rib. In patients undergoing thoracoabdominal resection, the incision was extended across the costal margin to the abdominal midline with extension to the midpoint between the umbilicus and the pubic symphysis. In patients undergoing thoracoabdominal exposure, the diaphragm was divided in a circumferential fashion preserving as much muscle as possible. The left common femoral artery and vein were exposed at the groin. Following heparinization, the femoral artery was cannulated with a straight arterial cannula, 20F or 22F. A 28F to 32F long venous cannula was inserted into the right atrium via the left common femoral vein. Following heparinization, high flow cardiopulmonary bypass 2.0 to 2.2 $L \cdot min^{-1} \cdot min^{-2}$ immediate cooling was used. Rectal and esophageal probes were used to monitor temperature. A cell-saver device was employed to remove all shed blood in the field in all patients. Dissection of the aneurysm was kept to a minimum and no dissection of the proximal extent of the aneurysm was performed. A Y-connector and additional line were placed in the arterial line for dual perfusion. The electroencephalogram was monitored in all patients using a 10-lead montage (14). All patients were cooled until the electroencephalogram was isoelectric. The period of cooling averaged 30 min. Ventricular fibrillation generally occurs between 26° and 28 °C. In no patient was left ventricular venting necessary. The left lung was collapsed and gently retracted with specific efforts directed toward minimalizing manipulation of the lung to reduce the risk of potential parenchymal hemorrhage. Cardioplegia for myocardial protection was not employed in any patient. Proximal aortic cross-clamping was not required. Cerebrospinal fluid drainage was not utilized nor was monitoring of somatosensory or motor-evoked potentials.

Once patients had reached a temperature consistent with electrocerebral silence, they were placed in a steep Trendelenburg position. Distal cross-clamping of the aorta where feasible was carried out and circulatory arrest was initiated. In patients in whom distal clamping was possible, a low flow 500 to 1000 cc/min was instituted. The aneurysm distal to the left subclavian artery was then opened longitudinally with extension of the incision in the aorta into the transverse aortic arch dictated by the proximal extent of the disease process. Proximal anastomosis at the level of the transverse aortic arch was carried out either as an end-to-end technique in the ascending aorta with arch vessels reattached to an oval opening in the transverse aortic arch, or, alternatively, a bevel anastomosis was carried out at the level of the transverse aortic arch underneath the brachiocephalic vessels. All anastomoses were carried out using 3-0 monofilament continuous suture. Following completion of the proximal reconstruction, a cannula was placed in the aortic graft immediately distal to the proximal anastomosis. Cardiopulmonary bypass was then reinstituted flushing the graft and aorta of air and debris. A clamp was then positioned on the graft distal to the arterial cannulation of the graft, allowing for perfusion of the heart and lungs, and distribution of the brachiocephalic arterial circulation. Distal arterial perfusion was discontinued. The distal aortic clamp was removed and the aneurysm was opened to its full extent. Rewarming was initiated.

When the extent of the aneurysmal process involved the thoracoabdominal aorta, intercostal arteries (if patent) were reattached to an oval opening in the graft. Cross-clamping of the graft was positioned distal to the intercostal reattachment to restore circulation to the spinal cord prior to reattachment of the visceral arteries in patients undergoing thoracoabdominal aortic aneurysm repair. Visceral vessel and distal aortic reconstruction dictated by distal extent of the disease, and a deliberate effort to reattach all patent intercostal and lumbar arteries below the 6th intercostal space was carried out.

In all patients a collagen impregnated woven Dacron graft to minimize the intraoperative loss of blood was used. Rewarming was ultimately carried to 36 °C rectally in all patients. During the period of rewarming distal aortic perfusion was not resumed in order to take advantage of the lower body hypothermia during the distal aortic reconstruction.

Patients

During the period between January 11, 1986, and September 6, 1995, the author treated 861 patients with aortic aneurysm by resection and graft replacement via the left chest, i.e., left thoracotomy or left thoracoabdominal aortic exposure. Of these, 619 were thoracoabdominal aortic aneurysms; the remaining 242 were descending thoracic aortic aneurysms (Table 1). Simple aortic clamping was used in 690 patients (80.1 %), and distal aortic bypass without oxygenation was employed in 134 patients (15.6 %) (Table 2). In a select group of high risk patients in whom, for anatomic reasons (large size, or proximal extent involving all or part of the transverse aorta arch), proximal aortic clamping was not feasible, and, consequently, the proximal anastomosis was carried out using femorofemoral cardiopulmonary bypass to allow for deep hypothermic circulatory arrest (HCA). Circulatory arrest was used in 37 patients (4.3 %), 26 males and 11 female, with exposure through the left chest. Of these 37 patients, distal aortic involvement extended to all of the descending aorta in 23 patients, only the distal aortic arch was replaced in 7 patients, and there were 7 patients with thoracoabdominal aortic aneurysms (Crawford extent I, 3

Table 1. Thoracic aortic aneurysms, 861 patients

	#Patients	Circ Arrest	ATR	Simple Clamp
ARH/DES	242 (28.1 %)	30 (12.4 %)	31 (12.8 %)	181 (74.8 %)
TAAA I	218 (25.3 %)	3 (1.4 %)	35 (16.1 %)	180 (82.6 %)
TAAA II	175 (20.3 %)	4 (2.3 %)	63 (36.0 %)	108 (61.7 %)
TAAA III	110 (12.8 %)	0 (0.0 %)	4 (3.6 %)	106 (96.4 %)
TAAA IV	116 (13.5 %)	0 (0.0 %)	1 (0.9 %)	115 (99.1 %)
TOTAL	861 (100 %)	37 (4.3 %)	134 (15.6 %)	690 (80.1 %)

ARH/DES = arch/descending thoracic aneurysm
TAAA = thoracoabdominal aortic aneurysm

Table 2. Thoracic Aortic Aneurysms, 861 Patients

Technique	# Patients	PAR/PLG
Circulatory Arrest	37 (4.3 %)	2 (5.4 %)
ATR	134 (15.6 %)	6 (4.5 %)
Simple Clamp	690 (80.1 %)	33 (4.8 %)

ATR = atriofemoral bypass

Table 3. Mortality

Patient	Cause	P/O Day
Arch	ARDS	# 8
Arch	ARDS, Pneumonia	# 58
Descending	Pulmonary Failure	# 189
Descending	Pneumonia	# 8
Thoracoabdominal	Myocardial Infarction	Intraoperative

patients; and Crawford extent II, 4 patients). Three patients had Marfan syndrome and 4 were treated for rupture. Aortic pathology and etiology included 5 patients with acute dissection, 14 patients with chronic dissection, and 18 patients with fusiform medial degenerative disease.

There was one intraoperative death secondary to myocardial infarction. No patient was returned to the operating room for postoperative hemorrhage. There were no hepatic or intestinal complications. The in-hospital mortality was 5 patients (13.5 %), and 2 patients (5.4 %) suffered postoperative stroke, one with full recovery and one with partial. For the group, the cardiopulmonary bypass time ranged from 29 to 188 min (mean 120, median 117), and the circulatory arrest time ranged from 13 to 79 min (mean 40, median 38). Two patients, one with descending aortic replacement and one with thoracoabdominal aortic replacement, developed postoperative paraparesis (5.4 %) Both patients were operated upon emergently, one secondary to acute dissection and one with rupture and hypotension. Postoperative hemodialysis was necessary in four patients (10.8 %), being temporary in two (5.4 %). The cause of death was pulmonary in four patients (Table 3).

Discussion

The first report of the successful use of deep hypothermic circulatory arrest through the left chest for complex aortic pathology was the repair of a posttraumatic fistula between the aortic arch and innominate vein fistula of the aortic arch by Borst in 1964 (15). The fistula was closed during a period of circulatory arrest lasting 15 min, and the patient recovered uneventfully.

Crawford et al. in 1987 reported upon the use of hypothermic circulatory arrest through a left thoracotomy and left thoracoabdominal approach in a clinical series of 25 patients (1). There were four postoperative deaths (16 %) in that series--one from bleeding, two from myocardial infarction, and one from pulmonary embolism. The indications for the use of hypothermic circulatory arrest were primarily for technical reasons, including proximal aortic involvement into the transverse aortic arch in patients with descending thoracic and thoracoabdominal aneurysms, injury to the proximal aorta during cross-clamping, ruptured aneurysms, and large aneurysms whose size prohibited proximal clamping. A high incidence of pulmonary complications was reported and included intrapulmonary bleeding during operation on the side of operation (the left lung) in five patients, secondary to retraction injury of the lung. Acute respiratory distress syndrome developed postoperatively in two of these patients, as well as in an additional three, requiring prolonged ventilatory support. Nine patients (36 %) required postoperative tracheostomy. Despite hypothermia, two (11 %) of 18 patients at risk for ischemic spinal cord injury developed paraplegia immediately following operation.

More recently, Kouchoukos and associates has reported upon the use of HCA as a technique for spinal cord and renal protection during operations upon the thoracoabdominal aorta (3, 4). They emphasized its use as a method to increase the tolerable duration of spinal cord ischemia to allow for the additional time necessary to reattach intercostal and lumbar arteries and to reestablish critical arterial blood flow prior to the onset of permanent spinal cord injury. Additionally, the hypothermia provides protection to the kidney preserving renal function by eliminating warm ischemic time. They reported upon the use of HCA in 51 patients, 19 with descending thoracic and 32 with thoracoabdominal aortic aneurysms (3). In only 8 patients in this series was the location, extent, or severity of disease precluding placement of a proximal aortic clamp. The remaining 43 patients underwent HCA for organ protection, primarily spinal cord and renal, due to perceived high risk of ischemia to these organs secondary to the extent of complex aortic pathology. The 30-day mortality was 9.8 % (5 patients) and in-hospital mortality, 11.8 % (6 patients). Paraplegia occurred in 2 patients, and 2 patients (4.3 % of 46 30-day survivors) suffered stroke. Additionally, paraparesis occurred in 1 of the 46 30-day survivors (total paraplegia/paraparesis, 6.5 %). Renal failure requiring hemodialysis occurred in 1 (2.2 %) of the 30-day survivors. Both incidences of paraplegia occurred in patients with thoracoabdominal aortic aneurysms, one with Crawford extent I (1/12, 8 %) and one of 5 with Crawford extent III (20 %).

Kieffer et al. reported upon 15 (17 %) of 87 patients treated for aneurysmal disease of the descending thoracic and thoracoabdominal aorta utilizing hypothermic circulatory arrest (5). Of these, there were four early deaths (26.7 %), two intraoperative (one from bleeding and one from left ventricular failure) and two early postoperative deaths (one from coagulopathy and another from aortic rupture). One patient developed delayed onset paraplegia despite hypothermia, emphasizing the complexity of postoperative neurological deficits in patients with extensive aortic aneurysmal disease.

The cannulation technique in the current series involves femoro-femoral partial cardiopulmonary bypass with systemic cooling to levels of deep hypothermia. Most authors have used complicated cannulation techniques that have included left ventricular decompression. The current experience reconfirms the effectiveness of this simple method without left ventricular decompression as described by Lillehei and associates (16). Left ventricular and general cardiac dilatation is limited by an intact pericardium. An alternative cannulation technique with venous return from the right atrium through the internal jugular vein and arterial return to the aortic arch has been described by Westaby (2). He successfully employed the technique in 6 patients for replacement of the descending thoracic and thoracoabdominal aorta. One patient suffered early paraparesis and eventually died of multisystem organ failure. A second elderly patient with severe chronic obstructive pulmonary disease died of respiratory failure 11 days postoperatively, for an overall mortality rate of 33.3 %.

In the current series, hypothermic circulatory arrest was not employed specifically for spinal cord or other organ (kidney, liver, bowel, etc.) protection. Rather, the technique was used primarily for cerebral protection when proximal aortic cross clamping was not feasible for anatomic reasons, aortic size too large for clamping, transverse aortic arch involvement, false aneurysm, dense scar tissue secondary to prior proximal aortic surgery, and friable aortic wall not amenable to safe clamping. As a group, these patients are anatomically more complex and are very likely to be at increased risk for morbidity (particularly stroke) and operative mortality than patients from other series selected solely for peripheral organ protection. Additionally, the technique eliminates the need for proximal aortic dissection reducing, if not eliminating, risk to the esophagus, pulmonary artery, vagus, and recurrent laryngeal nerves. Access to the entire transverse aortic arch and most of the ascending aorta allows for treatment of the proximal extent of disease with replacement of these segments. The surgeon is allowed reconstruction and replacement of the proximal aorta in an anatomic fashion with a quiet, bloodless surgical field. Risk of stroke is reduced as a consequence of the elimination of manipulation of the brachiocephalic vessels and transverse aortic arch, provided proper de-airing techniques are employed. The simple clamping of the transverse aortic arch in patients with friable intimal atherosclerosis or laminated luminal thrombus places such patients at extreme risk for embolic stroke. Calcified, "eggshell" arteries may be easily fractured or disrupted with even the most gentle clamp placement. These conditions can be detected preoperatively with proper evaluation, i.e., CT scan, MRI scan, transthoracic and transesophageal echocardiography, and arteriography.

In summary, the use of cardiopulmonary bypass with hypothermic circulatory arrest allows for the safe treatment of patients undergoing thoracoabdominal and descending thoracic aortic replacement with involvement of the transverse aortic arch. Since the etiology of spinal cord ischemia in such patients is multifactorial, despite the fact that profound hypothermia may provide a prolonged safe period of ischemia to the spinal cord, reimplantation of critical intercostal and lumbar arteries retaining direct circulation to the spinal cord remains imperative. Postoperative pulmonary problems remain the most common source of morbidity and mortality particularly in patients with poor preoperative pulmonary function. Despite the inherent limitations, the technique deserves further evaluation and should be included in the armamentarium of cardiovascular surgeons treating complex aortic pathology.

References

1. Crawford ES, Coselli JS, Safi HJ (1987) Partial cardiopulmonary bypass, hypothermic circulatory arrest, and posterolateral exposure for thoracic aortic aneurysm operation. J Thorac Cardiovasc Surg 94: 824–7
2. Westaby S (1992) Hypothermic thoracic and thoracoabdominal aneurysm operation: A central cannulation technique. Ann Thorac Surg 54: 253–8
3. Kouchoukos NT, Daily BB, Rokkas, CK, Murphy SF, Bauer S, Abboud N (1995) Hypothermic bypass and circulatory arrest for operations on the descending thoracic and thoracoabdominal aorta. Ann Thorac Surg 60: 67–77
4. Kouchoukos NT, Wareing TH, Izumoto H, Klausing W, Abboud, N (1990) Elective hypothermic cardiopulmonary bypass and circulatory arrest for spinal cord protection during operations on the thoracoabdominal aorta. J Thorac Cardiovasc Surg 99: 659–64
5. Kieffer E, Koskas F, Walden R et al. (1994) Hypothermic circulatory arrest for thoracic aneurysmectomy through left-sided thoracotomy. J Vasc Surg 19: 457–64
6. Mahfood S, Qazi A, Garcia J, Mispireta L, Corso P, Smyth N (1985) Management of aortic arch aneurysm using profound hypothermia and circulatory arrest. Ann Thorac Surg 39: 412–7
7. Massimo CG, Poma AG, Viligiardi RR, Duranti A, Colucci M, Favi PP (1986) Simultaneous total aortic arch replacement from arch to bifurcation: Experience with six cases. J Tex Heart Inst 13: 147–51
8. Szentpetery S, Crisler C, Grinnan GLB (1993) Deep hypothermic arrest and left thoracotomy for repair of difficult thoracic aneurysms. Ann Thorac Surg 55: 830–3
9. Coselli JS (1992) Suprarenal Aortic Reconstruction: Perioperative Management: Patient Selection, Patient Workup, Operative Management, and Postoperative Management. Sem Vasc Surg 5 (3): 146–156
10. Coselli JS (1992) Suprarenal Aortic Reconstruction: Endovascular Repair. Sem Vasc Surg 5 (3): 180–191
11. Coselli JS (1994) Thoracoabdominal Aortic Aneurysm. In: Rutherford RB, ed. *Vascular Surgery*, 4th Ed. Philadelphia, PA: W.B. Saunders Company: 1069–87
12. Coselli JS (1994) Thoracoabdominal aortic aneurysms: experience with 372 patients. J Card Surg 9: 638–47

13. Coselli JS (1995) Surgical Technique, Preoperative and Intraoperative Management of Thoracoabdominal Aortic Aneurysm. In: Yao JST and Pearce WH, eds. *Arterial Surgery: Management of Challenging Problems*. Norwalk, CT: Appleton & Lange: 223–35
14. Coselli JS, Crawford ES, Beall AC Jr, Mizrahi EM, Hess KR, Patel VM (1988) Determination of brain temperatures for safe circulatory arrest during cardiovascular operation. Ann Thorac Surg 45: 638–42
15. Borst HG, Schaudig A, Rudolph W (1964) Arteriovenous fistula of the aortic arch: Repair during deep hypothermia and circulatory arrest. J Thorac Cardiovasc Surg 48: 443–7
16. Lillehei CW, Todd DB Jr, Levy MJ, Ellis RJ (1969) Partial cardiopulmonary bypass, hypothermia and total circulatory arrest. J Thorac Cardiovasc Surg 58: 530–44

Author's address:
Joseph S. Coselli, M.D.
6560 Fannin, #1144
Houston, TX 77030
USA

Retrograde cerebral perfusion in surgery for aortic arch aneurysms

J. S. Coselli

The Methodist Hospital/Baylor College of Medicine, Houston, Texas, USA

Introduction

The first successful replacement of an aortic arch aneurysm was carried out in Houston, Texas, by DeBakey in 1957 using an aortic homograft (1). For many years to follow, the morbidity and mortality for the treatment of aortic pathology in the transverse arch location remained unacceptably high. Most early operations were carried out using one of two methods (2, 3). One technique was to establish circulation to the brachiocephalic vessels by placement of temporary bypass grafts originating off the proximal ascending aorta to be taken down at the completion of arch replacement. A second was antegrade direct perfusion of the brachiocephalic vessels using cardiopulmonary bypass. In each instance extensive dissection and mobilization of the cerebral arterial circulation was required. Both procedures met with an excessively high risk of stroke and mortality.

Griepp and associates in 1975 demonstrated that the use of profound hypothermia and circulatory arrest for cerebral protection during aortic arch repair in adult patients provided a far simpler and safer approach to the treatment of aortic arch pathology (4). The advantages of the hypothermic technique were immediately apparent and included a quiet, dry, motionless surgical field, which was unencumbered by temporary bypass grafts or perfusion cannulae. Excessive dissection and manipulation of the brachiocephalic vessels was no longer necessary with the routine replacement/repair conducted within the walls of the aneurysm. The prolonged periods of circulatory arrest occasionally required for the surgical treatment of complex pathology of the transverse aortic arch, particularly those involving reoperation, continued to remain a significant challenge. Diffuse cerebral injury with circulatory arrest periods beyond 60 min was confirmed in a clinical series by Griepp and associates (5). In the largest clinical experience reported to date, involving 656 patients treated by Crawford, it was found that there was an increased risk of stroke in patients treated with periods of circulatory arrest greater than 40 min and an increased early mortality for circulatory arrest periods beyond 65 min (6).

In an effort to extend the safe period of hypothermic circulatory arrest in adults requiring aortic arch replacement, Ueda and associates employed the use of retrograde cerebral perfusion via the superior vena caval cannula in a report in 1991 (7). Initially, retrograde cerebral perfusion via the superior vena caval cannula was employed as a treatment for massive air embolism occuring during cardiopulmonary bypass by Mills and Oschner in 1980 (8). Lemole and associates describe the use of retrograde cerebral perfusion as a form of cerebral protection during aortic arch repair in a report in 1982 (9). Lemole's initial description employed the technique used in an intermittent fashion, 2 minutes out of every 10 minutes of circulatory arrest. Ueda described retrograde cerebral perfusion via the superior vena caval cannula as a continuous flow during the period of circulatory arrest (7). The theoretical advantages of retrograde cerebral perfusion employed in this manner have been described to include the potential delivery of metabolic substrates to the cerebral tissues including oxygen and nutrients (10). Additionally, there is the potential for maintenance of cerebral hypothermia avoiding an upward drift in temperature as well as homogeneous cooling unaffected by arterial occlusive disease. Additional benefits have included a reduced risk of embolism of both air and particulate microemboli as a result of the backflow of perfusate through the cerebral arterial circulation with a washout of potential emboli (11, 12). Since 1991 the author has routinely employed a continuous retrograde cerebral perfusion technique in a large clinical series of patients; an evaluation of the results of this experience has identified a reduction in both early mortality and incidence of cerebrovascular accidents.

Patients

During the period from January 13, 1987, through August 15, 1995, 437 patients were treated surgically by the author for pathology involving the ascending and/or transverse aortic arch (Fig. 1). Of these, 361 patients required surgical repair via a median sternotomy, which due to the etiology of disease or extent of replacement required the use of profound hypothermic circulatory arrest. Of these, there were 216 male patients (59.8 %) and 145 female patients (40.2 %). The median age of this series was 66 years. Their ages ranged from 14 to 86 years. The etiology of the aortic pathology involved in this series was acute aortic dissection in 75 patients (20.8 %), chronic dissection in 100 patients (27.7 %), and fusiform aneurysmal disease or false aneurysm in 186 patients (51.5 %). Marfan syndrome was present in 23 patients and aortitis in 13 patients. Retrograde cerebral perfusion via the superior vena caval cannula continuously during the circulatory arrest period was employed for cerebral protection in 214 patients (59 %) and was not used in 158 patients (41 %). The presenting symptoms and associated diseases are outlined in Tables 1 and 2. Previous aortic surgery via a median sternotomy had been carried out in 148 patients (41 %), 67 undergoing retrograde cerebral perfusion and 81 without. The procedures employed in previous aortic and cardiac surgery are listed in Table 3.

Table 1. Causes of in-house mortality

	RCP (n = 213)	NO RCP (n = 148)	TOTAL (n = 361)
Stroke	0	4	4 (1.1 %)
Respiratory failure	1	2	3 (0.8 %)
Cardiac failure	1	11	12 (3.3 %)
Multiple organ failure	1	1	2 (0.6 %)
Pulmonary embolus	1	1	2 (0.6 %)
Intraoperative bronchial rupture	0	1	1 (0.3 %)
Aortic rupture	0	1	1 (0.3 %)
TOTAL	4	21	25 (6.9 %)

RCP = Reverse cerebral perfusion

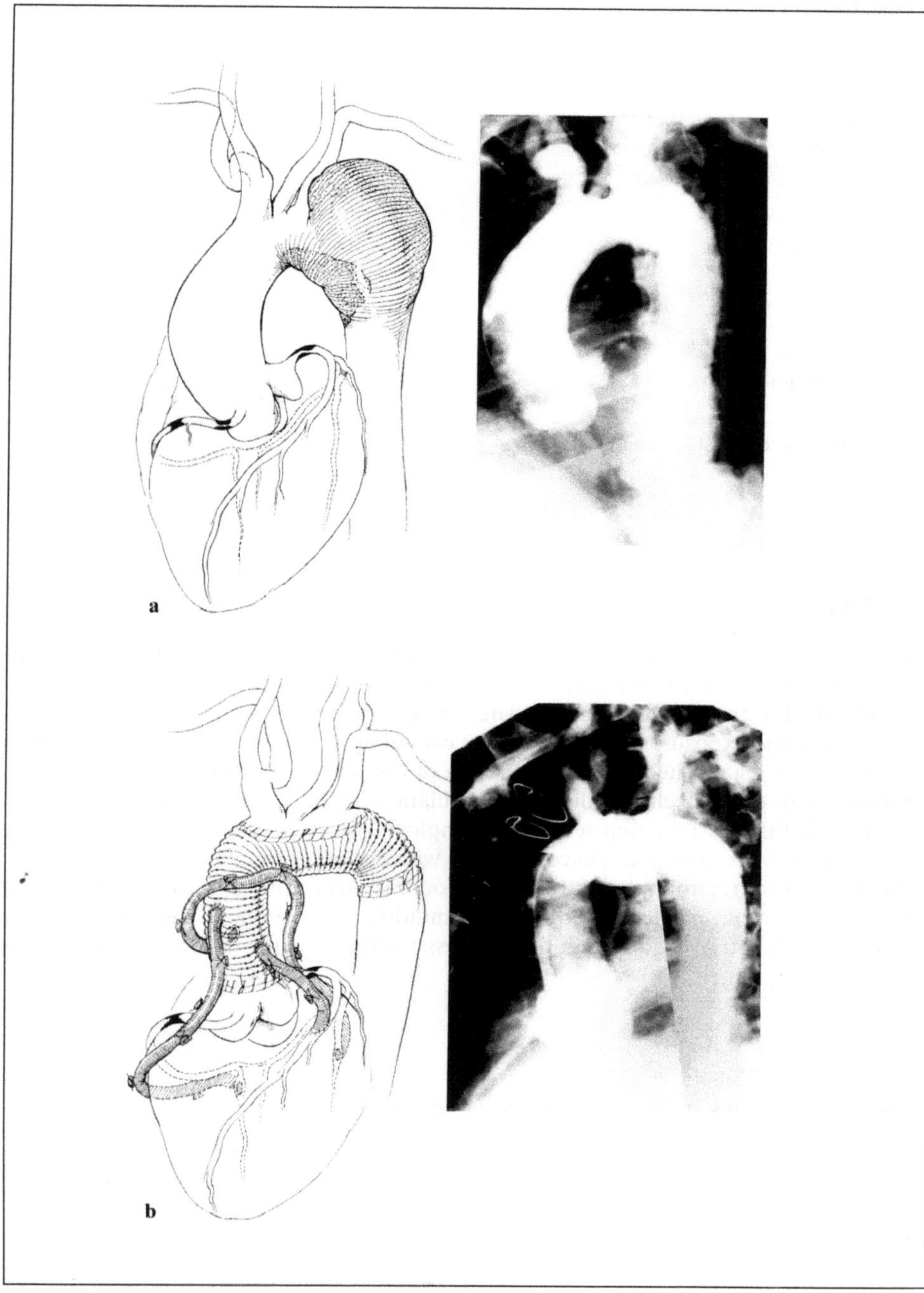

Fig. 1. A) Preoperative drawing and aortogram of patient with aneurysmal disease involving the ascending aorta, transverse aortic arch, and proximal descending thoracic aorta. Concomitant coronary artery occlusive disease with unstable angina is present, as well as intrascapular back pain secondary to symptomatic descending thoracic aortic component. **B)** Postoperative drawing and aortogram following resection and replacement of ascending aorta, transverse aortic arch, proximal descending thoracic aorta, and concomitant coronary artery bypass grafting.

Table 2. Early complications

	RCP (n = 213)	NO RCP (n = 148)	TOTAL (n = 361)
Stroke	3	10	13 (3.6%)
Pulmonary complications	89	64	153 (42.4%)
Cardiac complications	19	17	36 (10.0%)
Renal complications	11	14	25 (6.9%)
Wound dehiscence	4	5	9 (2.5%)
Vocal cord paralysis	19	19	38 (10.5%)
Fever	13	12	25 (6.9%)
Sepsis	4	8	12 (3.3%)
Encephalopathy	3	10	13 (3.6%)
Pericardial effusion	3	5	8 (2.2%)
Coagulopathy	11	17	28 (7.8%)
Reopening for bleeding	3	6	9 (2.5%)
TOTAL	182	187	369

RCP = Reverse cerebral perfusion

Technique

The essentials and details of the author's approach to retrograde cerebral perfusion and its application to aortic arch surgery have previously been reported in the literature in some detail (10–12). In all patients reported herein, a median sternotomy was employed for cardiac and aortic exposure (Fig. 2). Cardiac cannulation for cardiopulmonary bypass was preferentially established using cannulation of one of the femoral arteries; however, in patients with distal occlusive disease, cannulation of the ascending aorta or transverse aortic arch for arterial pump return was employed when necessary to establish bypass. Separate bicaval cannulation, in conjunction with occluding caval tapes, was utilized in all patients in whom retrograde cerebral perfusion was carried out (Fig. 3). In patients undergoing reoperation, particularly those with multiple prior surgeries, in whom extensive scarring in the atrial region prohibited access for the placement of both a superior and

Table 3. Previous aortic surgery on ascending aorta and aortic arch

	RCP (n = 213)	NO RCP (n = 148)	TOTAL (n = 361)
Coronary artery bypass	22	29	51
Ascending aortic graft replacement	16	16	32
Ascending and aortic arch graft replacement	1	2	3
Composite valve graft replacement	7	11	18
Aortic valve replacement	14	12	26
Ascending aortic graft replacement and aortic valve resuspension	3	0	3
Ascending aortic graft replacement and separate aortic valve replacement	4	11	15
TOTAL	67	81	148

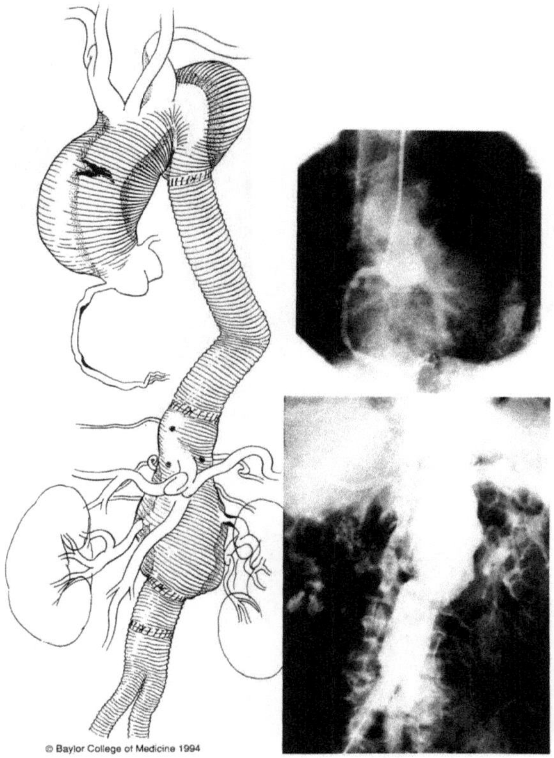

Fig. 2. A) Arteriogram and drawing of patient with coronary artery disease, ascending, arch, and proximal descending thoracic aortic aneurysms secondary to aortic dissection. Patient is status post descending thoracic aortic replacement and infrarenal abdominal aortic replacement.

inferior vena caval cannula, a single dual-stage venous cannula or femoro-femoral bypass was alternatively utilized. Naturally, these patients did not undergo retrograde cerebral perfusion via a superior vena caval cannula. In all patients, heparinization was monitored using activated clotting times. In all elective cases and most emergency cases, EEG monitoring was routinely employed. Circulatory arrest was not initiated until electrocerebral silence was achieved (13, 14). For all patients, pH control was carried out using the alpha-stat method, with the pH uncorrected for temperature and kept at 7.4. Mannitol 0.5 mg/kg was routinely administered intravenously by anesthesia prior to circulatory arrest but after electrocerebral silence. Steroids were routinely avoided. Although circulatory arrest was based upon EEG monitoring, the nasopharyngeal and rectal temperatures were constantly monitored. The inspired oxygen concentration was kept at 100 %, keeping the arterial PO2 in a range from 300 to 600 mm Hg and the PCO2 between 35 and 45 mm Hg. A membrane oxygenator and a centrifugal pump were used in all cases. Rapid cooling was carried out against a water bath of 0 °C after the initiation of cardiopulmonary bypass, with arterial inflow to a low temperature of 8 °C. Electrocerebral silence was

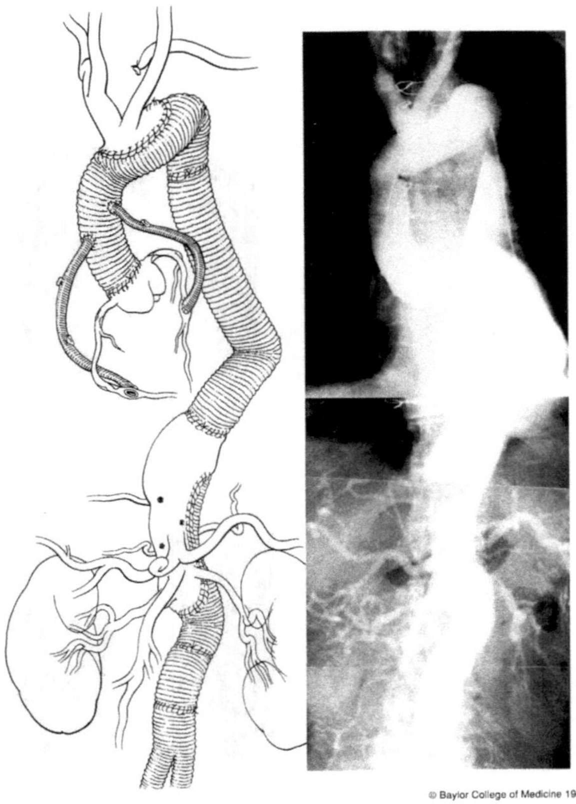

Fig. 2. B) Aortogram and drawing following resection and replacement of ascending aorta, transverse aortic arch, and proximal descending thoracic aorta as well as concomitant coronary artery bypass grafting.

achieved on an average of 26 min and a range of 12 to 96 min. The rectal temperature at the point of electrocerebral silence averaged 18.5 °C and the nasopharyngeal temperature averaged 14.5 °C. Myocardial protection was routinely achieved using cold dilute hyperkalemic blood cardioplegic solution directly into the coronary artery origins when available and, in the presence of diffuse coronary artery disease, retrograde cardioplegia via the coronary sinus.

In the bypass circuit, a Y-connector is attached to the superior vena caval cannula and a Y-connector to the arterial inflow line allowing for communication between these two (Fig. 4). After the initiation of circulatory arrest, arterial inflow at a low of 8 °C is routed only into the superior vena caval cannula (Fig. 5). Flow is adjusted to maintain a proximal venous pressure, monitored either via an internal jugular vein catheter or directly from the arterial line, to range between 15 and 25 mm Hg. Flows through the superior vena caval cannula during periods of circulatory arrest range between 150 and 500 mL/min. Perfusion through the superior vena caval cannula during the period of arrest was carried out in a

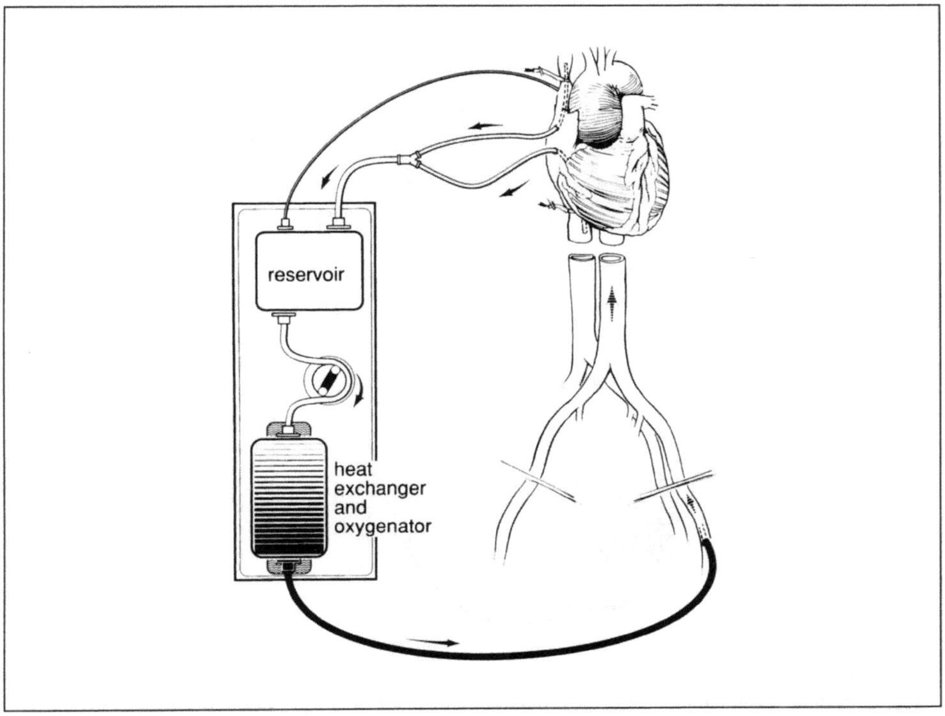

Fig. 3. Routine cardiopulmonary bypass circuitry for transverse aortic arch aneurysm repair using bicaval cannulation and femoral arterial perfusion for pump return.

continuous fashion. Additionally, drainage is persistently allowed from the inferior vena cava into the reservoir for the pump oxygenator. Following completion of the aortic arch repair, venous drainage was reinstituted utilizing both caval cannulae, and arterial inflow was reestablished via either the femoral artery cannula or, in those patients in whom intimal disease involving the descending thoracic or thoracoabdominal aorta places the patient at increased risk for embolization, arterial inflow is established via direct cannulation of the aortic graft in the transverse aortic arch for antegrade perfusion. Rewarming is begun and ultimately carried to 37° – 37.5 °C as measured rectally. During the initial period of rewarming proximal aortic repair is carried out based upon that which is necessary to correct aortic root pathology, aortic valve disease, and/or coronary artery occlusive disease. In this series, the time required for rewarming averaged 90 min and ranged from 40 to 222 min.

Results of treatment

The overall in-hospital survival was 93.1 %, 336 of 361 patients. The causes of in-house mortality are listed in Table 1. The in-hospital mortality for those patients receiving retro-

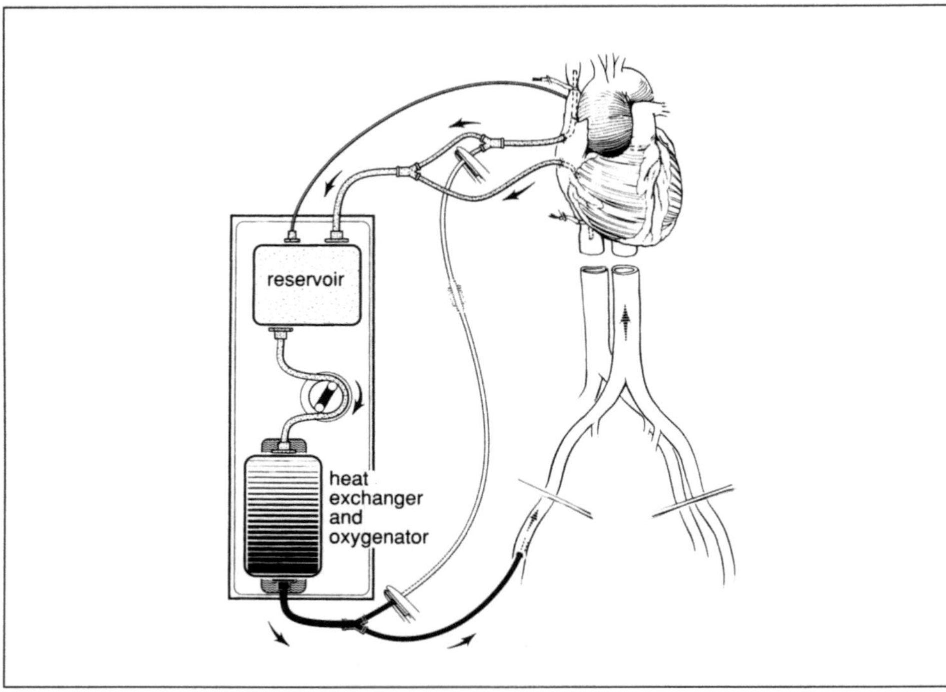

Fig. 4. Modified cardiopulmonary bypass circuitry for reverse cerebral perfusion with a Y-connection placed in the arterial line and in the line from the superior vena caval cannula.

grade cerebral perfusion was 1.9 % (4 of 213 patients) versus 14.2 % (21 or 148 patients) for those patients not receiving retrograde cerebral perfusion. The period of retrograde cerebral perfusion averaged 30.2 min and ranged from 10 to 79 min. The period of circulatory arrest for those patients without retrograde cerebral perfusion averaged 33.35 min and ranged from 8 to 124 min. Early complications were predominantly pulmonary, cardiac, and renal and are listed in Table 2.

Saccular aneurysms of the transverse aortic arch were treated with a simple patch graft repair in 9 patients. A total arch repair with reattachment of all the brachiocephalic vessels was carried out in 68 patients; of these, an elephant trunk repair for mega aorta was employed in 45 patients. A bevelled hemi-arch repair was employed in 271 patients. There was statistically significant difference in the in-house mortality and stroke rate for each of these approaches to transverse aortic arch reconstruction.

A thorough physical and neurological examination was carried out on all patients preoperatively and postoperatively. Strokes were defined as those events which included any new clinically evident neurological injury that was motor or sensory, focal or diffuse. Patients identified as having neurological deficits were further evaluated with EEG and CT or MRI scanning. Of the 144 patients surviving operation without retrograde cerebral perfusion, there were 10 strokes (6.9 %) versus 3 strokes in the 213 patients surviving operation in whom retrograde cerebral perfusion was employed (1.4 %, p-value = 0.006).

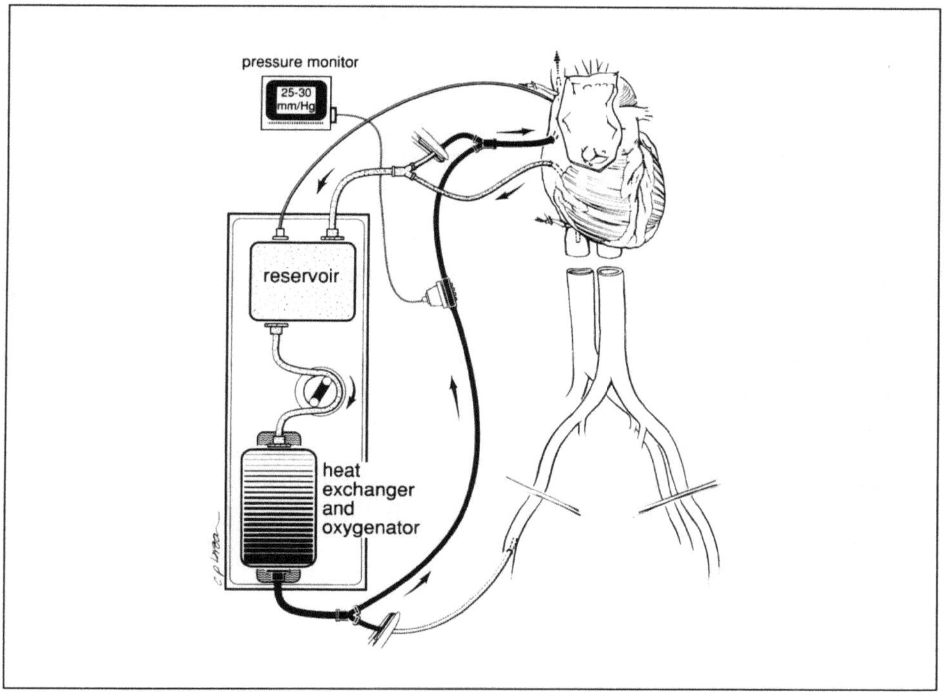

Fig. 5. During circulatory arrest, reverse cerebral perfusion is established by clamping the arterial line to the common femoral artery and the drainage of the superior vena caval cannula distal to the Y-connection. Oxygenated reverse cerebral perfusion via the superior venal caval cannula is regulated to keep the proximal central venous pressure less than 20 mm Hg. Central venous pressures are monitored either directly or from the arterial line.

Comments

This clinical evaluation of the use of retrograde cerebral perfusion establishes that the technique, as described herein, is safe, and has a favorable influence on reducing both early mortality and the significant morbidity of stroke in high-risk patients. Debate on the effectiveness of retrograde cerebral perfusion and the technique's ability to deliver blood with oxygen and nutrients to brain tissue has in part centered on competent valves in the venous circulation as well as dominant collateral circulation circumventing brain tissue. Clinical and metabolic studies have demonstrated that after 20 % of the blood perfused to the superior vena cava returns to the carotid arteries, the remaining is drained through collateral venous circulation into the inferior vena caval system (15, 16). With the concomitant use of deep hypothermia, this low flow, low perfusion of brain tissue may be sufficient to provide an extended safe period of hypothermic circulatory arrest for complex aortic arch repair. Boeckxstaens and Flameng found in the nonhuman primate model of retrograde cerebral perfusion that no significant perfusion of the brain occurred in their experimental model (16); however, Jean-Louis DeBrux, in a study of adult human cadavers in which the superior vena caval was injected with blue colored latex, was able to show anatomic evidence for real perfusion of brain tissue during retrograde cerebral perfusion via the superior vena caval cannula in a model similar to that used in the clinical series described herein (17). In a dog model study by Imamaki and associates that included microscopic evaluation, retrograde cerebral perfusion at 10° to 14 °C provided significantly greater brain protection during 120 min post circulatory arrest at 20 °C nasopharyngeal temperature when compared to no retrograde cerebral perfusion and retrograde cerebral perfusion at 18° to 20 °C (18).

Pagano and associates reported the results in three humans in which cerebral perfusion during RCP was demonstrated with technetium Te 99m-labeled brain perfusion agent d.L-hexamethyl propylene amine oxime and a portable gamma camera in the operating room (19).

The question of whether or not RCP can meet the metabolic demands of cerebral tissue is unresolved. However, Lin et al. have suggested that with RCP deep hypothermia may not be necessary and have applied the technique in a successful clinical series with a rectal temperature of only 21.7° ± 0.8 °C (n = 8 patients) (20).

Although the benefits of retrograde cerebral perfusion for brain protection during circulatory arrest will continue to be debated, there is accumulating evidence that its use is safe and its impact favorable (21, 22). Consequently, the technique is justifiable in patients requiring circulatory arrest for aortic arch surgery.

References

1. DeBakey ME, Crawford ES, Cooley DA, Morris GC (1957) Successful resection of fusiform aneurysm of aortic arch with replacement of homograft. Surg Gynecol Obstet 105: 657
2. Griepp RB, Stinson EB, Hollingsworth JF, Buehler D (1975) Prosthetic replacement of the aortic arch. J Thorac Cardiovasc Surg 70: 1051–63
3. DeBakey ME, Henly WS, Cooley DA, Crawford ES, Morris GC, Beall AC (1962) Aneurysms of the aortic arch: factors influencing operative risk. The Surgical Clinics of North America 42 (6): 1543–54
4. DeBakey ME (1979) The development of vascular surgery. Am J Surg 173 (June): 697–738
5. Griepp RB, Ergin MA, Lansman JL, Gall JD,Rogo G (1991) The physiology of hypothermic circulatory arrest. Semin Thorac Cardiovasc Surg 3: 188–93
6. Svensson LG, Crawford ES, Hess KR et al. (1993) Deep hypothermia with circulatory arrest determinants of stroke and early mortality in 656 patients. J Thorac Cardiovasc Surg 106 (1): 19–31
7. Ueda Y, Miki S, Kusuhara K, Okita Y, Tahata T, Yamanaka K (1990) Surgical treatment of aneurysm or dissection involving the ascending aorta and aortic arch, utilizing circulatory arrest and retrograde cerebral perfusion. J Cardiovasc Surg 31: 553–8
8. Mills NL, Ochsner JL (1980) Massive air emboli during cardiopulmonary bypass. J Thorac Cardiovasc Surg 80: 708–17
9. Lemole GM, Strong MD, Spagna PM, Karmilowicz NP (1982) Improved results for dissecting aneurysms: intraluminal sutureless prosthesis. J Thorac Cardiovasc Surg 83: 249–55
10. Coselli JS (1994) Retrograde cerebral perfusion via superior vena caval cannula for aortic arch aneurysm surgery. Ann Thorac Surg 57: 1668–9
11. Coselli JS, Büket S, Djukanovic B (1995) Aortic arch surgery: current treatment and results. Ann Thorac Surg 59: 19–27
12. Raskin SA, Coselli JS (1995) Retrograde cerebral perfusion: overview, techniques and results. Perfusion 10: 3–9
13. Coselli JS, Crawford ES, Beall AC Jr, Mizrahi EM, Hess KR, Patel VM (1988) Determination of brain temperatures for safe circulatory arrest during cardiovascular operation. Ann Thorac Surg 45: 638–42
14. Mizrahi EM, Patel VM, Crawford ES, Coselli JS, Hess KR (1989) Hypothermic-induced electrocerebral silence, prolonged circulatory arrest, and cerebral protection during cardiovascular surgery. Electroencephalogr Clin Neurophysiol 72: 81–85
15. Usui A, Hotta T, Hiroura M et al. (1992) Retrograde cerebral perfusion through a superior vena caval cannula protects the brain. Ann Thorac Surg 53: 47–53

16. Boeckxstaens CJ, Flameng WJ (1995) Retrograde cerebral perfusion does not perfuse the brain in non-human primates. Ann Thorac Surg 60: 319–28
17. DeBrux J-L, Subayi J-B, Pegis J-D, Pillet J (1995) Retrograde cerebral perfusion: anatomic study of the distribution of blood to the brain. Ann Thorac Surg 60: 1294–8
18. Imamaki M, Koyanagi H, Hashimoto A, Aomi S, Hachida M (1995) Retrograde cerebral perfusion with hypothermic blood provides efficient protection of the brain: A neuropathological study. J Card Surg 10: 325–333
19. Pagano D, Boivin CM, Faroqui MH, Bonser RS (1996) Retrograde perfusion through the superior vena cava perfuses the brain in human beings. J Thorac Cardiovasc Surg 111 (1): 270–2
20. Lin PJ, Chang C-H, Tan PPC et al. (1994) Protection of the brain by retrograde cerebral perfusion during circulatory arrest. J Thorac Cardiovasc Surg 108: 969–74
21. Pagano D, Carey JA, Patel RL et al. (1995) Retrograde cerebral perfusion: Clinical experience in emergency and elective aortic operations. Ann Thorac Surg 59: 393–7
22. Coselli JS, Büket S, Djukanovic B (1995) Aortic Arch Surgery: Current Treatment and Results. Ann Thor Surg 59: 19–27

Author's address:
Joseph S. Coselli, M.D.
6560 Fannin, #1144
Houston, TX 77030
USA

Chronic dissecting aneurysm of the innominate artery, surgical treatment under retrograde cerebral perfusion

L. Camilleri, B. Legault, D. Carrié, I. Brazzalotto, P. Bailly, L. Boyer, Ch. de Riberolles

Department of Cardiovascular Surgery, G. Montpied Hospital, C.H.U., Clermont-Ferrand, France

Introduction

Innominate artery aneurysm is uncommon. Most often, it is atherosclerotic in origin, frequently associated with aortic lesions (1). Given the propensity of this aneurysm to enlarge, rupture or embolize, surgical treatment is strongly recommended (3).

A chronic dissecting aneurysm of the innominate artery, 10 months after surgical repair of a DeBakey type I acute aortic dissection, was successfully operated on using retrograde cerebral perfusion as a method of cerebral protection.

Case report

Severe chest pain and stroke revealed a type I aortic dissection in a 62-year-old man. Transesophageal echocardiography visualized a mildly incompetent aortic valve. Ascending aorta, aortic arch and innominate artery were found dissected. During a 90-min circulatory arrest, cerebral protection was achieved using 18 °C hypothermia and cerebral retrograde perfusion at a mean jugular venous pression of 15 mm Hg. Two intimal tears located one on the ascending aorta and the other at the isthmus level were resected. Replacement of the ascending aorta and aortic arch were realized (Fig. 3). Paraparesia of the left upper extremity disappeared in 2 weeks.

Ten months later, an amaurosis fugax revealed a redissection of right common carotid and innominate arteries. By MRI (Fig. 1) and angiography (Fig. 2), the innominate artery was found dissected and, moreover, aneurysmal (35 mm). The right common carotid artery was dissected and seemed to be perfused only by the false channel. Given the aneurysmal change of the innominate artery, surgical replacement was recommended. The aorta was cannulated into the distal portion of the arch. The patient was cooled to a core temperature of 18 °C. During cooling and before circulatory arrest, a bifurcated 16/8 mm Dacron prosthesis was sewn to a 26-mm sleeve Dacron graft to allow replacement of the arch, carotid, subclavian and innominate arteries. During a 30-min circulatory arrest and cerebral retrograde perfusion at a mean jugular venous pression of 30 mm Hg, the proximal segment of the aortic arch including the origin of the innominate artery was resected. The distal anastomosis was constructed on an unclamped aortic arch, just above the left common carotid artery. Then the aortic cross-clamp was applied to the graft and anterograde C.B.P. was resumed, thus perfusing distal aorta and left common carotid artery. Successively, right common carotid artery, subclavian artery and proximal aorta were anastomosed and reperfused. Neurologic follow-up was uneventful but ventilatory assist was required for 16 days, due to phrenic nerve palsy.

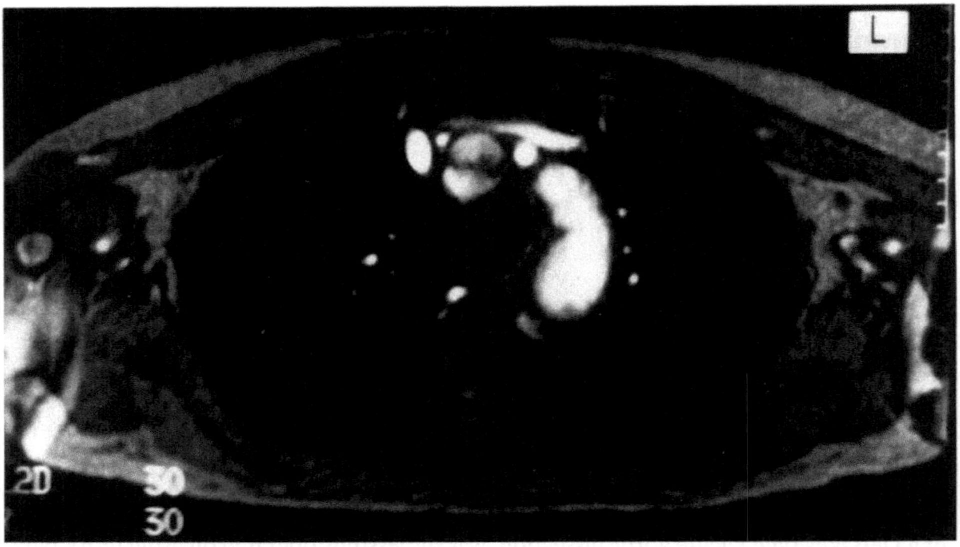

Fig. 1. Preoperative M.R.I.
F.L.A.S.H. gradient echo in axial plane. Enlarged innominate artery with linear intimal flap between two flowing channels.

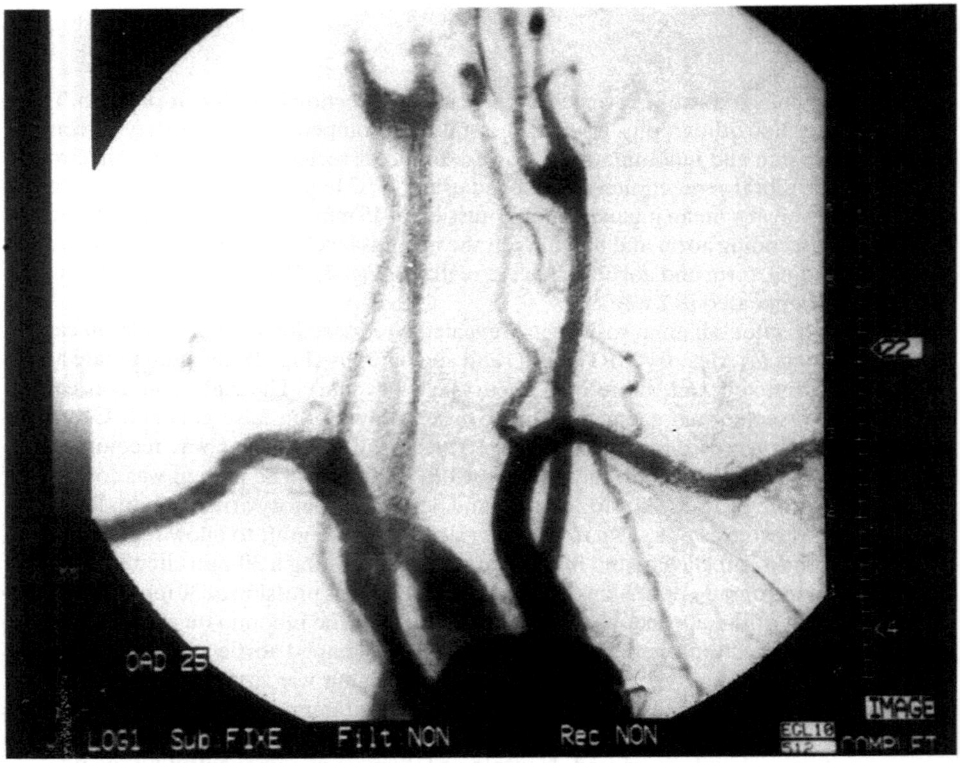

Fig. 2. Aortic arch angiography.
Enlarged and dissected innominate artery. Extension of the dissection onto the common carotid artery.

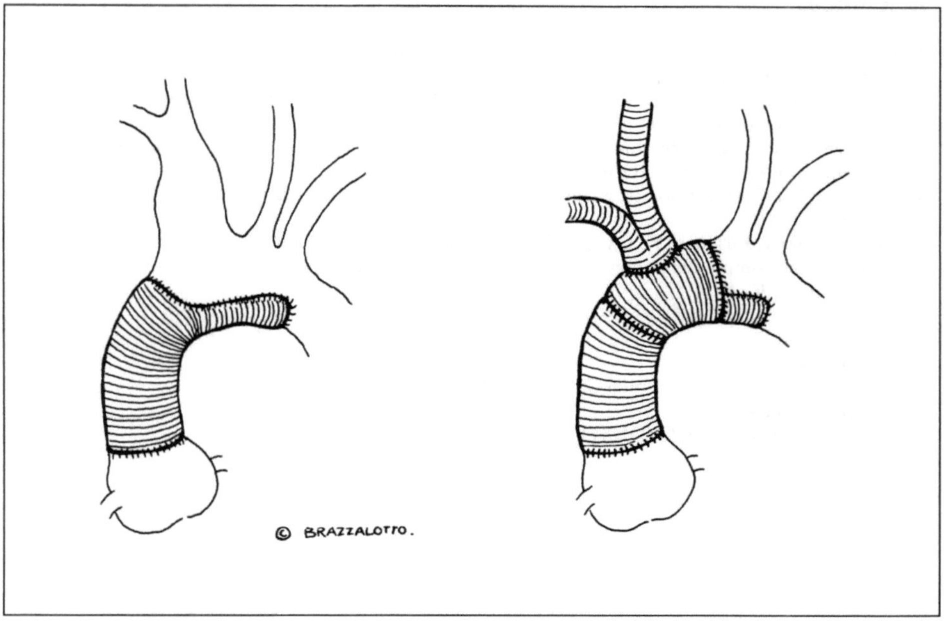

Fig. 3. Schematic drawing of the two procedures.
First operation: replacement of ascending aorta and aortic arch. Redo-operation: replacement of aortic arch and innominate artery.

Discussion

Although atherosclerosis, trauma, and infection are the usual causes of innominate artery aneurysmal formation (2, 4), this may occur as an evolutionary complication of aortic dissection (2).

Aneurysms of the innominate artery should be treated when diagnosed to prevent rupture or embolization (3). Ocular symptoms due to embolism are a particularly common manifestation of innominate artery disease (2).

An excellent exposure of the innominate artery and its bifurcation is obtained by a direct trans-sternal approach (4). Anatomic graft reconstruction seems to be the method of choice in innominate artery aneurysm (1, 2).

The major concern during repair is cerebral protection. As dissection, cross-clamping, direct cannulation or direct perfusion through the lumen of subclavian and carotid arteries seemed to be either source of discomfort in the operation field or even dangerous; we preferred to use retrograde cerebral perfusion.

This technique, besides being quite simple to accomplish, affords in addition to deep hypothermia, circulatory arrest, cerebral protection and comfortable operative conditions (5). It allowed us: completion of the distal anostomosis in an open manner, complete resection of the origin of the innominate artery where the intimal tear is located, and anatomical reconstruction of the common carotid, subclavian and innominate arteries.

References

1. Bower TC, Pairolero PC, Hallett JW, Toomey BJ, Gloviczki P, Cherry KJ (1991) Anévrysmes des troncs supra-aortiques: Importance d'un Diagnostic et d'un traitement Précoces. Ann Chir Vasc 5: 125–132
2. Brewster DC, Moncure AC, Darling C, Ambrosino JJ, Abbott WM (1985) Innominate artery lesions: Problems encountered and lessons learned. J Vasc Surg 2: 99–112
3. Ketonen P, Meurala H, Mattila S, Ketonen L (1983) Management of arteriosclerotic aneurysms of the innominate and subclavian arteries. Scand J Thor Cardiovasc Surg 17: 129–133
4. Thomas VT (1972) Intrathoracic aneurysms of the innominate and subclavian arteries. J Thorac Cardiovasc Surg 63: 461–471
5. Ueda Y, Miki S, Kusuhara K, Okita Y, Tahata T, Yamanaka K (1992) Deep hypothermic systemic circulatory arrest and continuous retrograde cerebral perfusion for surgery of aortic arch aneurysm. Eur J Cardiothorac Surg 6: 36–41

Author's address:
Dr. L. Camilleri
Chirurgie Cardiovasculaire, Hôpital Gabriel Montpied
Place Henri Dunant
F-63003 Clermont-Ferrand, CEDEX, France

Retrograde cerebral perfusion – An experimental study to evaluate brain perfusion in non-human primates

Chr. J. Boeckxstaens[1], V. van Hoof[1], R. Vanmaele[1], W. J. Flameng[2]

[1] University Hospital of Antwerp, Belgium
[2] Department of Cardiac Surgery, University Hospital Leuven, Belgium

Introduction

Lesions of the aorta, as well as the ascending, the aortic arch or the descending aorta have been recognized as far back as the sixteenth century (6). However, inspite of the development of cardiopulmonary bypass, the knowledge of different types of lesions and their etiologies, and the development of grafts and the various techniques, aortic surgery has remained an intriguing part of the cardiovascular surgery. The localization of the disease dictates the management of the operation, that, is, when the ascending aorta without the cerebral vessels is involved, or the aortic arch, or the descending or abdominal aorta different approaches with different precautions are necessary. Involvement of the aortic arch is the most challenging aspect of aortic surgery since the blood supply to the brain is affected, limiting the tolerance of normothermic total ischemia to 4 min (27). This tolerance is greatly improved during hypothermic conditions, hence, together with the development of cardiopulmonary bypass, techniques for deep hypothermia and circulatory arrest were introduced. In 1964, Borst (1) first described a successful intervention on the cerebral vessels with deep hypothermia at a nasopharyngeal temperature of 18 °C, using circulatory arrest for 16 min, a procedure which was devised by Griepp (9) and published in 1975. Nevertheless, even under deep hypothermia, circulatory arrest is limited to 45 min (10). The repair of an aortic arch in such a short time requires fast and skillful surgery without hesitation, putting the surgical team under considerable stress. Therefore, it is necessary to prolong the tolerance to circulatory arrest, using alternatives such as retrograde cerebral perfusion, first described in 1988 by our Japanese colleague Ueda (22) as a very promising technique. They reported an intervention on the aorta using circulatory arrest and "retrograde cerebral perfusion". During the circulatory arrest period, the brain was perfused via the superior caval vein. Many clinical studies followed with satisfactory results. However, despite some experimental data (23), real investigation to maintain structural integrity of the brain and extensive studies on tissue perfusion were not reported until this year (15, 18). Extrapolation of these results is somewhat controversial, while these studies are performed on pigs or dogs. So we designed an animal study using non-human primates for investigation of tissue perfusion during retrograde cerebral perfusion.

Material and methods

All animals received humane care in compliance with the "Guide for the Care and Use of Laboratory animals" published by the National Institute for Health in 1985.

Nineteen baboons, subtype papio Hamadryas, all young males, with an average weight of 9.3 kg (in the range 7 – 15 kg), were premedicated with ketamine (Ketalar, Parke Davis) 10 mg/kg intramuscularly. An intravenous infusion line was placed and 25 mg/kg of pentobarbital (Nembutal, Abott) was administered. The animal was intubated and mechanically ventilated using room air, enriched with oxygen to maintain adequate blood gases. pH was kept in the range of 7.38 – 7.45, pO^2 above 200 mm Hg, pCO^2 in the range of 35 – 45 mm Hg, and the oxygen saturation around 99 %. Anesthesia was maintained with fentanyl 0.03 mg/kg/30 min (Fentanyl, Jansen Pharmaceutica, Belgium) and with pancuronium 0.1 mg/kg/hour (Pavulon, Organon Technika).

The animals were divided in three subgroups according to the protocol (see Fig. 1): a control group (n = 6) was submitted to a period of 1 h of circulatory arrest at a rectal temperature of 18 °C, followed by 3 h of reperfusion; a second group, using retrograde cerebral perfusion (RCP) in the same conditions as in the first group, was submitted to 1 h of RCP followed by 3 h of reperfusion, and a third group was used to perform extensive flow studies using colored microspheres.

The surgical procedure was the same in all subgroups. When anesthesia was completed monitoring catheters were placed in the groin for arterial and venous pressure monitoring. The internal jugular vein was isolated in the neck for bloodsampling to follow enzyme release during the experiment. A temperature probe was inserted in the rectum and for brain temperature monitoring a probe was inserted in the parietal cerebral cortex via a small bore hole in the skull. After all these procedures a sternotomy was performed, with dissection of the heart, the aortic arch and the cerebral vessels. After heparinization of the animal (300 IU/kg) the bypass circuit was installed (see Fig. 2). The cardiopulmonary bypass was constructed with a Biomedicus BP 50 (Medtronic) centrifugal pump and a Minimax (Medtronic) oxygenator. The priming fluid was 250 ml Geloplasma (Merieux, Benelux) and 250 ml Plasmalyt A (Baxter) including 1000 IU of heparin. Cardiopulmo-

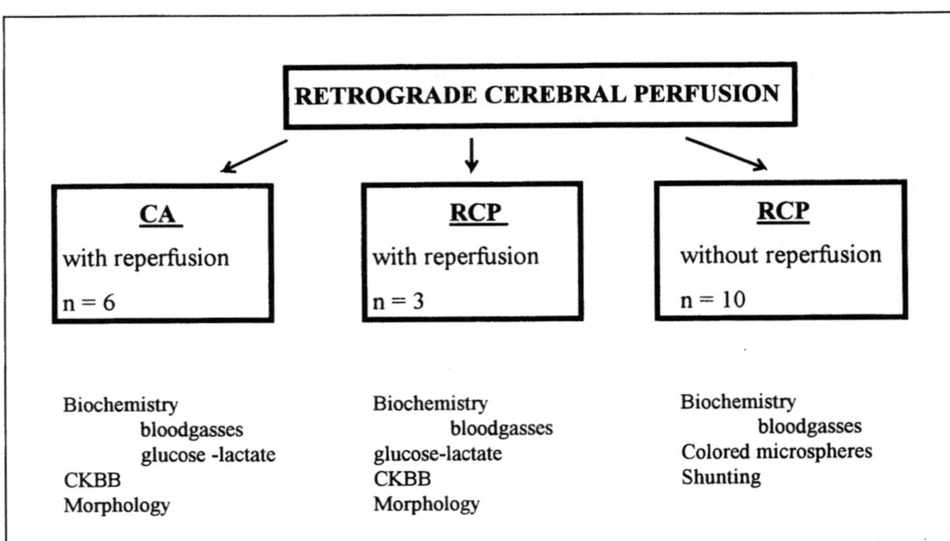

Fig. 1. Experimental protocol. CA = circulatory arrest, RCP = retrograde cerebral perfusion

nary bypass flow rate was 2.4 l/m^2 and mean arterial pressure was kept constant between 50 and 60 mm Hg. Central venous pressure was below zero during antegrade flow. During retrograde perfusion a central venous pressure of 20 mm Hg was not exceeded. The left ventricle was vented via the apex of the heart. After a period of 10 min of stabilization, cooling was started to a rectal temperature of 18 °C. During cooling cerebral and rectal temperature were monitored. Blood gas management during cooling and rewarming was "alpha stat". After cooling, a period of 1 h of circulatory arrest or retrograde cerebral perfusion was introduced according to the subgroup of experiments (see Fig. 1). A reperfusion period of 3 h followed CA or RCP in subgroup one and two. In these two subgroups at fixed intervals bloodsamples were taken for glucose and lactate (an arterial and venous

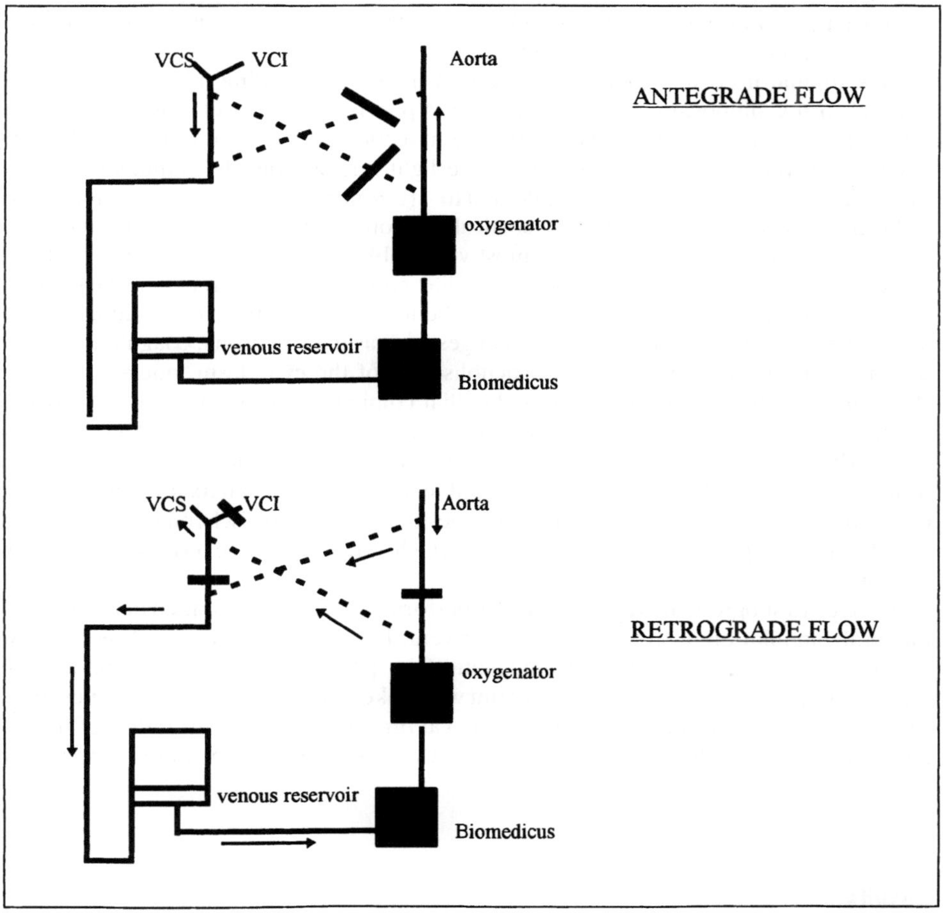

Fig. 2. Schematic overview of the cardiopulmonary bypass circuit during antegrade and retrograde flow. VCS superior caval vein, VCI inferior caval vein.
⟶ indicates the flow directions
▬ clamps placed on the circuit to switch the flow
...... extra bypass circuit for retrograde perfusion via the superior caval vein

sample) and for CK-BB release (venous sample). Blood gases were followed in arterial and venous blood. The arterial blood sample was taken out of the arterial line, the venous blood out of the internal jugular vein. The arterio-venous gradient (arterial value minus venous value) was calculated out of the arterial and venous levels of glucose and lactate. Glucose and lactate gradients were compared. Organ blood flow was measured with colored microspheres at 18° hypothermia before CA or RCP. Two other injections were given during RCP. Colored microspheres (Triton Technology Inc., San Diego, CA) were injected in the cardiopulmonary bypass at 50 cm distance of the tip of the flow line. Reference samples were taken from the femoral artery and, during RCP, out of the inflow line just before entering the animal. Samples were handled as described previously (15).

After the experiment the animal was sacrificed and the brain was fixated using the perfusion fixation technique with Karnowsky solution (2 % paraformaldehyde and 2.5 % gluteraldehyde in Sörensen buffer 0.1 M). At the end of the experiment, the subclavian arteries are ligated and the brain was flushed via the aortic arch with saline for about 1 min until the returning fluid was clear. Than the perfusate was switched to the fixative maintaining a perfusion pressure of 50 mm Hg. After this procedure an immersion fixation of the head was performed for at least 3 h.

Nine standardized specimens were taken of the brain including frontal, temporal and parietal cortex, hippocampus and cerebellum. A post fixation in OsO4 and routine embedding in Epon were performed, whereafter 2-μm sections were stained with toluidine blue. Unaware of the protocol, the sections were light microscopically examined. Different ischemic lesions were scored on a scale of 0 to 4 (0 = normal, 4 = maximal damage). The following items were investigated: cortical neurons, cortical glial compartment, hippocampal CA1/CA4 layer being the most vulnerable cell-layers for ischemia of the hippocampus, gyrus dentatus, hippocampal glial compartment, cerebellar Purkinje and granular cells, glial compartment of the cerebellum, white matter and vascular compartment. Attention was given to cellular changes such as dark neurons, coagulative cellular degeneration, cellular edema, microvacuolisation of the cytoplasm, nuclear chromatin clumping and nuclear shrinkage. For the glial compartment, edema and "status spongiosus" due to astroglial swelling by ischemia were scored in a similar way. Destabilization of the white matter and edema were also graded from 0 to 4. In the vascular compartment residual red blood cells were traced as a possible indication of a bad fixation, as well as vascular collapse and edema surrounding the vessels as a sign of ischemia. After all these investigations a global grading was made, which reflected the severity of the cerebral damage.

In the third subgroup no reperfusion was performed. RCP was installed in this group via bilateral cannulation of the internal jugular vein. Extensive monitoring of the flows was performed using calibrated electromagnetic flow probes. Colored microspheres were injected and samples for microsphere count were taken in the in- and outflow lines. Extensive bloodgas monitoring was also performed at three different places: inflow of the internal jugular vein, outflow of the aortic arch and venous return via the inferior caval vein.

Results

Temperature evolution

In the first subgroups temperature was registered every 10 min. Rectal temperature as well as cerebral temperature reacted in the same way in both groups. Evolution in brain temperature during cooling, RCP or CA period and reperfusion are depicted in Fig. 3. Although brain temperature was slightly lower in the RCP group there was no statistical difference in temperature evolution between both groups (ANOVA for repeated measurements $p > 0.05$).

Metabolic results

Cooling was associated with a rise in glucose and lactate levels, but with an arteriovenous difference close to zero (see Fig. 4, only the data of the RCP group are presented because of the similarity between both groups). At the end of CA and RCP the gradient becomes more pronounced with a more positive arteriovenous difference in glucose and a more negative one in lactate. Resuming the circulation, during reperfusion the gradient disappears with reappearance of the gradient but to a lesser extent after rewarming of the animal. This feature was the same in the control as well as the RCP group (ANOVA for repeated measurements $p > 0.05$).

Enzymatic results

CK-BB release in the internal jugular vein was followed as a marker for brain ischemia. The consecutive results of both groups are presented in Table 1. After starting the cardiopulmonary bypass a significant rise in CK-BB is noted (ANOVA for repeated measurements $p < 0.05$). This rise continues and becomes more pronounced after CA and RCP,

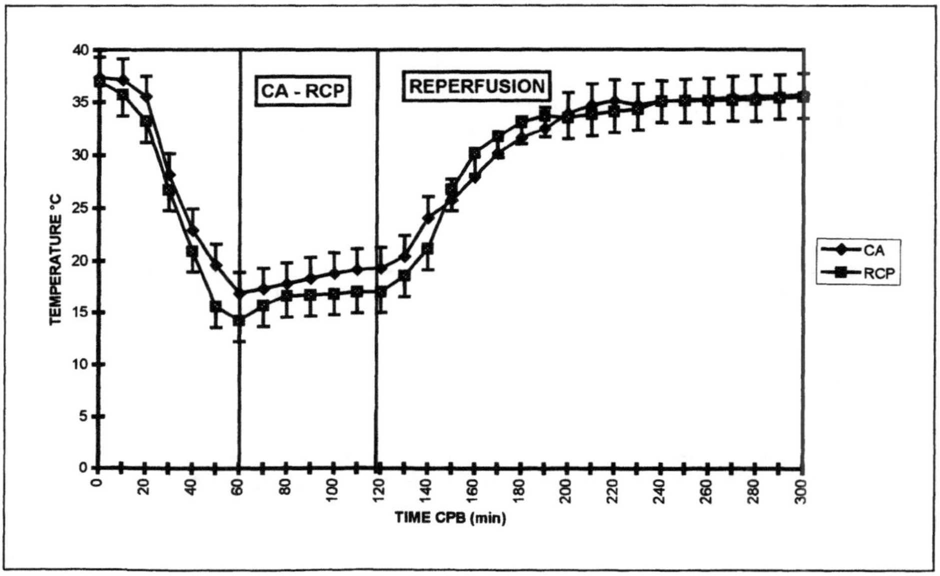

Fig. 3. Temperature evolution during the two first experimental groups: controlgroup, CA (circulatory arrest), and RCP (retrograde cerebral perfusion) with reperfusion. Values are presented as means ± SD. No statistical difference was noted between both groups ($p < 0.05$, ANOVA for repeated measurements).

with peak concentrations of 123 ± 97 U/L in the CA group and 164 ± 88 U/L in the RCP group. The enzymatic release although is in the same extent in both groups (ANOVA for repeated measurements $p > 0.05$).

Flow distribution during cooling and RCP

The results of the microsphere injections during RCP are presented in Fig. 5.

Note that microspheres are traced in all organs of the body. Flow calculations resulted in almost no flow in all subregions of the brain during RCP. As comparison the flow on CPB at deep hypothermia (18 °C) is presented in Table 2. A marked flow reduction of global brain flow of 31 ml/min/100 gr tissue at 18 °C to 0.5 ml/min/100 gr tissue during RCP ($p < 0.05$) is noteworthy. When the different samples are compared the largest amount of microspheres is even found in non-cerebral regions.

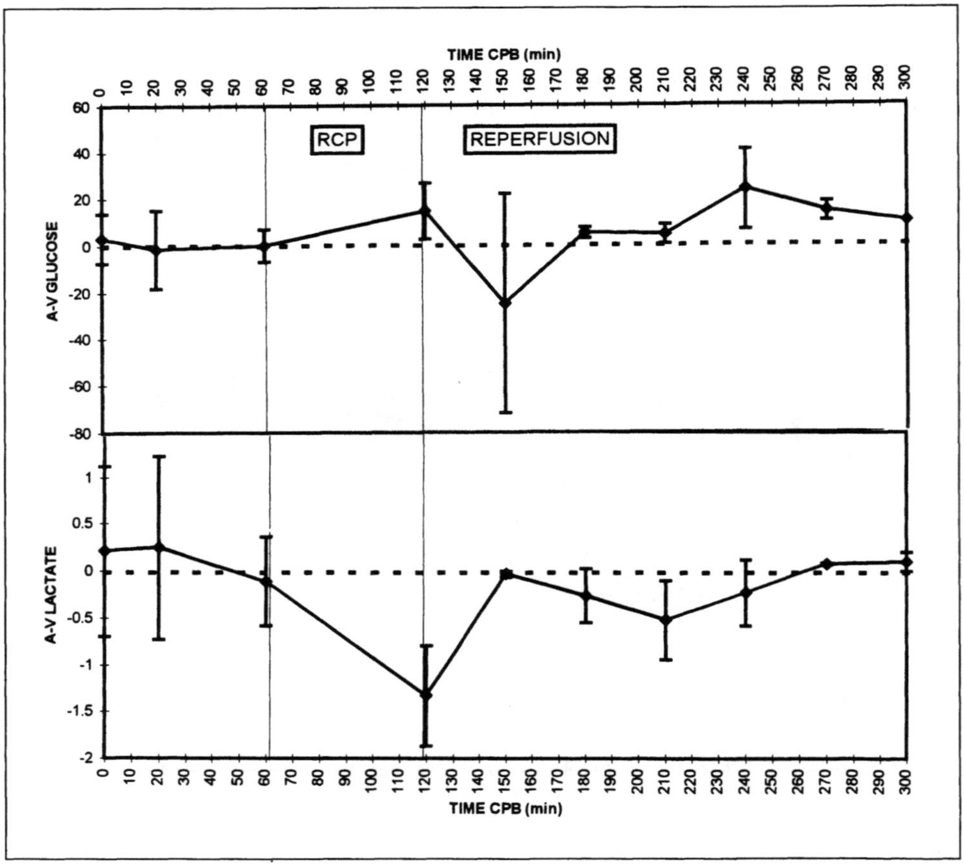

Fig. 4. Glucose and lactate gradient (arterio-venous difference) during RCP. Values are presented as means ± SD. After retrograde cerebral perfusion (RCP) the gradient in glucose becomes more positive due to possible glucose uptake, while the lactate difference becomes more negative, sign of production of lactate, due to anaerobic metabolism.

Shunting during RCP

One of the most striking features during RCP was that almost 90 % of the infused blood returned via the inferior caval vein, and that the return via the aortic arch was always less

Table 1. CK-BB values at fixed intervals during the experimental period; Values are presented as mean ± SD. Time indicates the duration of cardiopulmonary bypass (CPB). CA (circulatory arrest) and RCP (retrograde cerebral perfusion) was performed between 60 min and 120 min of the CPB.

TIME CPB (min.)	CK-BB U/L (mean ± SD) CA (60 – 120 min)	CK-BB U/L (mean ± SD) RCP (60 – 120 min)
0 min	21 ± 13	21 ± 13
20 min	23 ± 13	23 ± 13
60 min	49 ± 22	49 ± 22
120 min	68 ± 40	104 ± 45
150 min	96 ± 67	81 ± 19
180 min	123 ± 97	93 ± 40
210 min	111 ± 79	153 ± 94
240 min	84 ± 46	154 ± 71
270 min	118 ± 24	163 ± 88
300 min	182 ± 74	154 ± 94

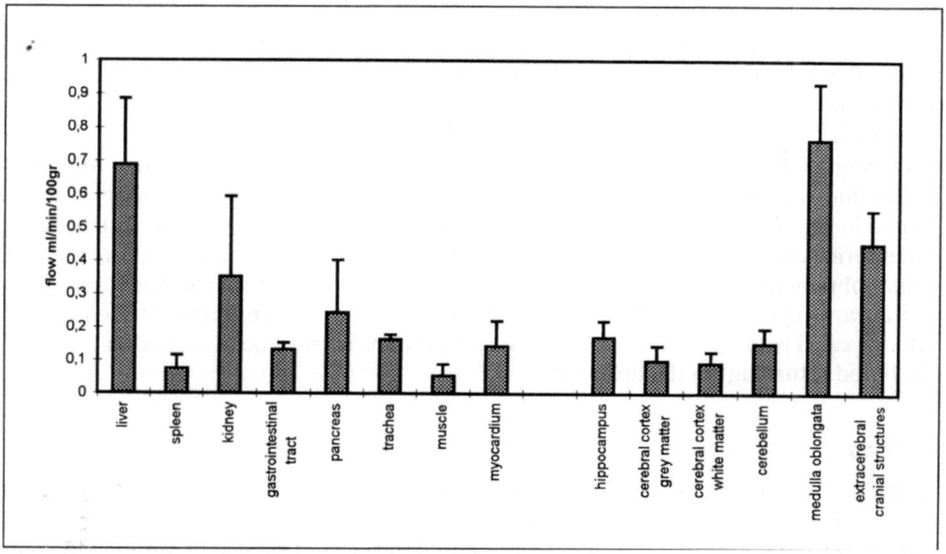

Fig. 5. Organ blood flow during RCP (retrograde cerebral perfusion). Flow values in ml/min/100 gr tissue mean ± SD

Table 2. Regional organ flow measured with colored microsphere technique. Values are presented as mean ± SD. Values obtained after injection at 18 °C antagrade flow are presented in the first column, RCP values as comparison are given in the second column.

Organ	Flow ml/min/100 gr 18 °C rectal temperature mean ± SD	Flow ml/min/100 gr RCP 18 °C mean ± SD
liver	38.72 ± 32.72	0.69 ± 0.19
spleen	69.29 ± 67.01	0.07 ± 0.04
kidney	219.67 ± 123.36	0.35 ± 0.24
gastro-intestinal tract	33.58 ± 30.54	0.13 ± 0.2
pancreas	68.33 ± 33.79	0.24 ± 0.16
trachea	17.10 ± 7.93	0.16 ± 0.01
muscle	7.18 ± 4.85	0.05 ± 0.03
myocardium	125.00 ± 78.88	0.14 ± 0.07
Brain		
hippocampus	33.63 ± 11.03	0.17 ± 0.05
cerebral cortex grey matter	20.83 ± 7.20	0.10 ± 0.05
cerebral cortex white matter	18.49 ± 9.68	0.09 ± 0.03
cerebellum	41.41 ± 25.93	0.15 ± 0.04
medulla oblongata	44.39 ± 32.26	0.76 ± 0.17

than 1 % (see Fig. 6). Injection of microspheres in the inflow line resulted in an equilibrium of circulating microspheres of 100 % in in- and outflow of the inferior caval vein. Investigation of the blood returning via the aortic arch showed minimal presence of microspheres (20 – 100 microspheres/ml).

During RCP bloodgases were taken at three different sites: a first sample out of the inflow line, a second in the inferior caval vein and a third in the aortic arch. Results are presented in Fig. 7. Comparable values are found in inflow of the RCP circuit and outflow of the inferior caval vein (statistical analyses with paired *t*-test showed no difference). The values obtained in the aortic arch showed significant difference in pH and pO2; pCO2 was not always significantly different, only at 20, 30, 50 min a significant difference in the inferior caval vein was noted. The most striking difference was the massive desaturation of the blood returning via the aortic arch.

Histology

In the first subgroups histological examination of the brain was performed. A semiquantitative analyses of the structural changes was done and afterwards the two groups were statistically compared. The results are presented in Fig. 8. The lesions were divided into four groups: the cellular changes, changes in the glial compartment, the damage to the white matter and to the vascular compartment. Different items were investigated in each subgroup. For cellular changes we scored in order of severity the appearance of dark neurons, the presence of microvacuolisation, cellular edema, clumping of chromatin, nuclear shrinking and picnosis of the cell. All of these features scored very minimal and in the same extent in both groups. The glial compartment showed higher scores in the three items investigated, namely chromatin clumping, edema and status spongiosus (also a sign of pronounced edema). None of these scores was a sign of real lethal damage. Between both groups only a statistical difference ($p < 0.05$) was found in the presence of status spongiosus in the disadvantage of RCP. The white matter showed no lethal damage of the myelin, but edema was present. The same edema was found around the blood vessels, with collaps of the blood vessels, although again to the same extent in both groups. Figure 9 shows representative light microscopical views representative for both subgroups. The most striking characteristics is the sponge like aspect of the cerebral cortex in the RCP group.

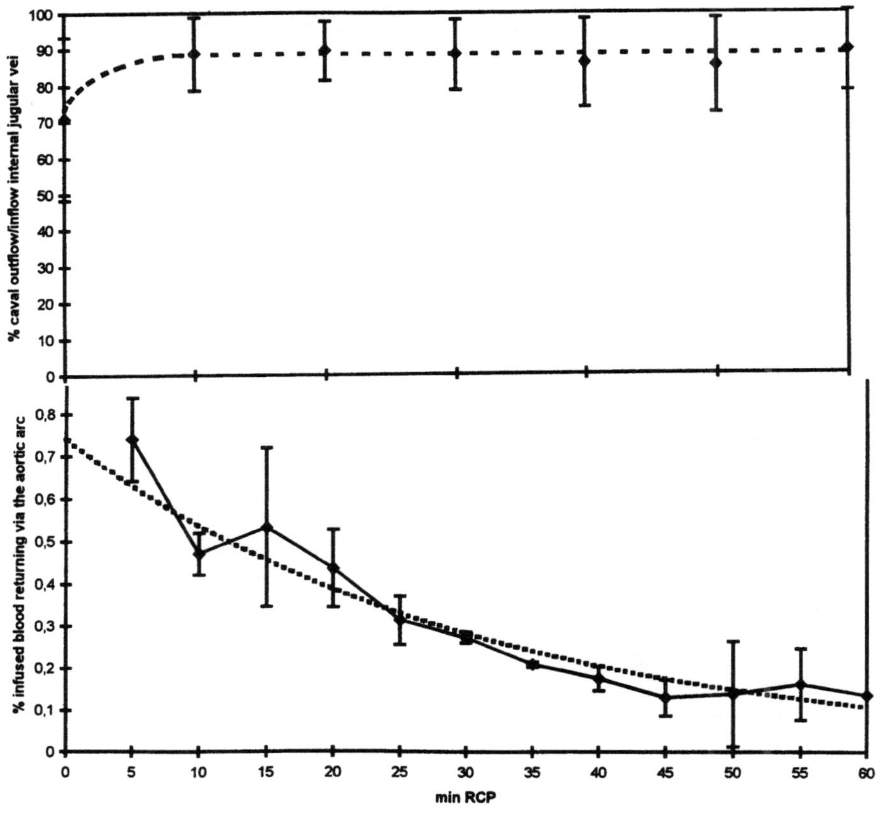

Fig. 6. Outflow during RCP. The different values are presented as % of the inflow in the internal jugular vein (value = mean ± SD). Upper panel: outflow via the inferior caval vein; lower panel: outflow via the aortic arch

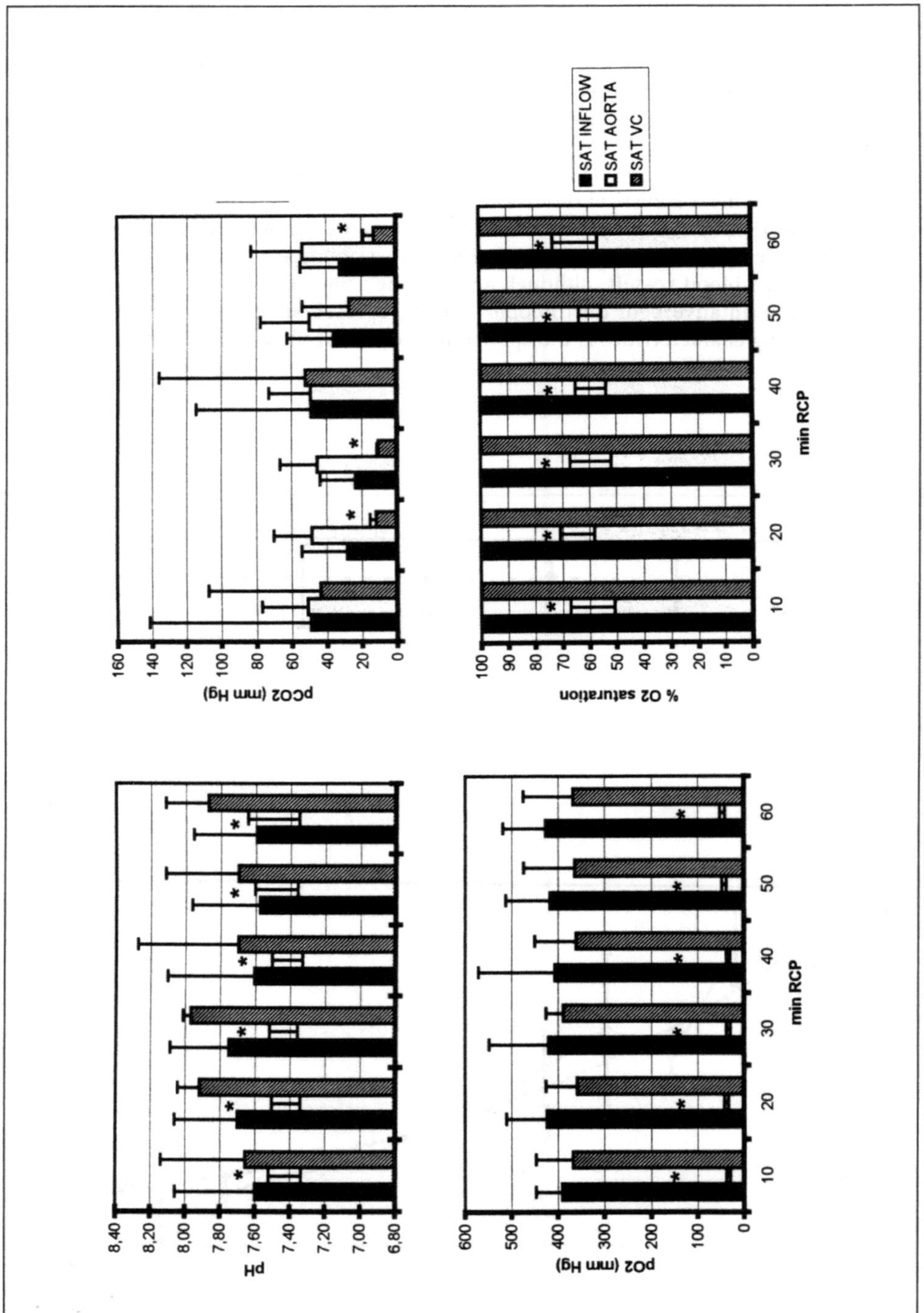

Fig. 7. Bloodgas analyses during RCP (retrograde cerebral perfusion). Inflow = inflow in both internal jugular veins, aorta = outflow aortic arch, VC, outflow inferior caval vein. Values are presented as means ± SD. *indicates $p < 0.05$ paired t-test

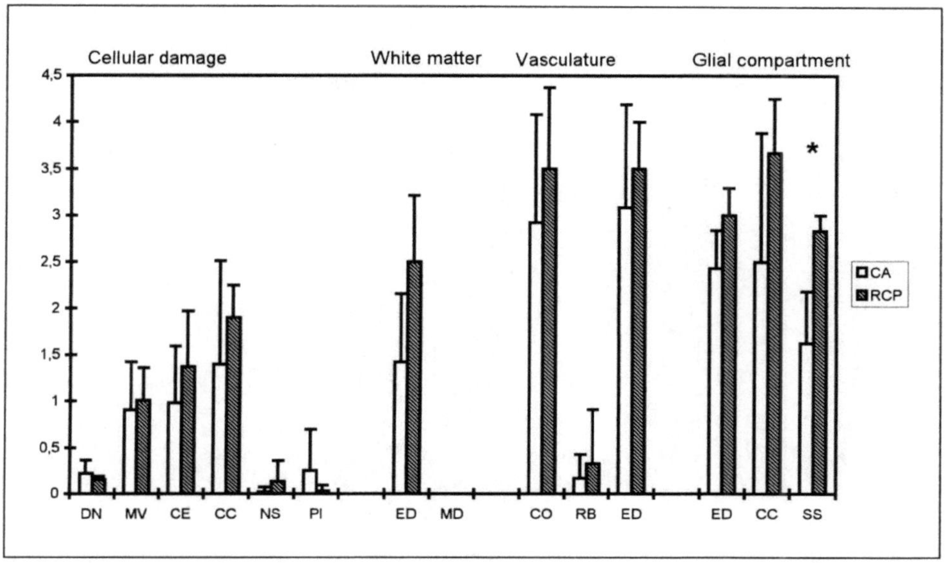

Fig. 8. Semiquantitative quotation of histological damage after one hour of hypothermic circulatory arrest (CA) or retrograde cerebral perfusion (RCP). Values are presented as means + SD, *indicates $p < 0.05$. (DN dark neurons, MV microvacuolisation, CE cellular edema, CC coagulative celchanges, NS nuclear shrinking, PI picnosis,ED edema, MD myeline destruction, CO collapse of the vessel, RB remaining red blood cells, SS status spongiosus)

Discussion

This study is far from complete. Neurological monitoring, such as electroencephalographic registration with evoked potentials was not included. Survival studies with postoperative neurological scores of the animal were not performed. Our special aim was to investigate if real *tissue perfusion* existed during RCP, therefore we have chosen the colored microsphere technique to estimate the blood flow in all regions of the brain. Biochemical, enzymatic and morphological studies were included to complete our findings. We have chosen a non-human primate as animal model, because in cerebral anatomy primates are completely different from other species.

Temperature evolution during RCP

The temperature evolution during RCP is quite similar as during CA even with a similar rise of approximately 2° during RCP or CA period. The speculation that with RCP the hypothermia is better maintained could not be confirmed.

Metabolic findings

Brain ischemia induces an anaerobic metabolism of glucose associated with the production of lactate. This production of lactate is an indirect marker of brain ischemia (2). In our

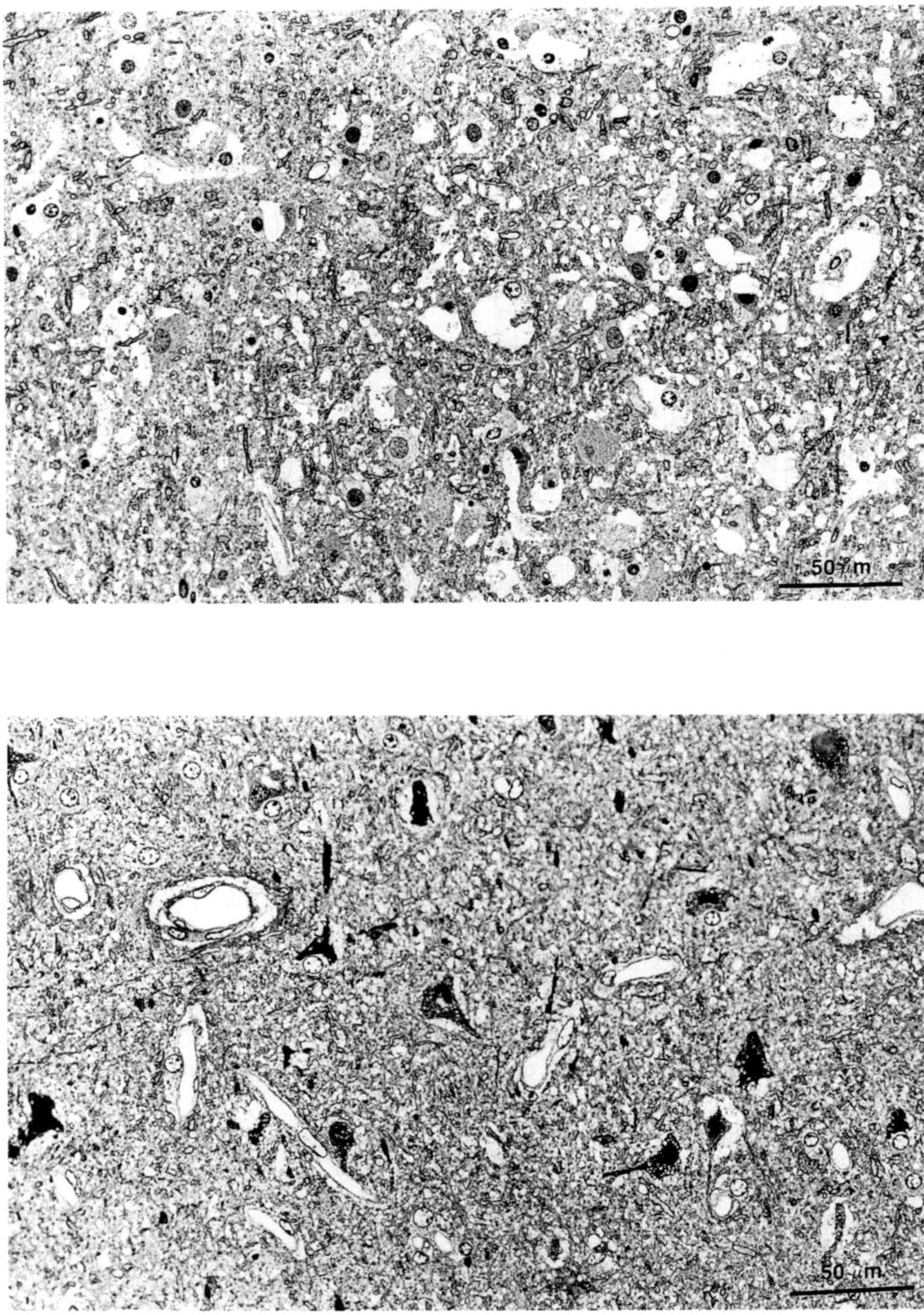

Fig. 9. Light microscopical view of parietal cortex after one hour of CA (circulatory arrest) upper panel, or RCP (retrograde cerebral perfusion) lower panel, followed by 3 hours of reperfusion. Magnification factor 400×. In the upper panel dark neurons with microvacuolisation are present. In the lower panel, after RCP, the edema is more pronounced.

experiments glucose uptake and lactate production can be demonstrated when we study the arteriovenous gradients of glucose and lactate. By sampling of the blood at the cerebral inflow (arterial line) and the cerebral outflow (internal jugular vein) an estimation of cerebral metabolism can be obtained. After circulatory arrest and retrograde cerebral perfusion the arteriovenous difference in glucose becomes more positive, which can be a sign of glucose uptake during the CA or RCP period. This more positive arteriovenous difference in glucose is associated with a more negative difference in lactate (venous lactate levels are higher than the arterial ones). So together with the uptake of glucose lactate production occurs, which is a sign of anaerobic metabolism. This feature is found to the same extent in both groups. From a metabolic point of view one cannot conclude that during RCP the brain is supplied with a sufficient amount of blood to avoid anaerobic metabolism.

Enzymatic release during RCP

CK-BB can be used as a specific marker of brain damage (2). Normally CK-BB cannot be traced in the blood. It appears in the cerebrospinal fluid and passes the blood brain barrier when cerebral damage occurs. There is a positive correlation between the extent of the injury and the appearance of the enzyme in the serum. CK-BB appears also in the serum in normal routine coronary bypass surgery (28). An explanation for this feature is not yet found. In congenital surgery peak concentrations of the enzyme are found after 127 to 180 min after circulatory arrest (5). Also a positive correlation was made between the extent of the arrest and the concentration of the enzyme. CK-BB release revealed in our study minor cerebral damage. Upon the first rise of the enzyme after starting the cardiopulmonary bypass a second rise was noted after the circulatory arrest period. The peak concentration was found approximately 90 min after the event, with a plateau until the end of the experiment. Although this rise is significant for brain damage the extent of the damage is not so pronounced as when real cell death occurs (19). When comparing the results in CK-BB release after CA or RCP, no positive conclusions can be made about the benefit for RCP: the release is to the same extent in both groups.

Histology

As metabolic and enzymatic parameters already indicate, histology could not reveal any difference between CA or RCP. Using perfusion fixation technique, we searched for minor changes which could indicate minimal to severe brain damage (24). Neuronal cells show coagulative changes to ischemic aggression such as in order of severity the appearance of dark neurons, cellular edema, clumping of chromatin and nuclear shrinkage with at the end picnosis of the cell. Dark neurons together with microvascualisation of the cytoplasm which is a sign of hypermetabolism are present. To a larger extent cellular edema and coagulative cell changes are present. All these changes are reversible. The category of severe cell damage such as nuclear shrinkage and picnosis are almost absent. The reaction of the glial compartment is characterized by edema. The damage to the glial compartment scores relatively higher than the damage on the neurons. Edema is also present in the white matter and around the blood vessels. All scores for edema are relatively high but probably this will disappear with longer reperfusion. Our histological findings correspond with earlier studies which report also minor cell changes after circulatory arrest (7).

The most striking feature was that, although not statistically different, the scores in the RCP group were relatively higher than those of the CA group except for pronounced edema "status spongious" where real statistical difference was found in the disadvantage of RCP.

Flow studies

Although a large amount of blood, up to 1 l per minute, could be perfused retrogradely in the internal jugular vein without increase of the central venous pressure above 20 mm Hg, no brain flow values above 2 ml/min/100 gr tissue could be detected with colored microsphere technique. In hypothermic conditions the brain still needs approximately 30 ml/100 gr/min. Our findings are contradicted by other studies, using hydrogen clearance (23) or colored microspheres (15). Hydrogen clearance measurements in dogs mentioned values up to 20 ml/min/100 gr tissue during retrograde cerebral perfusion at a pressure of 25 mm of Hg. Hydrogen clearance is however not the perfect method for measuring cerebral bloodflow. Flow is only measured in a very small part of the brain. The values obtained can be false high due to the hyperemia of introducing the electrode, or false low, by the edema around the electrode. Microsphere technique on the other hand is a widely accepted technique for regional blood flow studies in laboratory conditions. Introduced in 1968 (17), many investigators have worked out this technique to become an almost perfect instrument. Colored micropheres were used in RCP in dogs resulting in flow measurement varying from 10 to 25 ml/min/100 gr tissue (15). This study compared the findings obtained with hydrogen clearance with colored microsphere technique. Some remarks have to be made. The investigators used 50 μm microspheres, a size of microspheres that has not been used for quite some years (11), while one of the most important requirements concerning microsphere technique are not fulfilled: the density, the size and rheological characteristics of 50 μ spheres are too different from those of red blood cells, which means that they do not react as red blood cells and are trapped mainly because of their size before the end capillaries. Fifty micron spheres are mostly used to investigate the size of shunts. Using these microspheres false results can be obtained and not real tissue flow.

A second remark can be made on the experimental data obtained by other investigators (18, 22, 23). Extrapolation of flow measurements obtained in dogs or pigs to humans is a little bit controversial. Anatomically, primates and non-primates have a very different cerebral circulation. The cerebral circulation of primates is characterized by a complete double system with vessels for the blood supply of the brain, and vessels for the facial structures. Although pigs have also a double system without any venous valves, the proportion of bloodvessels supplying the brain is opposite to primates (8). Dogs, moreover, have not the complete double system (13). The internal maxillary vein is the major venous return of the whole head, cerebrum as well as snout structures. Veno-venous connections at different levels in the head are present in primates, and to a lesser extent in pigs and dogs. The complexity of the venous sinus system is also unique in primates. Although the same classification exists in the porcine and the carnivore brain, primates have a well developed nearly circular system, which is drained via the internal jugular vein to the superior caval vein.

Installing RCP via the superior caval vein is somewhat contradictory. Several studies revealed the presence of competent venous valves in the jugular vein in 80 % of the humans (12). The physiological meaning of these valves is discussed, but reports exist that they can stand pressures up to 40 mm Hg (4) and they have a protective purpose to prevent high pressures in the cerebral venous system caused by coughing. Even a disaster (23) in RCP is reported due to the existence of this valve. To avoid this problem canulation of the internal jugular vein was performed in the third experimental group.

The most remarkable finding installing RCP was that the largest amount of infused blood returned via the inferior caval vein. Veno-venous connections are widely present in the body, and especially in the head (see Fig. 10). Even direct connections intracranially and extracranially localized are being described extensively in anatomy books (20). So the infused blood does not follow the conventional expected way of vein, venules, capillary, arterioles, artery. But even so, tissue perfusion could be present. This was however not proved by microsphere count. The highest amount of microspheres was found in the cardiopulmonary bypass circuit, reaching an equilibrium of circulating microspheres in- and outflow after about 10 min, an equilibrium of 100 %. Flow measurements, comparing infused volume via the internal jugular vein and blood returning via the inferior caval vein showed also a stabilization of in- and outflow of approximately 90 % after 10 min. The microspheres were not found in the tissue, so tissue perfusion was absent.

Although in our study we could not show real tissue perfusion, the possible benefit of RCP is already shown in several clinical reports (3, 16). Clinical reports show better neurological outcome using this technique instead of classical circulatory arrest. These investigators try also to prove that the blood is reaching the brain. Undoubtedly, there is blood in the skull when perfusion via the superior caval vein is performed, but the proof of real "tissue perfusion" cannot be given. So as reported in earlier studies (14, 25), the benefit of retrograde cerebral perfusion has to be sought in wash-out of debris or prevention of air emboli, which remain two of the major risk of complications during aortic arch surgery.

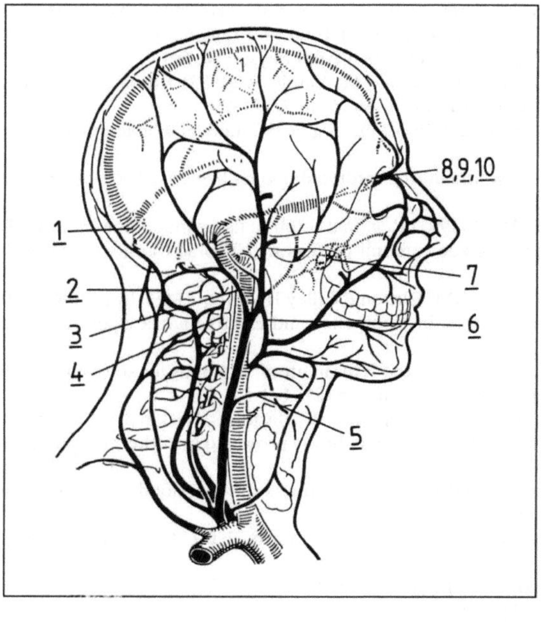

Fig. 10. Schematic overview of the connections between intra-cranial and extra-cranial venous system. The most important connections are: 1) vena emissaria, 2) plexus suboccipitalis, 3) vena auricularis posterior, 4) plexus spinalis, 5) vena retromandibularis, 6) ramus communicans juguli (anastomotic vein between int and ext jug vein), 7) plexus pterigoideus.

In conclusion, we can say that with our experimental setting we could not prove tissue perfusion during retrograde cerebral perfusion. Histologically and biochemically, there was no major difference between circulatory arrest and retrograde cerebral perfusion when performed for 1 h.

References

1. Borst HG, Shaudig A, Rudolph W (1964) Arteriovenous fistula of the aortic arch: repair during deep hypothermia and circulatory arrest. J Thorac Cardiovasc Surg 48: 443–47
2. Bradley HE, Fitch W (1994) Biochemical markers of cerebral ischemia. In: Sebel PS, Fitch W (eds) Monitoring the central nervous system. Blackwell, London, pp 26–50
3. Deeb GM, Jenkins E, Bolling SF, Brunsting LA, Williams DM, Quint LE, Deeb ND (1995) Retrograde cerebral perfusion during hypothermic circulatory arrest reduce morbidity. J Thorac Cardiovasc Surg 109: 259–68
4. Dresser LP, McKinney WM (1987) Anatomic and Pathophysiologic studies of the human internal jugular valve. Am J Surg 154: 220–224
5. Ekroth R, Thompson RJ, Lincoln C, Scallan M, Rossi R, Tsang V (1989) Elective deep hypothermia with total circulatory arrest: changes in plasma creatine kinase BB, blood glucose, and clinical variables. J Thorac Cardiovasc Surg 97: 30–5
6. Fernelius, cited by Scarpa A. A treatise on the anatomy, pathology and surgical treatment of aneurysm. Edinburgh, 1808. In: De Bakery ME, McCollum CH, Crawford ES et al. (1982) Dissection and dissecting aneurysms of the aorta: Twenty year follow up of five hundred twenty seven patients treated surgically. Surgery 92: 1118–33
7. Fessatidis IT, Thomas VL, Shore DF, Sedgwick ME, Hunt RH, Weller RO (1993) Brain damage after profoundly hypothermic circulatory arrest: correlation between neurophysiologic and neuropathologic findings. J Thorac Cardiovasc Surg 106: 32–41
8. Getty R (1975) The anatomy of domestic animals, 5th ed. WB Saunders, Philadelphia, pp 164–189
9. Griepp RB, Stinson EB, Hollingsworth JF (1975) Prosthetic replacement of the aortic arch. J Thorac Cardiovasc Surg 70: 1051–1093
10. Kirklin JW, Barratt-Boyes BG (1993) Cardiac Surgery, 2nd ed., Churchill Livingstone, New York
11. Markus ML, Heistad DD, Ehrhardt JC, Abboud FM (1976) Total and regional cerebral blood flow measurement with 7-, 10-, 15-, 25-, and 50-μm microspheres. J Appl Physiol 40: 501–7
12. Midy D, Le Huec JC, Dumont D, Cauveaux D, Cabanie H, Laude M (1988) Etude anatomique et histologique des valves des veines jugulaires internes. Bull Ass Anat 77: 21–29
13. Miller ME, Christensen GC, Evans HE (1964) Anatomy of the dog. WB Saunders, Philadelphia, pp 389–401
14. Mills NL, Ochsner JL (1980) Massive air embolism during cardiopulmonary bypass. J Thorac Cardiovasc Surg 80: 708–17
15. Oohara K, Usui A, Murase M, Tanaka M, Abe T (1995) Regional cerebral tissue blood flow measured by the colored microsphere method during retrograde cerebral perfusion. J Thorac Cardiovasc Surg 109: 772–9
16. Pagano D, Carey JA, Patel RL, Allen SM, Tsang GM, Hutton P, Lilley JP, Faroqui MH, Bonser RS (1995) Retrograde cerebral perfusion: clinical experience in emergency and elective aortic operations; Ann Thorac Surg 59: 393–97
17. Rudolph AM, Heymann MA (1967) The circulation of the fetus in utero: Methods for studying distribution of blood flow, cardiac output and organ blood flow. Circ Res 21: 163–84
18. Safi HJ, Iliopoulos DC, Gopinath SP, Hess KR, Asimacopoulos PJ, Bartoli S, Raskin SA, Shaibani AT, Leveque CM, Yawn DH (1995) Retrograde cerebral perfusion during profound hypothermia and circulatory arrest in pigs. Ann Thorac Surg 59: 1107–12
19. Sommer H, Kaste M, Troupp H, Kontinnen A (1975) Brain creatine kinase in blood after acute brain injury. J Neurol Neurosurg Psychiatr 38: 572–576
20. Töndury G (1970) Angewandte und topographische Anatomie: Ein Lehrbuch für Studierende und Ärzte, 3. Auflage. Thieme, Stuttgart, S 329–31
21. Tsuchida K, Hashimoto A, Yamaki F, Koyanagi H (1993) Cerebral death-like conditions after aortic aneurysm surgery using retrograde cerebral perfusion. Cardiovasc Surg 1: 701–3

22. Ueda Y, Miki S, Kusuhara K, Okita Y, Tahata T, Yamanaka K (1990) Surgical treatment of the aneurysm dissection involving ascending aorta and aortic arch utilizing circulatory arrest and retrograde perfusion. J Cardiovasc Surg 31: 553–8
23. Usui A, Oohara K, Lui T, Murase M, Tanaka M, Takeuchi E, Abe T (1994) Determination of optimum retrograde cerebral perfusion conditions. J Thorac Cardiovasc Surg 107: 300–8
24. Van Reempts J (1984) The hypoxic brain: histological and ultrastructural aspects. Behav Brain Res 14: 99–108
25. Watanabe M, Shimasaki T, Kuraoka S, Abe H, Iijima Y, Washio M (1992) Retrograde cerebral perfusion against massive air embolism during cardiopulmonary bypass. J Thorac Cardiovasc Surg 104: 532–33
26. Wieland W, Wouters RF, Van Aken H, Flameng W (1993) Measurement of organ blood flow with colored microspheres: a first time saving improvement using automated spectrophotometry. In: (no ed) Computers in Cardiology 1993, IEEE Computer Society Press, Los Alamitos USA, pp 691–94
27. Willner A (1993) Cerebral damage before and after cardiac surgery, Kluwer, Dordrecht, pp 15–37
28. Zweig MH, Van Steirteghem AC (1979) Increased CK-BB concentrations in serum following cardiac surgery. Clin Chim 93: 29–33

Authors' address:
Dr. C. Boeckxstaens
Department of Cardiac Surgery
University Hospital of Antwerp
Wilrijkstraat 10
2650 Edegem, Belgium

Is there a conflict between clinical and experimental evidence on the benefit of retrograde cerebral perfusion?

T. Treasure

Professor of Cardiothoracic Surgery, St. George's Hospital Medical School and Consultant Cardiothoracic Surgeon, St. George's Hospital, London, England

Introduction

In the papers presented in this symposium, on the subject of retrograde cerebral perfusion, there was a striking difference between acceptance of the usefulness of this technique from clinical surgeons (2, 4) and scepticism from basic scientists, based on experimental evidence that it offered no protection from the effects of circulatory arrest in carefully performed studies in a non-human primate (1). The surgical experts, presented with this divergence of opinion were prepared to accept the middle ground, that venous perfusion might not protect the brain in metabolic terms but would at least have a useful role in flushing the arterial system of air, particles, and atheromatous debris. The basic contradiction between practice and scientific evidence remained unresolved. This overview is written in the hope of finding evidence on which to base practice and to focus future research.

It must be acknowledged that there are times when it is difficult to know which of our surgical practices are of real benefit and which are part of ritual, without a firm basis. Retrograde cerebral perfusion is a particularly good example.

Clinical research is beset with difficulties:

1) It is difficult to obtain homogeneous groups of patients with aortic disease in whom a planned period of hypothermic circulatory arrest might be subjected to a consistent protocol in order to test a single hypothesis. The patients have a range of ages and pathologies, and the operations required vary in time and complexity.

2) It is difficult to identify cause and effect when the measures of outcome are influenced by several factors. We would like to study the time related damage of circulatory arrest, and its possible amelioration by retrograde perfusion, but in the background are the effects of cerebrovascular disease, dissection flaps, and preoperative events, and a number of other factors and events which may result in stroke independently of our operative strategy.

3) There is a limit to the type of data we can collect, and its completeness and consistency, when our first responsibility is to perform an expeditious and safe operation.

4) Finally, and inescapably, once there is a belief that a given strategy offers important benefit (such as saving life and preventing stroke and brain damage in this instance) it becomes impossible to deliberately deny the perceived advantage to our patients.

In spite of these difficulties, we have to proceed somehow. We have to devise the best studies we can in patients and in animals. Clinical research should be based on reasonable hypotheses, compatible with basic science, often derived in the animal laboratory. We should then return to the laboratory as necessary to test parts of our clinical practice in the more controlled environment which it offers, and so we should move intelligently between the two. In this instance there seemed to me to be an important mismatch between the evidence offered from these two domains. The clinical practice (2, 4) was contradicted (or at least challenged) by the laboratory work (1) and yet there was some doubt as to whether the laboratory work had sufficient credibility to alter practice. In all logic one should either alter clinical practice, or devise a more apposite experiment. While the pragmatic stance on the middle ground avoids unseemly dissension, it is not intellectually secure!

Clinical experience

Ueda and colleagues published their experimental work in rats in the journal, Stroke, in the late 1980s. Their clinical experience (11) was reported to the European Association for Cardio-thoracic surgery in the London meeting in 1992 when they described its application in ten patients. Safi et al. in 1993 (10) reported from The Methodist Hospital, Houston, Texas, their early experience with retrograde cerebral perfusion in 11 cases, during arrest for 11 to 71 min at 15 °C to 24 °C. It was obviously a workable technique but with so few patients, there were no statistical grounds to claim benefit.

Bonser's group in Birmingham, England have described their experience in 23 cases undergoing a range of elective and emergency operations during planned circulatory arrest at 15 °C with good results (9). The median arrest time was 21 min with a maximum of 51 min so most of these cases were comfortably within the low risk time at that temperature, and no benefit could be ascribed to the technique itself.

Lin and colleagues from Taiwan (5) report good clinical results in a series of 29 patients, 23 of whom had retrograde perfusion at arrest at temperatures of 15 °C or 22 °C. The authors argue that patients who had retrograde perfusion also had longer periods of arrest (up to 93 min) and some were at warmer temperatures, and yet they did well. Similarly, Deeb and colleagues from Ann Arbor, Michigan reported on 35 patients (3) with longer retrograde perfusion times up to 128 min, with the majority (30/35) arrested for more than 45 min. The results were excellent with only one stroke in the 34 surgical survivors. They monitored cerebral oxygenation with near-infrared spectroscopy and the combination of preserved cerebral oxygenation, and impressive outcome with arrest times into the danger zone, added impressive evidence to the arguments in favour of this technique.

In this book the very much larger clinical experience of Coselli (2) and Hetzer (4) supports this clinical belief that retrograde cerebral perfusion extends the time during which we can deprive the brain of its normal arterial flow and yet these results are from outstanding and enormously experienced surgeons and it is possible that these clinical results, reported as they are against historical experience, may be attributable to factors other than the beneficial effects of retrograde perfusion.

The only clinical evidence that the blood infused into the superior vena cava reaches the brain itself comes from Bonser's group (8) who reported homogeneous regional cerebral perfusion as determined by Technetium labelling. The evidence seemed good. All the surgeons who have used the technique are struck by the trickle of deoxygenated blood coming from the open arch vessels and I had accepted Bonser's data as supporting the belief that this is blood returning from the brain, having given up metabolically useful oxygen. It therefore came as a surprise and seemed to fly in the face of other evidence, when Flameng's colleagues (1) showed that retrograde perfusion of the superior vena cava in baboons, did not benefit the brain.

Laboratory evidence

Boeckxstaens (1) reported that although in excess of a litre per minute could be perfused into the SVC, never more than 2 ml/min/100 gr reached the brain. She and colleagues from Flameng's laboratory have used a primate, the baboon, in order to model as closely as possible the effects that might be expected in humans. They conclude that the explanation of perceived benefit in humans (if it is indeed a real benefit) must be due to flushing out potential emboli, rather than a true metabolic benefit due to perfusion of the brain itself.

The specific issue of the use of retrograde perfusion to reduce damage caused by arterial embolisation was addressed in a study in pigs by Griepp's group (13). The animals were at 20 °C but none in any of the four experimental groups were subjected to circulatory arrest. The study animals (20/30) were given an infusion containing 200 mg of microspheres measuring 250–270 μm. In half of the study animals (10/20) and half of the controls (5/10) the perfusion was converted after 5 min to retrograde SVC perfusion (azygos ligated) for a further 25 min, the flow governed by sagittal sinus pressure. The animals were allowed to recover.

More of the embolised animals died (3/20) compared with controls (0/10, $p = 0.28$ by Fisher's test) and more had behavioural scores below the expected recovery limit (6/20) compared with controls (0/10, $p = 0.06$ by Fisher's test). Within the limits of the statistical power of the study, and the limits of assessing function in postoperative pigs, these data support the proposition that this dose of particulate emboli damage the brain. What now was to be established was whether, between the embolised groups, subsequent retrograde perfusion saved the brain from the injury or ameliorated it.

For the 20 pigs who were embolised, you will recall that ten were perfused retrogradely and in the other ten antegrade perfusion continued. They were scored for function on a scale of 0–9 where better than 7 is regarded as compatible with complete functional recovery.

At 1 day their scores were as follows:

Embolised and continued antegrade	0,2,2,2,2,3,3,4,4,5
Embolised and then retrograde	0,4,5,5,6,6,6,6,6,8

If we simply look at the data, it comes as no surprise to learn that this shows significantly higher scores for the retrograde perfusion group ($p < 0.01$ by unpaired Wilcoxon).

However at 5 days the difference had disappeared:

Embolised and continued antegrade	0,1,5,6,6,6,6,7,8,8
Embolised and then retrograde	0,0,4,4,6,6,8,8,9,9

By 5 days, the antegrade group had improved, and some of the retrograde group deteriorated enough to lose any difference of statistical significance.

The observation that the SVC pressure ranged widely and were as high as 95 mmHg seemed of possible importance. The group went on to study more animals to help explain the wide variation in functional outcome. When a further ten animals were added the pressures ranged from 29 mmHg to 107 mmHg (median 40 mmHg, interquartile range 36–55 mmHg) and the SVC pressure seems to correlate with functional outcome (Fig. 1) and all animals with perfusion pressures below about 40 mmHg did well scoring 8 or 9 at 5 days.

It should be noted that in the five animals that had retrograde perfusion without prior arterial embolisation all had excellent scores, even the two perfused retrogradely at 80 mmHg. The conclusions that can reasonably be drawn from the data are limited but it appears reasonable to say that particulate emboli produce a demonstrable brain injury in this experimental animal model, and that early functional recovery is ameliorated by

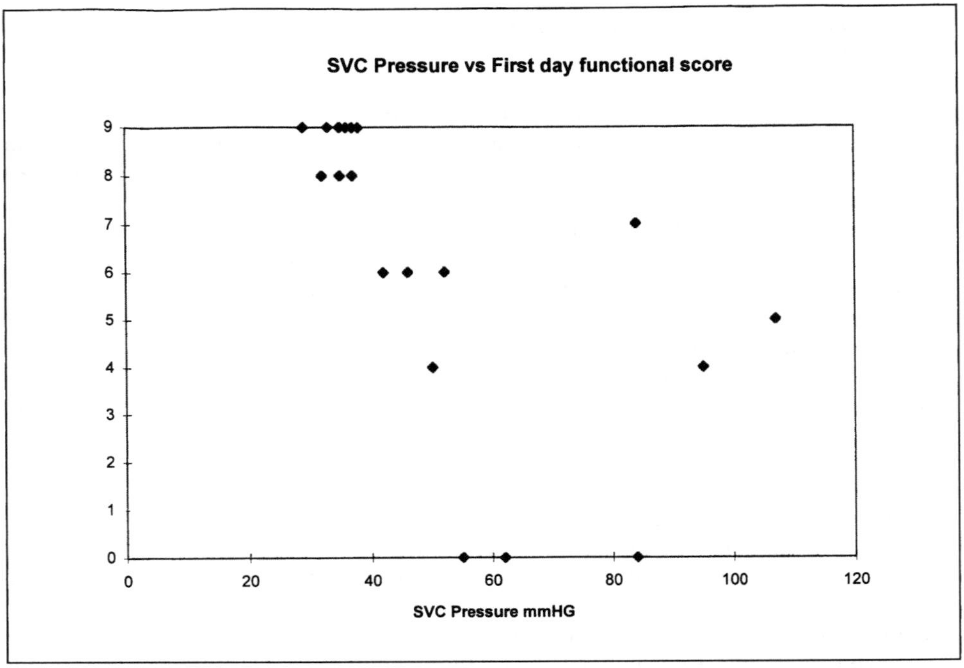

retrograde perfusion after embolisation. These benefits were not maintained at 5 days but one should note that high retrograde perfusion pressure may be damaging in itself.

In a study in dogs arrested at 20 °C for 60 min, Nojima et al. (7) explored the effect of retrograde perfusion at much lower pressures 10, 20 and 30 mmHg, of the order used in clinical practice. Flow doubled from around eight to about 16 ml/100 gm between the two lower flows and although a further small increase was achieved at 30 mmHg there was no further significant benefit in terms of oxygen consumption or carbon dioxide extraction. The fact that differences can be found between three flows, and in the absence of any source of antegrade embolisation, suggests that, in dogs, there is a beneficial metabolic effect on the brain.

Griepp's group (6) have studied, in their pig experiments, the effect of a period of circulatory arrest, known to be damaging at 20 °C, that is 90 min, about double the likely threshold for inevitable neuronal loss at this temperature. Retrograde cerebral perfusion showed undoubted benefit over sustained arrest. Interestingly, it was no better than the benefit obtained by packing the head in ice but again they used sagittal sinus monitoring and aimed for a pressure of 30 mmHg there. In order to achieve that the SVC pressures were as high as 65 mmHg, a pressure shown to be damaging in other work from that group (13).

Usui and colleagues (12) explored the changes in tissue oxygen and carbon dioxide, oxygen consumption, ATP, and lactate:pyruvate ratio during an hour at 18 °C in the dog either with arrest or with retrograde perfusion. The cerebral tissue oxygen fell from about 50 mmHg (with a wide range) to 10 mmHg and carbon dioxide climbed from 30 mmHg to 140 mmHg. Tissue oxygen reached a nadir by 15 min. ATP fell from 0.75 mmol/g to 0.2 by about 30 min and then fell no further following a similar but inverse pattern to carbon dioxide and lactate. Metabolism is still occurring between 15 and 30 min and after that there is not much further change in these indices of metabolism.

In these dogs retrograde flow of 20 mls/100 g/min maintained a tissue oxygen of 30 mmHg, ameliorated the rise in carbon dioxide and the fall in ATP. They both continued to change in the second 30 min and were still short of the 30-min point associated with total circulatory arrest.

The other animal data are reasonably consistent but they conflict with Boeckxstaen's evidence. These conflicting data ask for further work, but on the evidence available, I believe that the question we should ask first before doubting the clinical experience, is whether the baboon circulation truly reflects what happens in the human. One's first assumption is that it would be more likely to represent human flow characteristics than the dog or the pig, but that is not necessarily correct. Meanwhile, the sum of clinical experience and laboratory data suggest we should continue to use this technically straightforward and safe technique, pending better evidence but that the pressure should probably be carefully limited.

References

1. Boeckxstaens et al., this volume
2. Coselli, this volume
3. Deeb GM, Jenkins E, Bolling SF, Brunsting LA, Williams DM, Quint LE, Deeb ND (1995) Retrograde cerebral perfusion during hypothermic circulatory arrest reduces neurological morbidity. Journal of Thoracic and Cardiovascular Surgery 109: 259–168
4. Hetzer, this volume
5. Lin PJ, Chau-Hsiung C, Tan PPC, Wang C-C, Chang J-P, Liu D-W, Chu J-J, Tsai K-T, Kao C-L, Hsieh M-J (1994) Protection of the brain by retrograde cerebral perfusion during circulatory arrest. Journal of Thoracic and Cardiovascular Surgery 108: 969–974
6. Midulla PS, Gandsas A, Sadeghi AM, Mezrow CK, Yerlioglu ME, Wang W, Wolfe D, Ergin MA, Griepp RB (1994) Comparison of retrograde cerebral perfusion to antegrade perfusion and circulatory arrest in a chronic porcine model. Journal of Cardiac Surgery 9: 560–575
7. Nojima T, Magara T, Nakjima Y, Waterida S, Onoe M, Sugita T, Mori A (1994) Optimal perfusion pressure for experimental retrograde cerebral perfusion. Journal of Cardiac Surgery 9: 548–559
8. Pagano D, Boivin C, Faroqui MH, Bonser RS (1996) Retrograde perfusion through the superior vena cava perfuses the brain in human beings. Journal of Thoracic and Cardiovascular Surgery 111: 270–272
9. Pagano D, Carey JA, Patel RL, Allen SM, Tsang GMK, Hutton P, Lilley JP, Faroqui MH, Bonser RS (1995) Retrograde cerebral perfusion: clinical experience in emergency and elective aortic operations. Annals of Thoracic Surgery 59: 393–397
10. Safi HJ, Brien HW, Winter JN, Thomas AC, Maulsby RL, Doerr HK, Svensson LG (1993) Brain protection via cerebral retograde perfusion during aortic arch aneurysm repair. Annals of Thoracic Surgery 56: 270–276
11. Ueda Y, Miki S, Kusuhara K, Okita Y, Tahata T, Yamanaka K (1992) Deep hypothermic systemic circulatory arrest and continuous retrograde cerebral perfusion for surgery of aortic arch aneurysm. European Journal of Cardiothoracic Surgery 6: 36–41
12. Usui A, Oohara K, Liu T-I, Murase M, Tanaka M, Takeuchi E, Abe T (1994) Comparative experimental study between retrograde cerebral perfusion and circulatory arrest. Journal of Thoracic and Cardiovascular Surgery 107: 1228–36
13. Yerlioglu, ME, Wolfe D, Mezrow CK, Weisz DJ, Midulla PS, Zhang N, Shiang HH, Bodian C, Griepp RB (1995) The effect of retrograde cerebral perfusion after particulate embolization to the brain. Journal of Thoracic and Cardiovascular Surgery 110: 1470–1485

Author's address:
Tom Treasure, MD MS FRCS
St. George's Hospital
London SW17 0QT, England

FSC
www.fsc.org
MIX
Papier aus verantwortungsvollen Quellen
Paper from responsible sources
FSC® C105338

If you have any concerns about our products,
you can contact us on
ProductSafety@springernature.com

In case Publisher is established outside the EU,
the EU authorized representative is:
Springer Nature Customer Service Center GmbH
Europaplatz 3, 69115 Heidelberg, Germany

Printed by Libri Plureos GmbH
in Hamburg, Germany